Acupuncture for Brain

Tianjun Wang

Acupuncture for Brain

Treatment for Neurological
and Psychologic Disorders

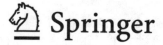 Springer

Tianjun Wang
TJ Acupuncture Academy
and UK Centre for Nanjing University
of Chinese Medicine
London
UK

ISBN 978-3-030-54668-7   ISBN 978-3-030-54666-3   (eBook)
https://doi.org/10.1007/978-3-030-54666-3

This Springer imprint is published by the registered company Springer Nature Switzerland AG
The registered company address is: Gewerbestrasse 11, 6330 Cham, Switzerland

Foreword

Acupuncture and the Brain

"Missing Links"

Early on in my acupuncture practice back in the 1990s, a patient of mine asked me to visit her father who was in hospital after suffering a serious stroke. I have not forgotten the dreary ward where he and other patients lay wretched and helpless, struggling to comprehend the terrible loss of physical feeling and control. My patient's father lit up at the possibility that the insertion of acupuncture needles might help in some as-yet unfathomable way. As I applied my traditional Chinese medicine (TCM) diagnosis of *"internal Liver wind"* and *"phlegm channel block-age"*, it struck me that there was a gaping hole in TCM organ physiology. How could a stroke, a condition that is essentially an injury of the central nervous system and thus of the Brain, not figure in TCM? Why was the Brain described as merely a *"Fu"*, or *"extra organ"*, of little consequence to either diagnosis or treatment? In the early days of practice, it was easy to gloss over such omissions and be smitten by the discovery of *"stagnations"*, *"deficiencies"* and *"excess"*, so eloquent in describing the symptoms that acupuncturists were taught to observe in their sick patients.

Acupuncture practice has evolved in many ways since then, but it remains the case that the language of TCM represents an expression of ideas that came long before the development of neuroanatomical and physiological knowledge.

I met Dr. Tianjun Wang in 1991 at Nanjing Jianye TCM Hospital, where a large proportion of the patients had suffered strokes. But here too, although I occasionally saw scalp acupuncture in use, there was never any mention of specific pathology relating to the Brain. That the patients' symptoms seemed to improve with the acupuncture they received was sufficient reason to dispel any need for further questioning.

Wang too was acutely aware of this gap and was intrigued to discover the work of Prof. Xuemin Shi at the Tianjin University of Chinese Medicine, pioneering a technique called *"Awake the Brain and Open Orifical"* in the early 1990s. Twenty years later, far away from China, Wang finally had an opportunity to put this technique to the test. A 31-year-old man had suffered a sudden stroke, leaving him in a Brain stem coma. His family had discovered that a similar case had been successfully treated with Shi's protocol in the USA. After much searching, they located Wang, now a London-based acupuncturist who was unusually familiar with Shi's unique treatment. Given acupuncture's lack of statutory regulation in the UK, there was initially much resistance to allowing an acupuncturist to work within the ICU of a London hospital. But thanks to pressure from the patient's family and Wang's impressive credentials, he was finally approved to apply Shi's treatment and scalp acupuncture at the patient's bedside. It was the ideal opportunity to employ the unique scalp acupuncture technique Wang had been long investigating. In so doing, he placed *"the Brain"* at the centre of TCM diagnosis and treatment, with its own unique set of differentiations.

It was essentially a novel set of acupuncture tools.

Much to the surprise of the hospital staff, the patient regained consciousness and made a gradual recovery.

The positive outcomes gained by this patient and others suffering from neurological conditions including depression—the subject matter of Wang's PhD—have created an urgency to disseminate this missing knowledge across the acupuncture profession at large—and that is the purpose of this book.

The text starts by delving into the history of the understanding of the Brain in TCM and raises the vexed question as to why, given that the concept of the Brain was mentioned as far back as *the Huangdi Neijing* more than 2000 years ago, there was no further development of treatment strategy. Wang has mused on the possibility that once the concept of *"the five elements"* was dominant, there would be simply no room in "the circle" for another organ. It was not until the 1980s that modern Western medical neurological knowledge combined with scalp acupuncture technique was introduced into the national TCM curriculum in China, along with the acknowledgement of the importance of the *Du Mai* as the key affiliated channel to the Brain. This was also a response to the increasing incidence of psychological disease in a developing China, where more societal competition and much higher levels of stress led to an increased interest in finding better ways to treat neurological and psychological conditions. However, the categorisation and application of *"the Brain"* in standard TCM teaching is largely missing from more recent Western textbooks and translations. Wang's book is the first to focus on the techniques and theories of the Brain for practitioners to put into therapeutic effect.

Wang has a great deal of clinical experience to share both from his early career as a senior acupuncturist in China to his subsequent career in the UK. As Course Leader of one of the UK's University BSc Acupuncture programmes, I recruited Wang as director of the university's busy teaching clinic, where Wang was able to build on his experience and research in China and begin the process of applying his newer techniques to the day-to-day clinical reality of practice in the West.

Treatments of patients suffering from stroke, Parkinson's, depression, anxiety, dementia, Alzheimer's, multiple sclerosis and other neurological conditions are described throughout this new book. Part 1 outlines the history, theory, research and specific new techniques in treating Brain disorders. Part 2 is organised into sections on specific diseases commonly seen in clinical practice. There is an introduction to each disease, aetiology, pathogenesis, modern treatment and TCM understanding with current syndrome-based treatment, but with the addition of unique protocols to treat newly discovered syndromes such as *"deficiency of bone marrow", "Brain Yang Qi"* and *"disorder of Brain Shen"*.

As practitioners, we are always looking for ways to expand the toolset of what we can offer our patients as we develop our practice over the years.

When I treated an elderly woman in clinic for depression, it became clear after a 10-session course of acupuncture that something was missing from her diagnosis. I had tackled every possible angle of her *Zang Fu*-based syndrome differentiation, utilising different point combinations and different modes of needling. There were no apparent lifestyle or emotional causes for her ailment, and even the application of counselling skills, which acupuncturists can sometimes usefully borrow from the school of psychotherapy, proved ineffective. I concluded that the grassroots, this particular problem was something much more "physical", not least because her symptoms were always worse in the morning, suggesting that overnight, *"stagnation"* had built up somewhere in the channel system. Fortunately, I had at the time been working with Wang's new differentiations and techniques and, after adding scalp acupuncture and points recommended to clear the *Du Mai*, her symptoms improved for the first time.

I hope this text can serve as the groundbreaking guide for all acupuncturists treating neurological and psychological disorders. It represents a welcome opportunity to expand our ideas and practice.

Cambridge, UK   Charmian Wylde

Foreword

Acupuncture for the Brain, Traditional and Modern

When I received the manuscript *Acupuncture for the Brain: Treatment of Neurological and Psychological Disorders* from Prof. Tianjun Wang on April 2020, my time with Prof. Xuemin Shi just came back to mind.

Due to his great achievements in acupuncture, especially in the creation of acupuncture Brain theory, Prof. Xuemin Shi was elected as member of the Chinese Academy of Engineering (CAE), the highest academic title in engineering science and technology in China and a lifelong honour, in 1999. I started my postdoctoral research under the guidance of Prof. Shi from 2002 at the Tianjin University of Chinese Medicine (TJUCM). During those 3 years of study and research with Prof. Shi, I gradually understood both him and his creation, the Xing Nao Kai Qiao acupuncture technique (XNKQ).

Traditionally, acupuncture treatment for acute strokes is mostly based on the principles of calming Liver Yang and extinguishing Liver wind. The main strategy for stabilising and steadying patients is to clear the channels. The selection of acupuncture points (acupoints) for treating apoplexy is mainly based on Yang meridians, particularly on the Yang-Ming meridians. In 1972, based on his own clinical experiences and studies, Dr. Xuemin Shi created and established his new acupuncture technique, Xing Nao Kai Qiao (XNKQ), which has demonstrated a completely new approach to treating stroke patients.

XNKQ is translated as "activating the Brain and opening the orifices" or "Awake the Brain, open the orifices". XNKQ mainly uses Yin meridians and the Du Mai points to activate the Brain, open the orifices and nourish the Liver and Kidney, along with smoothing the relevant meridians to promote Qi flow. The main acupoints of XNKQ are DU-26 Renzhong, PC-6 Neiguan and SP-6 Sanyinjiao, etc.

Since its commencement nearly 50 years ago, the application of XNKQ has gradually been improved through clinical practice, clinical trials and laboratory research, and it has been continuously applied to a wide spectrum of diseases, not only stroke, but also many other Brain-related disorders.

After completing my postdoctoral research with Prof. Shi in 2005, I came back to the Nanjing University of Chinese Medicine (NJUCM) where I gained my TCM education and PhD. I have worked there since and am currently a Professor and the Dean of the College of Acupuncture, Tuina Massage, Health Preservation and Rehabilitation.

Since 2017, I have been the Chairman of the Brain Science Committee of the China Association for Acupuncture and Moxibustion (CAAM). The main function of this committee is to focus on the acupuncture treatment and research on the Brain and its related disorders. The Brain has become one of the top subjects in acupuncture practice and research.

I met Tianjun Wang in 1984 in NJUCM, where we all studied TCM and acupuncture, and Tianjun arrived two years after me. We had more opportunities to discuss Brain-related subjects during his "acupuncture for depression" PhD research in NJUCM from 2005. After he moved to the UK, we have had some occasions to meet at various internationally conferences.

This book, *Acupuncture for the Brain: Treatment of Neurological and Psychological Disorders*, has many highlights and attractions for Western readers. Firstly, it has systematically reviewed the history, development and status quo of TCM Brain theory, techniques and their clinical practice. Secondly, Dao-qi acupuncture technique and its clinical application, particularly explained in detail on Du Mai and Ren Mail points, were for the first time completely introduced in Western publications. Thirdly, scalp acupuncture, which Tianjun and I studied at the university 30 years ago, has been fully revised. The newly created colourful illustrations of scalp acupuncture are distinctive and easy to follow and practise. Last but not least, the treatment of Brain-related disorders is the key part of the book. The major diseases, neurological diseases and psychological disorders are all covered with both modern medicine and Chinese medicine basic theory and general acupuncture. The aim of this book is to focus on the introduction of unique Brain acupuncture treatments, scalp acupuncture, Dao-qi technique and XNKQ and so forth.

I hope this book, *Acupuncture for the Brain: Treatment of Neurological and Psychological Disorders*, will introduce the TCM Brain theory and science to the West, and will benefit more Western practitioners and their patients.

Wishing you all success, Prof. Tianjun Wang.

Nanjing, China   Guangxia Ni, PhD

Acknowledgements

Firstly, I would like to express my sincere thanks to my family, teachers, colleagues, students, patients and friends.

In particular, I would like to thank Prof. LingLing Wang from the Nanjing University of Chinese Medicine, my PhD supervisor, for her guidance and support during the three-plus years of full-time research.

I am very grateful to Prof. Ningsheng Wang, my boss and clinic practice supervisor in Nanjing China, for his continuing encouragement and support since my days as a junior doctor.

I feel so grateful to have received the two weeks of face-to-face direct training and advice from Prof. Shunfa Jiao, the inventor of scalp acupuncture; 30 years ago I started to learn and practise the unique technique as a university student in China.

I am indebted to Ms Charmian Wylde for her kind invitation to apply for and subsequently join the acupuncture programme team at the University of East London, and for much encouragement and support in making the transition to working life in the UK. In addition, thanks are due for her contribution to the wonderful foreword of this book.

I would also like to thank Prof. Jason-Jishun Hao and Dr. Linda Lingzhi Hao, co-authors of the widely accepted book *Chinese Scalp Acupuncture*, for their generous efforts in writing Chap. 10 on multiple sclerosis and Chap. 12 on autism. Both are very busy practitioners and lectures and I appreciated their encouragement through my writing process.

Many thanks to Dr. Liuzhong Ye, PhD, for his contribution in writing Chap. 16 on anxiety and other relevant support.

Many thanks to Prof. Guangxi Ni, Chairman of the Brain Science Committee of China Association for Acupuncture and Moxibustion (CAAM), for his contribution of the valuable preface.

Thanks to Ms Hai-Yen Hua-Stroefer for encouraging me to write the book and for her help with publishing.

Finally, many thanks to Mr Casey Choong, for his great ideas and techniques in creating useful illustrations.

About the Book

The Journey of My Interest in the Brain

As a typical traditional Chinese medicine (TCM) doctor, I completed my TCM education together with basic biomedicine training at the Nanjing University of Chinese Medicine (NJUCM) 31 years ago. During these combined medical studies, I was often confused between TCM Zangfu organs and channels and the organs in anatomy and physiology such as Shen (mind), or the questions of which organ controls Shen, namely the Heart or Brain? My lecturers said TCM and Western medicine can be two different systems but can frequently be interactively described and managed. The functions of the Brain in Western medicine are distributed across several Zangfu organs in TCM, and Brain issues can be diagnosed and treated according to related Zangfu pattern differentiations. I accepted this advice at that time but with a lingering underlying question: is it true?

My TCM university study was based on the foundation of TCM theory but focused on classic acupuncture method, meridians and collaterals, acupuncture points, needling techniques and moxibustion, Wuyun Liuqi (the five Movements and six climates), Ziwuliuzhu (the stems and branches theory), treatment of conditions and so on. There were brief introductions of some modern acupuncture needling techniques such as electric acupuncture, ear acupuncture, scalp acupuncture, wrist-ankle acupuncture, point-injection and more. I still remember one of the needling assessments, scalp acupuncture, required a rapid manipulation minimum of 200 movements per minute. It was quite painful.

The final year of our TCM education consisted of clinical practice in different TCM hospitals. My key supervisor was Dr. Su for acupuncture observation and practice specialised in strokes. One of his unique techniques was scalp acupuncture with two hands simultaneously moving needles over 200 times within a minute. I tried to follow his technique but with only a few successes. However, many of our patients showed very good improvement and some even fully recovered. This practical training left me with very deep memories and understanding of scalp acupuncture treating neurological diseases, particularly strokes.

In my early career as a junior TCM doctor in a TCM hospital in Nanjing, partly to fulfil the training requirement for a junior doctor, I took turns in different departments besides acupuncture, such as internal medicine, surgery, gynaecology, the paediatric department, the emergency department and so on. This training not only built up my fundamental knowledge of both TCM and Western medicine but also widened the opportunity for me to gain experience in a broad range of diseases. One of my achievements during the junior doctor rotation was that many severely ill and urgently ill patients, including some with early-stage stroke and Brain injuries, were helped effectively. Another achievement was a paper published regarding point injection on ST-37 (Shangjuxu) to treat diarrhoea, published in 1992, which was my first clinical study paper published.

From 1996, I was appointed Director of the Department of Acupuncture, Tuina Massage and Rehabilitation. We have an in-patient ward for severe patients, and half of them were suffering from neurological diseases such as different stages of stroke, Brain injuries, spinal diseases and Parkinson's disease. During that period, I visited the Tianjin University of Chinese Medicine and its affiliated hospital and attended many conferences to observe and discuss the newly developed acupuncture technique Xing Nao Kai Qiao (XNKQ) (awake Brain open orifices) by Prof. Xuemin Shi. XNKQ mainly focuses on the Brain and on regulating and controlling the Shen and its functions, in order to ameliorate Brain-related acute problems, especially for the early stages of stroke.

I started my PhD research subject "acupuncture for depression" supervised by Prof. Lingling Wang of NJUCM in 2005. The three years' full-time study involved literature review of TCM for depression and modern medicine for depression, including animal experiments, as well as eight months of clinical study in Nanjing Brain Hospital (NBH). In NBH, the hospitalised depression patients were all given usual care along with one of the selective serotonin reuptake inhibitor (SSRI) antidepressants, and then their interventions were randomised, being divided into a control group, which used SSRI only, and a treatment group, which used SSRI plus acupuncture. The main treatment principle was to use Du Mai points to stimulate Du Mai and regulate the Brain. The results indicated that acupuncture plus antidepressant treatment for depression patients was not only more effective than antidepressant use only, but it could also be rapidly therapeutic with fewer side effects.

From late 2007, I was employed as a Lecturer at the University of East London, UK (UEL), then Senior Lecturer and Director of the Acupuncture Clinic. During my teaching and clinical supervision, I realised that the Brain was missing from TCM education curricula in the West. Most of the key TCM textbook translations were based on Chinese TCM textbooks dating back 20–30 years ago and very few books explained the new TCM developments such as the Brain. In practice, there were very few neurological patients visiting the acupuncture clinic, besides one Chinese patient with a stroke issue. Many colleagues had never seen one single stroke patient in their 10 to 20 years of practice. Those Brain-related techniques, such as scalp acupuncture, XNKQ and Du Mai Dao-qi, were scarcely present in overseas TCM acupuncture training.

Therefore, I started to introduce this new and developing subject into Western acupuncture education. I have presented talks three times at the British Acupuncture

Council (BAcC) conferences in 2013, 2016 and 2019 with the topics "The new understanding of TCM Brain and its clinical practice", "Chinese scalp acupuncture" and "Du Mai is the channel of the Brain and Dao-qi technique", respectively. In 2014, part of my PhD clinical study results were published in the journal *Acupuncture in Medicine* 2014. In 2015, the case report of a brainstem haemorrhage coma patient successfully treated by my acupuncture in an NHS hospital was published in the journal *Acu*. In the same year, the paper "A new understanding of the Brain and its clinical application" was published in *EJOM*. In 2018, my research of "Developments in the understanding of the Brain in Chinese medicine" was updated and published.

Since moving to the UK 12 years ago, I have presented more than fifty conference talks, seminars and workshops worldwide promoting TCM Brain and its related theories, techniques and clinical practice.

In 2017, I was appointed one of the Vice Chairpersons of the 1st Board of the Special Committee of Head Acupuncture of the World Federation of Chinese Medicine Societies (WFCMS). In July 2018, Prof. Shunfa Jiao, the inventor of scalp acupuncture, came to the UK on my invitation to teach his own scalp acupuncture style, which was the first time for him to visit Europe.

As a result of the above promotions of TCM Brain theory and techniques, the number of colleagues interested in and practising TCM Brain theory and techniques has increased, and hence more patients have benefited from this method. It seemed to many that there was a demand for a book that would summarise systematically the developments of the TCM Brain. This situation became the starting point for the book: *Acupuncture for the Brain: Treatment of Neurological and Psychological Diseases*.

In the summer of 2018, Hai-Yen Hua-Stroefer invited me to Germany, to help her husband, a stroke patient. Hai-Yen is a writer herself and has published several books. She encouraged me to publish the present book to benefit more colleagues and patients, providing useful advice along the way.

In late 2018, I then had the opportunity to contact Springer to present my book proposal. To improve the quality and coverage of the book, I invited Prof. Jason-Jishun Hao, Dr. Linda Lingzhi Hao, Dr. Liuzhong Ye and Ms Charmian Wylde to join me as contributors in the writing. Prof. and Dr. Hao are the co-authors of the widely used book *Chinese Scalp Acupuncture* and are famous for neuro-acupuncture worldwide. Dr. Ye obtained his TCM PhD in China and regularly teaches at different colleges in the UK. Ms Wylde was the acupuncture course director at UEL. Prof. Guangxia Ni was my university mate at NJUCM, and now he is the Dean of the College of Acupuncture, Tuina Massage, Health Preservation and Rehabilitation of NJUCM. They are all my close friends, all are familiar with my ideas of TCM Brain, and I greatly appreciate their valuable contributions.

After many discussions and revisions, the Publishing Agreement was signed in April 2019, the day of my 54th birthday. The book, *Acupuncture for the Brain: Treatment of Neurological and Psychological Diseases*, was formally launched.

There are two major parts in the book, Part one is about TCM Brain theory and unique acupuncture techniques, and part two is about commonly seen Brain-related disorders and their acupuncture treatments.

The first chapter summarises in detail the history of TCM Brain, from the origin and arguments of the *Huangdi Neijing* to the developments in the last fifty years, TCM Brain theory, unique Brain-related techniques, etc. The second chapter introduces the Brain and Shen or mind. What is the meaning of Shen (mind) in TCM and what is the relationship between Shen and the Brain and the Brain's functions and Shen. The third chapter, Du Mai (Governor Vessel) is the channel of the Brain, introduces Du Mai, the modern research on the Du Mai and the Brain, the functions, the pathological changes and the clinical application of Du Mai and finally summarises the patterns of the Brain and their treatments which will be first published on academic books. Chapter 4 briefly reviews the acupuncture research on the Brain, focusing more on the two major areas: acupuncture influence central neurotransmitters and may remap the Brain, also mentioning the possible bias on languish publishing. Chapter 5 introduces in detail scalp acupuncture which is one of the unique techniques for Brain-related disorders. This chapter starts with explaining TCM Brain theory and practice including the channels and acupoints on the head, the channel diseases and treatment on the head and modern developments in head acupuncture. All the classic scalp acupuncture methods stimulate areas and indications explained with created colourful illustrations which are first published. Scalp acupuncture needling techniques and precautions are explained in this chapter. Another unique technique for Brain-related disorders, Dao-qi acupuncture technique, is introduced in detail in Chap. 6. The chapter starts from Dao-qi needling origin and development history and then explains the process of Dao-qi, followed with Shen (Mind) during Dao-qi needling and its precautions. Finally, it introduces commonly used Dao-qi acupoints, which are mostly on Du Mai and Ren Mai, and special Dao-qi needling on these points.

In Part two, from Chaps. 7, 8, 9, 10, 11, 12, 13, 14, 15, 16, 17 and 18, commonly seen neurological and psychological disorders will be introduced. They are stroke, Parkinson's disease (PD), Alzheimer's disease (AD) and other dementias, multiple sclerosis (MS), traumatic brain injuries (TBI), autism and cerebral palsy (CP), and some other neurological diseases, epilepsy, headache and pain-associated with neurological disorders, will be briefly introduced. Three most commonly seen mental disorders, depression, anxiety and bipolar disorder (BD), will be introduced in detail, and another three commonly seen disorders will be briefly explained, post-traumatic stress disorder (PTSD), insomnia and substance abuse.

There were two indexes followed by the main content. One is Index of Name of Channel and Point, which not only lists all the names of the channels and some sample acupoints, but also lists some commonly seen different Pinyin names of channel and points. Index two lists the translations of the name of the *Huangdi Neijing*.

The book, *Acupuncture for the Brain: Treatment for Neurological and Psychological Diseases*, is suitable for acupuncture practitioners, medics who are interested in acupuncture, acupuncture and TCM researchers, final year acupuncture students, interested public and so on.

Contents

List of Editors and Contributors

About the Author

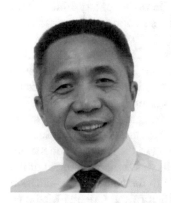

Tianjun Wang (王天俊) PhD, FHEA, MBAcC, is a guest professor of the Nanjing University of Chinese Medicine (NJUCM) and a PhD supervisor for overseas postgraduate students of NJUCM at its UK Centre. Dr. Wang is also the Principal of TJ Acupuncture Academy, London UK. After studying at NJUCM, Dr. Wang became a Medical Doctor and an Acupuncturist in Nanjing China for 18 years before moving to the UK and joined the University of East London, UK, as a Senior Lecturer and the Director of Acupuncture Clinic in 2007 until December 2014. Dr. Wang obtained his PhD from NJUCM in 2008 on acupuncture study for depression. From 2015 to 2017, Prof. Wang was the Acupuncture Course Director and Senior Lecturer at College of Naturopathic Medicine (CNM). Prof. Wang is the Vice President of the scalp acupuncture committee of the World Federation of Chinese Medicine Societies (WFCMS). He owns his TJ Acupuncture Clinic and Brain Care Centre in London, UK. Prof. Dr. Wang has published on a wide range of topics in acupuncture and Chinese medicine in both national and international periodicals and in both Chinese and English languages. As a well-known speaker, he has presented talks in a great number of international conferences and seminars.

Contributors

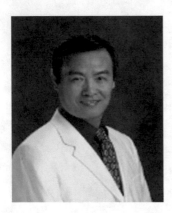

Jason Jishun Hao (郝吉顺) received his bachelor's and master's degrees of traditional Chinese Medicine from Heilongjiang University of TCM in Harbin, China, in 1982 and 1987, respectively. He received his MBA from the University of Phoenix in 2004.

Dr. Hao has been practising and researching scalp acupuncture for thirty-seven years and has been teaching classes and seminars in the USA and the West since 1989, including many cities in America, Canada, Australia, Netherlands, Italy, Denmark and Dubai. Many American newspapers, journals, television shows reported his successful cases and stories in the past 30 years. The documentary film on him and his wife, Linda Hao's treatments *Return to Life*, will be released on July 2020.

Jason Hao is editor in chief and translator in chief for the book *Acupuncture and Moxibustion* published by the World Federation of Chinese Medicine Society. Jason Hao currently serves as the vice-chairman for the education guiding committee at the World Federation of Chinese Medicine Society. Jason Hao is the president of the Neuro-Acupuncture Institute in the USA. He was former chairman of the acupuncture committee in the National Certification Commission of Acupuncture and Oriental Medicine in the USA. He is the co-author of the book, *Chinese Scalp Acupuncture.*

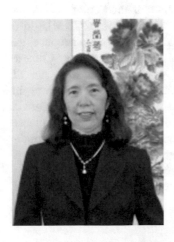

Linda Hao 史灵芝 PhD, received a Doctorate Degree in Chinese Medicine from China, with specialty in neuro-acupuncture. She is the co-founder and full professor at the Neuro-Acupuncture Institute in the USA. She serves as Vice President to Head Acupuncture Specialty Committee of the World Federation of Chinese Medicine Societies.

She is a pioneer in the neuro-acupuncture treatment of children with autism, ADHD and other Brain and neurological disorders, including cerebral palsy, trisomy18, strokes, TBI, and paralysis. Her patients come from all walks of life, among them celebrities in the USA and abroad. Her work garnered national and international fame, recognised locally and nationally by TV channels like Fox News and Action 7 News and newspapers. Documentary films by renowned producers highlight her accomplishments, helping to bring worldwide acceptance of neuro-acupuncture.

She lectures extensively domestically and internationally. Her published works include a prominent textbook *Chinese Scalp Acupuncture* and professional articles in English and Chinese.

Dr. Linda Hao was awarded one of the Top Ten Honorees of *Hundred Professionals Award* by the Academy of Science in Chinese Medicine 2016; Santa Fe Mayor Gonzales proclaimed 16 February 2018 *Dr. Jason and Linda Hao's Day* to acknowledge their significant contributions to medicine.

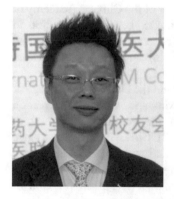

Liuzhong Ye (叶柳忠) PhD and Master of TCM achieved from Guangzhou University of TCM in 2003, started his practice of TCM as senior consultant in the UK after graduating from Guangzhou. He established his own clinic in Norwich, Hado, in 2008. And now he is the senior lecturer and module leader of several TCM colleges across Europe, including CNM, London, and Wroclaw Academy of Acupuncture, Poland. And he is appointed as supervisor professors of master's and PhD scheme of TCM at Shulan College Manchester, UK. He is also serving as the director of CAHMN (Chinese Acupuncture and Herbal Medicine Network) and the general Secretary of the British Institute of Scalp Acupuncture.

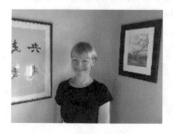

Charmian Wylde MA, MBAcC, FHEA, has practised acupuncture for over 30 years, having studied initially in London and Nanjing, China. She was Co-Founder and Director of the Birmingham Centre for Chinese Medicine and, using her previous experience as a lecturer in higher education, went on to design and run one of the UK's BSc Acupuncture degree programmes at the University of East London, where she was Course Leader and Senior Lecturer for 10 years. Charmian continues her interest in acupuncture education as a member of the

Accreditation Committee for the British Acupuncture Accreditation Board.

Having developed a specific interest in the development of acupuncture through its migration beyond China, particularly to Cuba and the UK, Charmian has an MA in intercultural communication and pursues research activities as Director of Research and Academic Affairs for Sietar (Society for Intercultural Education, Training and Research). She also maintains her own busy acupuncture practice near Cambridge.

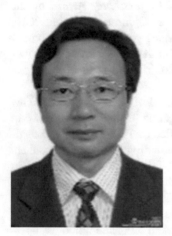

Guangxia Ni (倪光夏) PhD, received his bachelor and PhD degrees of TCM from the Nanjing University of Chinese Medicine, Nanjing, China, in 1987 and 2002, respectively. Dr. Ni started his postdoctoral research under the guidance of Prof. Xuemin Shi, the member of the Chinese Academy of Engineering (CAE), the highest academic title in engineering science and technology in China, and studied deeper on the Xingnao Kaiqiao acupuncture technique (XNKQ).

He is the Professor and the Dean of the College of Acupuncture, Tuina Massage, Health Preservation and Rehabilitation of the Nanjing University of Chinese Medicine (NJUCM). In addition, since 2017, he has been the Chairman of the Brain Science Committee of China Association for Acupuncture and Moxibustion (CAAM). The main function of this committee is to focus on the acupuncture treatment and research on the Brain and its related disorders. Prof. Ni has obtained many times national and local awards, published more than hundred academic papers and supervised 80 postgraduate students. As the vice chief editor, he has published eight key textbooks.

Abbreviations

5-HT	5-Hydroxytryptamine
ACTH	Adrenocorticotropic hormone
Acupoint	Acupuncture point
AD	Alzheimer's disease
ADL	Activities of daily living
ALFF	Amplitude of low-frequency fluctuations
ANS	Autonomic nervous system
CIs	Cholinesterase inhibitors
CNS	Central nervous system
CSF	Cerebrospinal fluid
CTS	Carpal tunnel syndrome
DALYs	Disability-adjusted life years
DOC	Disorders of consciousness
EA	Electro-acupuncture
EAE	Experimental autoimmune encephalitis
EDSS	Expanded disability status *scale*
ELISA	Enzyme-linked immunosorbent assay
EOC	Endogenous opioid circuit
FMF	Fine motor function
fMRI	Functional magnetic resonance imaging
FSS	Fatigue severity scale
GABA	Gamma-aminobutyric acid
GCS	Glasgow Coma Scale
GDNF	Glial cell line-derived neurotrophic factor
GMF	Gross motor function
HAMD-24	Hamilton Depression Scale-24
HDRS-17	Hamilton Depression Rating Scale
HPA	Hypothalamus–pituitary–adrenal axis
HPG	Hypothalamic pituitary–gonadal axis
IADL	Instrumental activities of daily living
IWG	International Working Group

LFF	Low-frequency fluctuation
MAS	Modified Ashworth Scale
MCI	Mild cognitive impairment
MOR	Mu-opioid receptors
mTBI	Mild trauma brain injury
NDS	Neurological function deficit scale
NGF	Nerve growth factor
NTF	Neurotrophic factors
PCS	Post-concussion syndrome
PET	Positron emission tomography
PTH	Post-traumatic headache
QoL	Quality of life
rACC	Rostral anterior cingulate cortex
RCT	Randomised controlled trial
rs-fMRI	Resting-state functional magnetic resonance imaging
rt PA	Recombinant tissue plasminogen activator
SDS	Self-Rating Depression Scale
SP	Substance P
SSRIs	Selective serotonin reuptake inhibitors
TBI	Trauma brain injury
TCM	Traditional Chinese medicine
TIA	Transient ischemic attack
VaD	Vascular dementias
VIP	Vasoactive intestinal peptide
WHO	World Health Organization

Part I
Acupuncture for the Brain, Introduction, Theory and Techniques

Chapter 1
Brain in TCM Origin and Short History

It is a common knowledge in modern science that the Brain is the major centre of control and regulation system of our human body, not only the physical and the neurological systems but also psychological system. In traditional Chinese medicine (TCM), Brain (Nao 脑) is not one of the major internal viscera and not play any important role of control or regulation. This contradiction has generated one of the major controversies between modern medicine and TCM.

Does TCM has no Brain, or is the Brain not an important organ in TCM? To answer this question, we should trace back to the origin of TCM theory.

Brain was one of the important internal organs in TCM going back 2000 years. There were the embryonic form, the basic physical function and pathologic changes of the Brain.

In this chapter, Huangdi Neijing, which translated as Yellow Emperor's Canon of Internal Medicine, or the Yellow Emperors Internal Classic, could be referred to as Neijing, or Internal Medicine. The first part of Neijing, Suwen, or Plain Questions, will be abbreviated as NJSW. The second part of Neijing, Lingsu, or Spiritual Pivot, would be abbreviated as NJLS.

1.1 Brain in Huangdi Neijing Era

Although there were little other literature mentioned about the Brain previously, the majority of texts were from Huangdi Neijing. As Ted J Kaptchuk introduced in his famous book "Chinese medicine: The Web that has no Weaver" states 'The Huang-di Nei-jing or Inner Classic of the Yellow Emperor (hereafter referred to as Nei Jing) is the source of all Chinese medical theory, the Chinese equivalent of the Hippocratic Corpus. Compiled by unknown authors between 300 and 100 B.C.E., is the oldest of the Chinese medical texts. The knowledge and the theoretical formulations it contains are the basic medical ideas developed and elaborated by later thinkers. …The Nei Jing has been called the bible of Chinese medicine. ' [1, p. 25].

© Springer Nature Switzerland AG 2021
T. Wang, *Acupuncture for Brain*, https://doi.org/10.1007/978-3-030-54666-3_1

As 'the bible of Chinese medicine', Neijing has many chapters discussing about the Brain, which will be described and summarized below.

1.1.1   Embryonic Form of the Brain

Similar to other TCM knowledge, 2000 years ago, ancient Chinese doctors had already understood the human body through autopsies, although limited. As "Neijing Lingshu Chapter 12-The Water of Channel" described 'to a dead body, one can examine it carefully by autopsy' [2, p. 578]. Based on these preliminary autopsy measurement, the ancient doctors had already gathered some basic knowledge about the anatomy, such as "Neijing-Lingshu Chapter 14-Measurement of the Bone" says 'The circumference of the skull when measuring on the level of the peaks of the ears is two feet and six inches…the length from the frontal hairline to the location of the neck covered by the hair is one foot and two inches' [2, p. 590].

Two thousand years ago, the Chinese master doctors had already dissected the dead body and examined the internal organs with some detail, including the Brain. The observations noted, thousands of years ago, are very close to modern analysis.

In terms of the Brain location and shape, as "Neijing Lingshu Chapter 33-On the Seas" says 'The Brain is the sea of marrow, Its transport (Openings) are in the upper region at the top of the skull and below the Fengfu Du 16 (opening)' [3, p. 345]. We can see at the time of Neijing, through autopsy, it has been realized that the Brain is located in the upper top of the skull and lower to the point of Fengfu DU-16.

In addition, Neijing already understood that the eyes is connect with the Brain and eyes is the monitor of spirit, as explained below:
"Neijing Lingshu Chapter 80-On Massive Confusion" [3, p. 711–712].

> The essence of the den of the qi [collects in] the white [parts of] eyes;
>   essence of the sinews and the flesh [collects in] the eyelids.
>
> The [eyelids] enclose the essence of the sinews and the bones, the blood
>   and the qi. They are tied to the vessels and form a connection that is linked
>   to the Brain and comes out in the nape.
>
> The eyes are [the den collecting] the essence of the five
>   long-term depots and six short-term repositories. The camp and the guard [qi], the
>   *hun* and the *po* souls pass through there continuously. That is where the spirit qi are
>   generated.

1.1.2   Argument on Physical Functions of the Brain

At the time of the Huang Di Nei Jing (The Yellow Emperors Internal Classic) there were different points of view on the Brain and its connections. The Su Wen (Plain Questions), in Chap. 11, talked about the different functions of the five-zang. Chapter 11 Further Discourse on the Five Depots (Wu zang bie lun pian) [4, p. 203].

Huang Di asked:
  "I have heard:
  of the prescription masters
  some consider the Brain and the marrow to be depots;
  others consider the intestines and the stomach to be depots;
  still others consider them to be palaces.
  May I ask about these contradictions;
  all say of themselves they are right.
  I do not know the Way of their [reasoning];
  I should like to hear an explanation for this."

In the above statement describes with explicity the time of Huang Di Nei Jing around 300 BC [5], the arguments about the characteristic of Brain, is it Zang or Fu organ, already existed, which is still argued till now.

1.1.3   The Importance of the Brain

'In the beginning of human life, the essence of life is formed first, then it develops Brain and spinal cord and Marrow, and finally, the human body is shaped. The skeletons are like the wooden pillars on the two sides of the wall, the channels are like the barracks connecting each other, the tendons are like the strings, the muscles are like the walls, and the skin and hair are protecting the bones, channels, tendons and muscles.' (Neijing-Ling Shu-Channel and Colleterals chapter 10) [2, p. 556]. This paragraph indicates that the Brain is formed first, before the other tissues and organs and therefore conditions the others. Similarly seen another chapter in NJSW [4, p. 280]:

As for the head,
  it is the palace of essence brilliance.
  When the head is bent and vision is in the depth,
  essence and spirit are about to be lost.

The Internal Classic believed that the Brain was related to mental activities, audio and visual senses, as well as certain functions of body movement. It also noticed in about the Discourse on Prohibitions in Piercing "Neijing Suwen Chapter 52-Discourse on Prohibitions in Piercing" [4, p. 745] 'If one, when piercing the head, hits the Brain's Door [hole], if [the needle] enters the Brain, [the patient] dies immediately.'

Huang Di asked:
  "I should like to hear about prohibited techniques [in piercing]."
  Qi Bo responded:
  "[Each] depot has an important [location where it can be] harmed;
  [these locations] must be inspected!
  When a piercing hits the heart, death occurs within one day.
  If the [heart] was [merely] excited, this causes belching.
  When a piercing hits the Liver, death occurs within five days.
  If the [Liver] was [merely] excited, this causes talkativeness.
  When a piercing hits the Kidneys, death occurs within six days.

> If the [Kidney] was [merely] excited, this causes sneezing.
> When a piercing hits the lung, death occurs within three days.
> If the [lung] was [merely] excited, this causes coughing.
> When a piercing hits the spleen, death occurs within ten days.
> If the [spleen] was [merely] excited, this causes swallowing.
> When a piercing hits the gallbladder, death occurs within one and a half days.
> If the [gallbladder] was [merely] excited, this causes vomiting.
> If one, when piercing the instep, hits the large vessel and if blood leaves [the body] and does not stop, [the patient will] die.
> If one, when piercing the face, hits the stream vessel, in unfortunate [cases this] causes blindness.
> If one, when piercing the head, hits the Brain's Door [hole], if [the needle] enters the Brain, [the patient] dies immediately."

If the patient was pierced on their Heart, death occurs within one day; on Liver five days, on Kidney six days, on Lung three days, Spleen ten days, Gallbladder one and half days, etc. Finally if the patient was pieced on the head and hit the Brain hole and enters the Brain, death is immediate.

Therefore, the Brain is considered to be of the utmost importance and a vital part of life. How important is the Brain for the life!

1.1.4   Brain and Marrow

Brain has a close relationship with Marrow, as Huangdi Neijing says: 'All marrow is tied to the Brain'. (Plain Questions, Chapter 10-The Generation and Completion of the Five Depots) [4, p. 190] and 'Brain is the sea of Marrow' (Lingshu Spiritual Pivot, Chapter 33-On the Seas) [3, p. 345], and NJLS Chapter 10 says [2, p. 556]: 'Once the essence has formed Brain and marrow are generated…'.

Marrow combines to form the Brain, which is contained in the cranial cavity. As the locations of Marrow are different, they each have their own names, the bone Marrow, the spinal Marrow and the Brain [6]. Brain is closely connected with Marrow, but different with other Marrow, as "NJSW Chapter 76-Discourse on Demonstrating a Natural Approach states" [4, p. 652]:

> The five depots and the six palaces,
> > the gallbladder, the stomach, the large and the small intestines,
> > the spleen, the uterus, and the urinary bladder,
> > the Brain, the marrow, the snivel, and the saliva,
> > weeping, sadness, and grief, as well as
> > the paths where the water moves,
> > all these together form the basis of human life.

"NJLS Chpater 30-Differentiation of the Qi" says: 'When the grains enter [the body] and fill it with the qi, then a viscous liquid pours into the bones, enabling the bone connections to bend and stretch. [The qi] flow out to fill the Brain with marrow and they provide the skin with dampness. That is what is called "*ye* liquid"'. [3, p. 336]. Ye liquid should receive the qi from the Brain and Marrow to dampen the skin.

When the Jin and Ye liquids of the five types of grain find together, they will generate a paste. Internally [this paste] will seep into the hollow spaces in the bones and supplement the Brain with bone Marrow, (NJLS Chapter 36-The Separation of the Five //Protuberance-Illnesses//Jin and Ye Liquids.) [3, p. 367]. Jin and Ye nourish the Brain with bone Marrow.

The joints of the bones are the places where the hollow space in the bones are filled and from where the Brain Marrow is augmented. (NJLS Chapter 59-Weiqi Shichang) [2, p. 512] and Marrow is what fills the bones. (NJSW Chapter 81-Jie jingwei Lun) [2, p. 725].

All above statements have clearly explained the relationship within the Brain and Marrow.

There are two other Marrows, spinal Marrow and bone Marrow. The spinal Marrow communicates with the Brain, flowing up to Brain and down to the coccyx, in other words corresponding to the cerebrospinal cord. The formation of Marrow is related to the congenital essence and acquired essence. Basically, Marrow is manufactured by the Kidney-essence. Kidney stores essence which manufactures Marrow. Furthermore, the essential substances produced from food and drink supply nourishment to the bone Marrow via the bone cavity, which reinforces the Brain. Thus, either insufficiency of congenital essence, or impairment of the acquired essence may affect Marrow formation [6].

1.1.5 Pathlogial Changes of the Brain

There were some preliminary statements about the pathologial changes of the Brain in Neijing.

"Suwen-Chapter 17-The Essential and Fundamentals of Diagnostic Palpation" states 'The head is where the spirit locates, if the head hangs down or tilts with eyes caving in, it shows the spirit will decline soon' [2, p. 88]. Brain with vision was explained in detail in NJLS Chapter 80 On Massive Confusion [3, p. 712]

> The fact is:
> When evil [qi] strike the nape, they will connect with the body's [regions of] depletion.
> When they enter deeply, then they follow the eye connection and enter the
> Brain. When they have entered the Brain, the Brain will rotate. When the Brain rotates
> it pulls the eye connection which will become tense. When the eye connection
> is tense, the eyes will be dizzy and [one feels as if they were] rotating. When the
> evil [qi strike] the essence, the essence is unable to remain concentrated where it
> was struck. Hence the essence dissipates. When the essence dissipates, one's vision
> separates into two directions. When the vision has separated into two directions,
> one sees the items twice. The eyes are [the den collecting] the essence of the five
> long-term depots and six short-term repositories. The camp and the guard [qi], the
> *hun* and the *po* souls pass through there continuously. That is where the spirit qi are
> generated.

There was one pathological pattern in Huangdi Neijing is in "NJLS-Chapter 33-On the Seas", 'When the sea of bone marrow has an insufficiency, then the Brain revolves, and there are noises in the ears. The lower legs cramp, and vision is dimmed. The eyes see nothing. [Patients] are relaxed and sleep peacefully.' [3, p. 348]

Although it limited, it has been there. In addition, we can understand from this pathologic description, the Marrow in Huangdi Neijing has not only included the spine Marrow, but mostly meaning the Brain Marrow, because the symptoms, such as turning, tinnitus, dizziness, impairment of vision, indolence and desire to sleep, are not directly related to the spinal cord and spine Marrow.

"Neijing Lingshu-Chapter 13-Jīng Jīn (The Tendons Distributed Along the Channels)" states: 'When the sinew channel of the left side head is injured, the right foot will not be able to move' [2, p. 583] which is very similar to the modern medical science about the central nervous system.

> Tears and snivel are Brain
>> The Brain is yin.
>> Marrow is what fills the bones.
>> Hence, when the Brain leaks, this generates snivel [4, p. 725].
>> Wang Bing: "The nose orifice communicates with the Brain. Hence, 'when the Brain leaks, this is snivel,' and it flows in the nose." [4, p. 725]

1.1.6 The Functions of the Brain

After the above analysis of the physiology and pathology of the Brain, it is not difficult to summarize the main functions of Brain as: To dominate the life; the centre of physical activities and to govern the mental activities (details of the Brain functions will be explained in Chap. 2 Sect. 2.3).

Brain is formed by the convergence of the Marrow produced by the Yuan Qi (Essential qi), the pathological mechanism of the Brain occurs when insufficient Yuan essence brings about a failure to produce the Marrow, and the deficiency of the Marrow fails to replenish Brain, leading to the decline of the Brain function. The manifested pathological changes include weakness of vitality, decline of intelligence, and abnormality in the ears and eyes, et al. The pathological mechanism is caused by debility of the body, overstrain of the Brain, or lack of proper care due to protracted illness.

1.1.7 Brain with Other Zangfu Organs

From classic TCM theory, the Brain is only one of the extraordinary Zangfu organs, there was a little introduction of physiological functions and pathological changes of the Brain. Most of these are scattered in Heart and other internal viscerals. In particularly, the Brain is more closed with the Heart, as "the Heart is a monarch" and houses the mind (NJSW Chapter 8-Discourse on the Hidden Canons in the

Numinous Orchid) [4, p. 155], and "Heart is the supereme monarch of all the organs" (NJLS Chapter 71-Evil visitors) [3, p. 603].

In the relations with different spirits, Heart stores the mind and dominates joy; Lung stores the soul and dominates grief; Spleen stores the inertia memory and dominates pensiveness; Liver stores the ethereal soul and dominates anger and Kidney stores the will and dominates fear [7, pp. 241–254].

However, Brain is the very first to be formed than the other tissues and organs and then conditions the others. Therefore the Brain control and regulate other Zangfu organs particularly when they are in a severe conditions or over a long term period with more organs involved [6].

1.2 TCM Brain After Huangdi Neijing

After the time of Huangdi Neijing, TCM theory of the Brain has slowly developed. Unfortunately it did not develope further more from than the following major TCM texts.

Zhang Zhong Jin in Han Danesty (AD 150–219) stated in the "Jinggui Yuhan Jing-general introduction of treatment" 'The head is the ruler of the body. It is the concentrate of Mind (Shen)'. Yang Shang Shan in Sui danesty (AD 575–670) said: "Head is the house of Heart and Mind".

Sun Si Miao in Tang Danesty (AD 581–682) has agreed similar meaning. In addition, in his book "Qianjin Yaofang" has listed one separate section 'Marrow deficiency and Excess' and provided two herbal formulas as well. 'If marrow deficiency, Brain pain and disturbed; If in excess fierce and over active.' 'All marrow deficiency and excess, belong to Liver and Gallbladder.' The treatment principle in his book were based on Liver and Gallbladder as well, but only prescription with herbs.

Song danesty "Lu Xing Jing-Foreword" stated 'Taiyi is original in the head, called Ni Wan. It controls all kinds of spirit (Shen)'. Song danesty Chen Wu Ze (1131–1189) stated "the head is the meeting area of all the Yang channels, upper Dan Tian is produced in Ni Wan palace, which is the governor of all spirits".

Ming danasty Li Shi Zhen (1518–1593) says, in his illustrious book "Ben Cao Gang Mu", 'The Brain is the house of Yuan Shen', also translated by Maciocia [7, p. 231] 'Brain is the palace of the original Shen'. The detail of Yuan Shen well be discusses in Chap. 2.

Qing dynasty Chen Meng Lei (1650–1741) stated "The Shen Qi of all Yang channel are meeting at head, all the essence of Marrow are meeting in the Brain, so the head is the palace of essences, marrow and spirits". Qing dynasty Wang Qing Ren (1768–1831) said manifestly "Intelligence and memory reside not in the Heart but in the Brain".

Unfortunately, above statements were unclear and very few acupuncture treatment strategies introduced.

1.3   Brain in the Last Fifty Years

The majority of TCM theories in the last two centuries still focus on five Zang and six Fu systems. The Brain is still only one extraordinary Fu with minimal introduction, little practice and very little research. Only from 1970s, there are some new thoughts on TCM Brain, particularly on acupuncture for the Brain conditions. There are several major thoughts listed below:

1.3.1   Xing Nao Kai Qiao Acupuncture Technique

Based on traditional Chinese medicine theory, modern medicine theory, and clinical treatment experience over 30 years, the Xing Nao Kai Qiao (XNKQ, Awake Brain and Open Orifices acupuncture) needling method was developed by Professor Xue-min Shi, an academician of the Chinese Academy of Engineering, in 1972 for the treatment of stroke, especially ischemic stroke. XNKQ acupuncture needling is a specific acupuncture therapy that acts to regulate and calm the Shen (vitality), and wake up a patient from unconsciousness through rigorous manipulation [8, 9].

Manipulation of the XNKQ needling method varies in accordance with the patient's condition. In general, the points PC-6 Neiguan, DU-26 Renzhong, SP-6 Sanyinjiao, HT-1 Jiquan, BL-40 Weizhong, and LU-5 Chize are the major points which involve therapeutic priority treatment; GB-20 Fengchi, SJ-17 Yifeng, and GB-12 Wangu are used for dysphagia; LI-4 Hegu is applied in patients with finger dysfunction; et al. The XNKQ needling method is now a widely accepted intervention for the treatment of acute ischemic stroke [10].

Since its inception 40 years ago, the application of XNKQ has gradually been improved through clinical practice, clinical trials, and laboratory research, and it is used to treat a continuously expanding spectrum of diseases [11].

1.3.2   Scalp Acupuncture

From early 1970s, based on the traditional TCM Brain theory, clinical practice and combination of modern western medicine neurological knowledge, there were several acupuncture practitioners that started to focus on the points or stimulation areas on the head to treat neurological or Brain related diseases and achieved better clinical results. After further research and study, scalp acupuncture has been formally published and promoted throughout China. From early 1980s this unique acupuncture technique has been included in the national text book for acupuncture higher education in almost all of the China TCM Universities or colleges [12, p. 81–84]. Scalp acupuncture will be explained in detail in Chap. 5.

1.3.3 Du Mai Dao-qi Technique

From 1980s, more research has focused on the relationship of Du Mai with the Brain. More Du Mai points are used in the treatment of Brain related conditions, particularly psychological conditions, such as depression, anxiety, etc., instead of Heart channel, Liver channel, Kidney channel points as traditionally used. The detail of Du Mai and Dao-qi technique will be discussed detailly in Chap. 6.

1.3.4 TCM Brain Science

After more than 30 years of practice and research, increasing experiences and evidences have led to updating of TCM Brain theory. There are many academic articles and books were published on this subject. The masterpiece of them is "Chinese Medicine Brain Science (中医脑病学)", which was edited by two national chief masters and academicians of the Chinese Academy of Engineering, professor Yongyan Wang and professor Boli Zhang, in 2007 [13].

The book, Chinese Medicine Brain Science (中医脑病学) (in Chinese), has three parts. First part: General introduction on Chinese medicine and western medicine on the Brain with 10 chapters, second part TCM conditions and treatments with 37 sections and third part western medicine diseases and treatments with 12 chapters and 48 diseases in total. It has summarized the origin of TCM theory and clinical application on commonly seen neurological and psychological conditions with majority of Chinese herb treatments and some acupuncture treatments, after traditional Chinese medicine pattern identifications.

1.4 Summary

TCM Brain theory was originally traced back to two millenniums. In the time of Huangdi Neijing, there were numerous statements about the embryonic form of the Brain, the arguments about the role of the Brain, Brain and Marrow, pathological change and function, the relationship with the Brain and other Zangfu organs.

There were limited developments after Huangdi Neijing. The more wider and deeper developments of the Brain were in the 1970s with focus on the area of acupuncture. Increasing interests focused on the functions of the Brain and its clinical practice. Several special acupuncture techniques on the Brain have been developed such as scalp acupuncture, Xing Nao Kai Qiao acupuncture technique (XNKQ), and Du Mai Dao-qi technique, etc. The Iconic book, Chinese Medicine Brain Science (中医脑病学) (in Chinese), was published in 2007 in China.

References

1. Kaptchuk T. Chinese medicine, the web that has no weaver. London: Rider; 2000.
2. Wang B, Wu LS, Wu Q (trans). Yellow emperors Cannon of internal medicine. Beijing: China Science & Technology Press; 1997.
3. Unschuld PU. Huang Di Nei Jing Ling Shu: the ancient classic on needle therapy. California: University of California Press; 2016. eBook.
4. Unschuld PU, Tessenow H, Zheng JS. Huang Di Nei Jing Su Wen: an annotated translation of Huang Di's inner classic – basic questions. California: University of California Press; 2011. eBook.
5. Curran J. The yellow emperor's classic of internal medicine. BMJ. 2008;336(7647):777. https://doi.org/10.1136/bmj.39527.472303.4E.
6. Wang TJ. A new understanding of the brain and its clinical application. EJOM. 2015;8:28–31.
7. Maciocia G. The foundations of Chinese medicine. 2nd ed. Edinburgh: Churchill Livingstone; 2005.
8. Shi XM. Stroke and awake the brain and open orifical acupuncture technique (中风病与醒脑开窍针刺法 in Chinese). Tianjin: Tianjin Science and Technology Press; 1998.
9. Shi XM. Clinical reseach on the treatment of 9005 cases of apoplexy with the acupuncture method of sharpening mind and inducing consciousness (Chinese with English abstract). Zhongyiyao Daobao. 2005;11(1):3–5.
10. Yang ZX, Xie JH, Liu YP, et al. Systematic review of long-term Xingnao Kaiqiao needling effcacy in ischemic stroke treatment. Neural Regen Res. 2015;10(4):583–8.
11. Zhao WL, Li JT, Wang YL, et al. Efficacy and safety of the "Xingnao Kaiqiao" acupuncture technique via intradermal needling to treat postoperative gastrointestinal dysfunction of laparoscopic surgery: study protocol for a randomized controlled trial. Trials. 2017;18:567.11 pages. https://doi.org/10.1186/s13063-017-2319-3.
12. Xi YJ, Situ L. Acupuncture and Moxibustion techniques (Chinese). Shanghai: Shanghai Science and Technology Press; 1985.
13. Wang YY, Zhang BL. Chinese medicine brain science (中医脑病学 in Chinese). Beijing: People's Health Publishes; 2007.

Chapter 2
Brain and Shen (Mind) 神

When talking about TCM Brain, Shen (神Mind) is the word we cannot avoid. There are many statements about Shen in ancient Chinese medicine classics, particularly 'the bible of Chinese medicine' [1, p. 25] Huangdi Neijing (黄帝内经 Yellow Emperor's Canon of Internal Medicine), shortly Neijing. Shen is very closely related to the Brain, although there are many reference about Shen with Heart and other Zangfu organs.

The meaning of Shen is diverse, could be very wide, or very narrow. Shen is one of the three treasures. Shen can be monitored.

In this chapter, Huangdi Neijing, which translated as Yellow Emperor's Canon of Internal Medicine, or the Yellow Emperors Internal Classic, could be referred to as Neijing, or Internal Medicine. The first part of Neijing, Suwen, or Plain Questions, will be abbreviated as NJSW. The second part of Neijing, Lingsu, or Spiritual Pivot, would be abbreviated as NJLS.

2.1 Shen (神Mind) in Chinese Medicine

2.1.1 The Meaning of Shen

The word Shen can be translated in different ways in English, such as spirit, mind, consciousness, vitality, expression, soul, energy, God, psyche or wisdom. From a grammatical point of view, it can be a noun, adjective or verb [2, p. 112]. Contemporary Chinese dictionaries translate Shen as: (1). 'divinity, god'; (2) 'spirit, mind'; (3) 'supernatural, magical'; (4) 'expression, look'; (5) 'vigorous, intelligent'; (6) 'vitality, energy' [3, p. 48].

In TCM there are two major meanings of Shen. The broader meaning refers to the general manifestations of life's activities, as essence and Qi are the substantial foundation of Shen. The narrower meaning relates only to the mind and mental

© Springer Nature Switzerland AG 2021
T. Wang, *Acupuncture for Brain*, https://doi.org/10.1007/978-3-030-54666-3_2

activities [4, p. 9]. In this book, we prefer to use Mind as the English name of the narrow meaning of Shen. In some references, Shen maybe translated as spirit as well.

2.1.2 Shen in Three Treasures

TCM considers Shen to be one of the 'three treasures' [2, p. 69] that constitute life: Jing, Qi and Shen (精、气、神) or, essence, the life force and the mind. The 'three treasures' represent three different states of condensation of Qi, ranging from Jing or essence which is more fluid and more material, to Qi, more rarefied, and Shen or Mind, even more rarefied, the subtlest and more immaterial.

Although Huangdi Neijing did not put "Jing, Qi and Shen" together, there are many statements that discuss about "Jing and Shen, or essence and mind" and "Jing and Qi, or essence and Qi". Such as "Neijing Suwen Chapter 3-Discourse on how the Generative Qi Communicates with Heaven" says 'When the yin and yang are balanced and sealed, then essence and spirit are in order. When yin and yang are dissociated, then the [flow of] essence qi is interrupted.' [5, p. 78] "Neijing Suwen Chapter 1-Discourse on the True [Qi Endowed by] Heaven in High Antiquity" says: 'They exhaled and inhaled essence qi. They stood for themselves and guarded their spirit.' [5, p. 42] "Neijing Linshu Chapter 8-To Consider the Spirit as the Foundation" says 'The origin of life is called essence. When two essences clash that is called spirit.' [6, p. 146]

The Essence and Qi are the fundamental basis of the Shen. Intellectual and emotional functioning are distributed throughout the body. Shen in an important integral part of health and wellbeing. Healthy Shen depends on the strength of Essence (stored in Kidney) and Qi (produced by Spleen and Stomach). Thus, Shen is dependent on the prenatal Jing and the postnatal Jing. If Essence and Qi are healthy, Shen will be nourished.

In pathological states, Mind may affect Qi and Essence. If the Mind is disturbed by emotional stress, becoming unhappy, depressed, or anxious, it will affect Qi or the Essence, or both. In most cases it will affect Qi first since all emotional stress upsets the normal functioning of Qi. Emotional stress will tend to weaken the Essence and wither when it is combined with overwork or excessive sexual activity, or both, or when the Fire generated by long-term emotional tensions injuries Yin and Essence [2, p. 69].

"Neijing Linshu Chapter 80-On Massive Confusion": 'The heart has what pleases it. The spirit has what it abhors. When suddenly both confuse each other, then the essence qi is disturbed. Vision is dimmed and hence one is confused. Once the spirit is directed to something else, recovery sets in' [6, p. 714].

Neijing has located different Essences with result Shen to different organs in "Suwen Chapter 23-Wide Promulgation of the Five Qi" [5, p. 404]:

The locations where the five essences collect:
When essence qi collects in the heart, joy results
When it collects in the lung, sadness results

> When it collects in the Liver, anxiety results
> When it collects in the spleen, fright results.
> When it collects in the Kidneys, fear results.
> These are the so-called "the five accumulations.
> {In cases of a depletion mutual accumulations occur}

2.1.3   Shen (Mind) with Zangfu Organs

Each Zangfu organ system in TCM is associated with an emotion and with a spirit or aspect of intellectual capacity. "NJLS Chapter 78-On the Nine Needles" [6, p. 694] says

> The five long-term depots:
>   The heart stores the spirit.
>   The lung stores the po soul.
>   The Liver stores the hun soul.
>   The spleen stores the intentions.
>   The Kidneys store the essence and the mind.

Traditionally, of all the organs, the Mind is most closely related to the Heart, which is said to be the Mind's 'residence'. "Suwen ('Simple Questions') in chapter 8-Discourse on the Hidden Canons in the Numinous Orchid [Chambers]" says 'The heart is the official functioning as ruler. Spirit brilliance originates in it.' [5, p. 155]. "NJLS Chapter 71-Evil Visitors" says: 'The heart is the big ruler among the five long-term depots and six short-term repositories. It is the place where the essence/spirit resides.' [6, p. 603]. "NJLS Chapter 80-On Massive Confusion" 'The heart is the residence of the spirit.' [6, p. 713]

2.1.4   Monitor of Shen

The state of Shen is said to be visible in the eyes [3, p. 50]. Healthy Shen produces bright, shining eyes, with vitality. As "NJLS Chapter 80-On Massive Confusion" says: 'All the essence qi of the five long-term depots and six short-term repositories pour upwards into the eyes and let them be clear' [6, p. 711]. Disturbed Shen produces dull eyes, which seem to have a curtain in front of them—as if no one were behind them. Disturbed Shen is often seen in those with long-term emotional problems or after serious shock (even a shock that occurred a long time ago). It is also stated in the same chapter as below [6, p. 712]:

> When the evil [qi strike] the essence, the essence is unable to remain concentrated where it
>   was struck. Hence the essence dissipates. When the essence dissipates, one's vision
>   separates into two directions. When the vision has separated into two directions,
>   one sees the items twice. The eyes are [the den collecting] the essence of the five
>   long-term depots and six short-term repositories. The camp and the guard [qi], the
>   hun and the po souls pass through there continuously. That is where the spirit qi are
>   generated.

2.2   Yuan Shen (元神)

Ming dynasty Li Shizhen (1518–1593), in his book "the Compendium of Materia Medica (Ben Cao Gang Mu)", pointed out: 'Brain is the residence of the Yuan Shen' explaining that the Brain is the source of mentality, consciousness, thought and mental activities. Maciocia [2, p. 112] stated that 'from the Ming dynasty (1368–1644) onwards some doctors attributed the 'residence' of mind to Brain rather than Heart.' However, the difference between Mind and original Mind was not explained. This is the very first statement about Yuan Shen (original mind) in TCM text.

2.2.1   What Is Yuan Shen (元神)

The character Yuan (元), stands for head, the origin, the source, the root, the original and the raw. Yuan Shen refers to the 'possession Shen' or 'prenatal Shen'. It is the source of all the other Shen. It is the largest and most honored Shen and dominates life. Yuan Shen is innate and governed by the Brain [7].

Yuan Shen is the original Shen, the raw material or original mind. It seems to be more of a mystical element to most because it is so vague and hard to understand or witness it. "Neijing Lingshu Chapter 10-To Consider the Spirit as the Foundation" says 'The origin of life is called essence. When two essences clash that is called spirit.' [6, p. 146] All the genetic information is included in the Yuan Shen, such as talents, major characteristics, et al., which will not be changed and controlled after birth.

2.2.2   Yuan Shen and Shen

In classic TCM theories postnatal Shen lives in the Heart. Shen is specifically said to live in the blood vessels (part of the system of the Heart) and to be nourished by Blood. In TCM pathology, therefore, deficient Blood may fail to nourish Shen. Alternatively, Heart may disturb Shen.

If we say five Zang organs and their Shen are batteries that storage energies; Qi and Blood, to maintaining the functions of each visceral, then the Yuan Shen is the power plant of the body. It generates all the energies and essences and delivers to the Zangfu organs. The Zang organs' Essences are received from the Yuan Shen, they are charged from Yuan Shen. On the other hand, the Zang organs absorb, digest and process the food, drink, air, and all the elements to nourish the Yuan Shen. This makes it the circulation of Yuan Shen-Essence-Zang organs-essence—Yuan Shen.

2.2.3 Yuan Shen and Brain

Yuan Shen is the prenatal Shen, which is resident in the Brain. This is the meaning of Li Shi Zhen's reference to the Brain is the residence of the Yuan Shen (Original Mind) [2, p. 842].

There has always been an argument of what attributed mental functions and consciousness, the Heart or the Brain. In Huangdi Neijing time, they were both existing. After that, the popular of five-element theory and it being widely applied in TCM, the Brain has no place in the close cycle of the five-element due to five Zangfu organs have already take their roles of each element. There were very few developments on the Brain and Shen for about 1500 years, until Ming dynasty the time of Li Shi Zhen's reference to the Brain being the residence of the Yuan Shen (Original Mind).

Yuan Shen, resident in the Brain, refers to possession Shen or prenatal Shen, which is innate and governed by the Brain. Postnatal Shen is resident in the Heart. Both prenatal Shen and postnatal Shen are all nourished by Blood.

2.3 Functions of the Brain

As Chap. 1 summarized, the main functions of Brain are: To dominate the life; to be the centre of physical activities and to govern the mental activities. The Brain is attributed to senses and mental activities.

2.3.1 To Dominate the Life

Even in the Huangdi Neijing time, about 2000 years ago, it has been in term of the importance of the Brain with life. In the "NJSW chapter 52-The Discourse on Prohibitions in Piercing" says 'If one, when piercing the head, hits the Brain's Door [hole], if [the needle] enters the Brain, [the patient] dies immediately.' [5, p. 745]. Compared with other Zangfu organs, the dangers of prohibitions in piercing, as described in Neijing same chapter and summary as below:

> If the patient was pierced on their Heart, death occurs within one day, on Liver five days, on Kidney six days, on Lung three days, Spleen ten days, Gallbladder one and half days, etc. Finally, if the patient was pieced on the head and hit the Brain hole and enters the Brain, will die immediately.

Therefore, the Brain is considered to be of utmost importance and a vital part of life. Without the function of the Brain, one should not be conscious. Consciousness indicates the totality of thoughts and perceptions as well as the state of being conscious. In the first sense, the Shen (Mind) is responsible for the recognition of thoughts, perceptions and feelings. In the latter sense, when the Shen is clear, we are conscious; if the Shen is obfuscated or suddenly depleted, we lose consciousness [2, p. 76].

2.3.2 Control Feeling and Physical Activities

There are many physical activities that are controlled by the Brain and related with other Zangfu organs. This session will focus on the senses: vision, hearing, smelling, taste and sound.

Ancient Chinese medicine books related the functions of sight, hearing, smell and taste to the 'Sea of Marrow', i.e. the Brain. Chapter 28 of the NJLS 'Spiritual Axis' says:

> When the qi above are insufficient, it is because of this that the Brain is not filled, that the ears suffer from hearing noises, that the head suffers from being bent to one side, and that the eyesight is dimmed. [6, p. 322]

Wang Qing Ren was even more explicit in "Correction of Medicine—Bain and Marrow" [8, p. 45]:

> The two ears communicate with the Brain and therefore hearing depends on the Brain; the two eyes form a system like a thread that connects them to the Brain and therefore sight depends on the Brain; the nose communicates with the Brain and therefore smell depends on the Brain … in small children the Brain grows gradually and that is why they can say a few words.

Therefore, the senses of sight, hearing, smell, taste and the function of speech all depend on the Brain.

2.3.2.1 Vision

There are many ancient classic TCM references that discuss in detail the vision and most of them are linked to the eyes and the Brain.

"NJLS chapter 80-On Massive Confusion" [6, p. 711] 'All the essence qi of the five long-term depots and six short-term repositories pour upwards into the eyes and let them be clear. The den where the essence collects are the eyes.'

> The essence of the bones [collects in] the pupils.
> The essence of the sinews [collects in] the black [parts of] the eyes.
> The essence of the blood [collects in] the network [vessels].
> The essence of the den of the qi [collects in] the white [parts of] eyes;
> Essence of the sinews and the flesh [collects in] the eyelids.
> The [eyelids] enclose the essence of the sinews and the bones, the blood and the qi. They are tied to the vessels and form a connection that is linked to the Brain and comes out in the nape.

"NJLS Chapter 33-On the Seas" [6, p. 348] 'When the sea of bone marrow has an insufficiency, then the Brain revolves, and there are noises in the ears. The lower legs cramp, and vision is dimmed. The eyes see nothing. [Patients] are relaxed and sleep peacefully.'

The above statements clearly explain that the vision function is closely related to the Brain and controlled by the Brain.

Same as Qinren Wang in Qin Dynasty "Correction of Medicine—Bain and Marrow" 'The two ocular connectors thin like thread from the Brain. The objects of sight attributable to the Brain' [8, p. 45]. The Brain and Marrow when sufficient, Brain functions healthy, then two eyes are fascinating, flexible, and clear.

2.3.2.2 Hearing

Hearing is very closed related with the Brain function, based on its channel connections with ears and the substances to nourish and support hearing.

There are lots of channels that connect ear and the Brain, such as Foot Yangming, Foot Shaoyang. As "NJLS Chapter 10-Conduit Vessel" [6, pp. 180–189]

'The foot major yang [conduit] vessels of the urinary bladder: They originate from the inner corner of the eye. They ascend at the forehead and cross on the skull. Their branches extend from the top of the skull to the upper corner of the ears. Their straight courses extend from the top of the skull into [the head] and connect with the Brain.'

'The hand minor yang [conduit] vessels of the triple burner: Their branches originate from the chest center and appear at the broken basin. They ascend along the nape and connect with the back of the ear. From there they ascend straight and appear at the upper corner of the ear. They bend downward and descend to the cheeks, reaching the bulging bones below the eye. Further branches extend from the back of the ear into the ear and appear in front of the ear. They pass in front of the ke zhu ren [opening], cross the cheek and reach the pointed corner of the eye.'

'The foot minor yang [conduit] vessels of the gall bladder: They originate from the pointed corner of the eye. They ascend through the temples and descend to behind the ears. They extend through the neck in front of the hand minor yang [conduits]. They reach the top of the shoulder where they turn around, cross each other and appear behind the hand minor yang [conduit]. They enter the broken basin.

Their branches extend from behind the ear into the center of the ear, and appear in front of the ear, from where they extend to behind the pointed corner of the eye. Further branches diverge from the outer corner of the eye and descend to the *da ying* [opening].'

As previously discussed, if the Brain is insufficient, then there are noises in the ears. "NJLS Chapter 33-On the Seas" [6, p. 348]: 'When the sea of bone marrow has an insufficiency, then the Brain revolves, and there are noises in the ears. The lower legs cramp, and vision is dimmed. The eyes see nothing. [Patients] are relaxed and sleep peacefully.' As well in "NJLS Chapter 28-Oral Inquiry" [6, p. 322]: 'When the qi above are insufficient, it is because of this that the Brain is not filled, that the ears suffer from hearing noises, that the head suffers from being bent to one side, and that the eyesight is dimmed.'

In addition, the substances, including Essence and Ye, are all related of hearing, as "NJLS Jueqi" [6, p. 337]: 'When the essence is lost, the ears are deaf.... When the *ye* liquids are lost, the bone connections cannot be bent and stretched freely, the complexion is one of early death, the Brain marrow melts, the lower legs have a blockage-illness, and the ears are filled with frequent noises.'

Similar with Qinren Wang "Correction of Medicine—Brain and Marrow" 'The two ears related to the Brain. The objects of hearing, attributed to the Brain' [8, p. 45].

Brain and Marrow when sufficient, the Brain functions healthy, then the two ears are smart and clear.

2.3.2.3 Olfactory

Nose is in charge of the olfactory, its function is controlled by the Brain.

As "NJSW Chapter 81—Discourse on Explaining the Subtleties of Essence" explains [5, p. VII 725]:

> Tears and snivel are Brain.
>> The Brain is yin.
>> Marrow is what fills the bones.
>> Hence, when the Brain leaks, this generates snivel
>> Wang Bing: "The nose orifice communicates with the Brain. Hence, 'when the Brain leaks, this is snivel,' and it flows in the nose.

Similar with Li Shi Zhen "Ben Cao Gang Mu 本草纲目—Xinyi" 'The nose is through the heaven; Heaven is the head" Same as Qinren Wang "Correction of Medicine-Brain and Marrow" 'The nose is connected with the Brain. The objects of smelling attributed to the Brain' [8, p. 45]

Only when Brain and Marrow sufficient, Brain functions healthy, then the nose uses its sense of smelling.

2.3.2.4 Taste and Sound

Tongue overseas or controls the taste, throat is in charge the sound, their function is controlled by the Brain. There are many channels connect tongue and throat to the Brain, most of them are described in "NJLS Chapter 10-Conduit Vessel" [6, p. 181]:

> The hand minor yin [conduit] vessels of the heart... Their branches originate from the heart connection and ascend along the esophagus until they link up with the eye connection [to the Brain].
>> The ceasing yin [qi] conduits of the Liver: ascend through the diaphragm, contact the ribs on the side, follow the back of the windpipe, ascend further and enter the upper denture. They link up with the eye connection, appear above at the forehead and merge on the head with the supervisor [conduit]... Their branches originate from the eye connection, descend into the cheek and wind around the lips.
>> The [vessel] diverging from the hand minor yin [conduit]... It connects with the basis of the tongue and links up with the eye connection.

When the Brain and Marrow are sufficient, the Brain functions healthy, then the tongue and throat smart of sound and tasting. If the Brain Qi is insufficient, the taste and sound will be impacted. 'When the sea of the qi has an insufficiency, then the [breath] qi will be diminished and are not enough to allow one to speak' [6, p. 347].

2.3.3   Governed Mental Activities

All the mental activities are governed by the Brain and associated with other internal organs, all memory, sleep or intelligence.

2.3.3.1   Memory

Memory is one of the major functions of the Brain, which implies recognising things and keeping them in mind, and retrieved when needed. It has two different meanings. On the one hand it indicates the capacity of memorizing data when one is studying or working, on the other, it is the ability to reminder past events [2, p. 70].

Memory can be divided by two terms: implicit memory and explicit memory. Implicit memory is revealed when performance on a task is facilitated in the absence of conscious recollection; explicit memory is revealed when performance on a task requires conscious recollection of previous experiences, or short-term memory and long-term memory [9]. As a sample of, swimming and cycling are implicit memory, and study and research are explicit memory.

In traditional Chinese medicine (TCM), long-term memory belongs to Heart, as the Heart houses the Mind and influences thinking. It is the sense of being able to think clearly when faced with life problems and it affects long-term memory of past events. While the short-term memory influences to the Kidneys as Kidneys nourish the Brain. In fact, in old age there is a decline of Kidney-Essence, which fails to nourish the Brain. It is important to remember that the decline in memory experienced by the elderly is also frequently caused by Phlegm or Blood stasis obstructing the Brain [10, p. 179].

Similar as Qinrn Wang, Qing dynasty (1830), dealt at length with the role of the Brain in relation to intelligence and memory. He believed that intelligence and memory are functions that depend on the Brain rather than the Heart. He said: 'Intelligence and memory reside in the Brain. Food generates Qi and Blood … the clear Essence is transformed into marrow which ascends along the spine to the Brain and is called Brain Marrow, or Sea of Marrow.' [8, p. 45]

We can say the memory in majority is related to the Brain, then Heart and Kidney are involved as well.

2.3.3.2   Sleep

A good night's sleep plays an extremely important role for man's health, which is close related to the state of Shen (Mind). If the Shen is peaceful, sleep well. On the other hand, if the Shen is disturbed or restless, poor sleep or even bad sleep occurs.

Good sleep relies on the healthy Qi, as "NJLS Chapter 18-Camp [Qi] and Guard [Qi]—Generation and Meeting" [6, p. 253] says:

> In strong [persons] the qi and the blood abound. Their muscles and their flesh are smooth and the paths of their qi are passable. The movement of their camp and guard [qi] never loses its regularity. Hence they are of a clear [mind] during daytime, and they close their

eyes at night. In old [persons] the qi and the blood are weak. Their muscles and their flesh wither and the paths of their qi are rough. The qi of the five long-term depots strike at each other. The camp qi is weak and diminished, and the guard qi attack their own interior. Hence they are not of a clear [mind] during daytime, and they do not close their eyes at night.

Sleep is also related to other Zangfu organs, mostly to Spleen, Kidney and Heart. As "NJLS Chapter 10-The Conduit Vessels" [6, p. 180–185] says: 'These are diseases generated by the spleen: …They cannot lie down/sleep…. These are diseases generated by the Kidneys, a desire to sleep'. Also seeing at "NJLS Chapter 35-On Swelling" [6, p. 359] 'in the case of a heart swelling [patients have] a vexed heart and they are short of [breath] qi. They cannot sleep peacefully…In the case of a spleen swelling [patients] tend to hiccup. The four limbs are agitated. The body feels heavy and cannot bear clothing. The sleep is uneasy.'

Outside evil Qi can impact sleep through disturb the Hun and Po souls. As "NJLS Chapter 43-Excess Evils Release Dreams" [6, p. 402] says: "Regular evil [qi]1 originate from outside and attack the inside. They do not settle at a specific location. When they, contrary to normal, spread to the long-term depots, they are still unable to remain at a specific location. They move together with the camp and guard [qi]; and they fly and rise into the air together with the *hun* and *po* souls. The result is that people do not sleep peacefully and tend to have dreams." Similar with "NJLS Chapter 80-On Massive Confusion" [6, p. 718] 'Evil qi remain in the upper burner. The upper burner is closed and not passable. If [that person] has eaten or drunk something hot, his guard qi will remain in the yin realm for long, and fail to move on. Hence he will suddenly sleep a lot.'

There is a commonly used reference in Huangdi Neijing to describe the pathology of the Brain, it is: "髓海不足, 则脑转耳鸣, 胫酸眩冒, 目无所见, 懈怠安卧". Unschuld translates it "NJLS Chapter 33—on the seas" [6, p. 180–189] 'When the sea of bone marrow has an insufficiency, then the Brain revolves, and there are noises in the ears. The lower legs cramp, and vision is dimmed. The eyes see nothing. [Patients] are relaxed and sleep peacefully.' The last word 'sleep peacefully' was directly translated from the Chinese characters 安卧, which looks right, but not the original meaning here. First, marrow insufficiency; how can the patient can sleep peacefully? Second, the 懈怠 in Chinese meaning is slack or slothful, but not meaning relax.

Let us compare another two translations for the same sentence. Chinese lecturers Mr.Wu and his son [11, p. 651] translated the same sentence as "when the sea of marrow is insufficient, one's Brain will feel like turning and he will have the syndromes of tinnitus, sore legs, dizziness, seeing nothing, slothful and sleepiness.". Maciocia's translation is "When the Sea of Marrow is deficient, there is dizziness, tinnitus, blurred vision, weak legs and desire to lie down." [2, p. 235]

We can see most of the words in these two translations are very similar to Unschuld, except the last one 懈怠安卧 "relaxed and sleep peacefully". I believe those translations are correct and reasonable, "slothful and sleepiness" or "desire to lie down". When the sea of Marrow (Brain) is insufficient, slothful and sleepiness, or desire to lie down, but not "relaxed and sleep peacefully".

A good night sleep is very important to health, but should be in balance. If too much sleep then this may damage health as well. As "NJLS Chapter 78-On the Nine Needles" says [6, p. 691] 'Long sleep harms the qi.'

2.3.3.3 Intelligence

Similar with memory and sleep, intelligence is also related to the Brain and Shen. The Brain, which is inside of the head, is where the spirit locates [11, p. 88]. It is the governor of Shen and relevant functions, which includes intelligence. Sufficient Brain and Marrow will generate bright intelligent. Insufficient Brain Shen will be related to slow and dull. As "NJLS-On the Seas" [6, p. 348] 'When the sea of bone marrow has an insufficiency, then the Brain revolves, and there are noises in the ears. The lower legs cramp, and vision is dimmed. The eyes see nothing.'

Although early traditional Chinese descriptions of the Brain (Nao) did not give it much attention compared to our modern-day understanding of its functions, later texts attributed more function and placed more attention and importance on the Brain [12, p. 135–136]. Summary the Brain functions, to dominate the life through consciousness; to control the five senses, vision, hearing, smelling, taste and sound; to regulate the mental activities such as sleeping, memory and intelligence. There is an overlap between the Heart and Brain with regards to these functions [2, p. 231]. However, based on recent research and discussions, mostly in China, in clinical practice, the relationship between the Brain and these functions, is more important than that of the Heart.

References

1. Kaptchuk T. Chinese medicine, the web that has no weaver. London: Rider; 2000.
2. Maciocia G. The foundations of Chinese medicine. 2nd ed. Edinburgh: Churchill Livingstone; 2005. eBook.
3. Rossi E. Shen: psycho-emotional aspects of Chinese medicine. Edinburgh: Churchill Livingstone; 2007.
4. Wang LF. Diagnostics of traditional Chinese medicine. Shanghai: Publishing House of Shanghai University of Traditional Chinese Medicine; 2002.
5. Unschuld PU, Tessenow H, Zheng JS. Huang Di Nei Jing Su Wen: An annotated translation of Huang Di's Inner Classic – basic questions. Berkeley: University of California Press; 2011. eBook.
6. Unschuld PU. Huang Di Nei Jing Ling Shu: the ancient classic on needle therapy. Berkeley: University of California Press; 2016. eBook.
7. Wang TJ. A new understanding of the brain and its clinical application. EJOM. 2015;8:28–31.
8. Wang QR. Yi Lin Gai Cuo-correcting the errors in the forest of medicine. Bilingual ed. Boulder: Blue Poppy Press; 2007.
9. Graf P, Schacter DL. Implicit and explicit memory for new associations in normal and amnesic subjects. J Exp Psychol Learn Mem Cogn. 1985;2(3):501–18.
10. Maciocia G. The psyche in Chinese medicine-treatment of emotional and mental disharmonies with acupuncture and Chinese herbs. Edinburgh: Churchill Livingstone; 2009. eBook.
11. Wang B, Wu LS, Wu Q (Trans). Yellow emperors cannon of internal medicine. Beijing: China Science & Technology Press; 1997.
12. Wingate DS. Healing brain injury with Chinese medical approaches: integrative approaches for practitioners. London: Singing Dragon; 2018. eBook.

Chapter 3
Du Mai (Governor Vessel) Is the Channel of the Brain

In 2015, TCM Brain theory has been described on European Journal of Oriental Medicine (EJOM) [1], which was the first to be published in English literatures. Recently there are some updates and develops in this area, particularly on the channel of the Brain.

In traditional Chinese medicine (TCM) basic theory, the Brain is only one of the extraordinary organs. Not like other regular Zangfu organs, Brian has no affiliated channel which results in exceedingly difficult for TCM treatments of the Brain related diseases, particularly for acupuncture. In the last three decades, TCM Brain theory has been developed rapidly. There are a great number of books and papers published in China and some in western literatures as well. As a sample, "Healing Brain Injury with Chinese Medical Approaches", in the Chap. 11 [2, p. 134] 'Nao, the Brain in Chinese medicine' mentioned some TCM theories of the Brain. Several Brain related theories and techniques, such as "Xing Nao Kai Qiao (Awake the Brain and Open orifical)" [3, p. 111], "Tong Du Tiao Shen (Dredging Governor Meridian and Regulating Shen)" [4], have provided strong support for the clinical practice of Brain diseases. Gradually the relationship between the Du Mai (Governor Vessel) and Brain have been realized and make up for the lack of information with TCM Brain theory.

3.1 Governor Vessel in Classic TCM Texts

The earliest and most complete TCM text to describe the Du Mai (Governor Vessel) was "Huang Di Nei Jing Su Wen (The Yellow Emperor's Internal Classic Plan Questions)". In the chapter 60 'Discourse on Bone Hollows' states [5, VII p. 79]

> As for the supervisor vessel (Du Mai), it emerges from the lower abdomen and then moves down to the centre of the [pubic] bone. In females it enters and ties up with the court cavity.
>
> Its network [vessels] follow the yin (i.e., sexual) organ [with the various branches] uniting again in the region of the perineum. They wind around to behind the perineum,

© Springer Nature Switzerland AG 2021
T. Wang, *Acupuncture for Brain*, https://doi.org/10.1007/978-3-030-54666-3_3

separating into branches winding around the buttocks and reaching the network [vessels] between the [foot] minor yin and the [foot] great yang [conduits]. They merge with the [foot] minor yin [conduit] and rise on the inner back edge of the upper thighs, penetrate the spine, are connected with the Kidneys, emerge together with the major yang [conduit] from the inner canthi of the eyes, rise to the forehead, intersecting [with the major yang conduit] **on the peak of the skull, enter and enclose the Brain**, return to the outside and branch out to descend along the nape, follow the inside of the shoulder blades, move on both sides of the spine and reach the centre of the lower back. They enter and follow the spinal column and enclose the Kidneys.

In males it follows the stalk and descends to the perineum; [their further course] equals that in females. That course of it which rises straight upwards from the lower abdomen, it penetrates the navel centre, rises and penetrates the heart, enters the throat, rises to the lower cheek, winds around the lips, rises and ties up with the centre below both eyes.

This paragraph clearly described the rout of Du Mai's trunk and branches, and the major Zangfu organs which are connected. Mostly importantly The Yellow Emperor's Internal Classic has already clearly proposed that the 'Du Mai (Governor Vessel) ......enters and encloses the Brain'

"Nanjing (Yellow Emperor's Canon on Eighty-One Difficult Issues)" in its Chapter 28 states 'Governor vessel starts from lower abdomen, merge in the inner of spinal, up to Fengfu (DU-16), enters and affiliates to the Brain' [6, p. 327]. Relative to Neijing "Du Mai, enter and enclose the Brain", Nanjing directly point out that "Du Mai, enters and affiliates to the Brain".

There are some other TCM classic description about Du Mai (Governor Vessel), "Su wen. chapter 59-Discourse of Qi Palace" states: 'There are 28 holes on the supervisor vessel where the qi is effused: Two in the centre of the nape. Eight in the centre backwards from the hairline. Three in the face. And 15 holes from the great hammer down to the sacrum and on the side. {Down to the sacrum there are altogether 21 joints. This is the law of [determining holes according to] the vertebrae.}' [5, VII p. 69].

In the "Yellow Emperor's Cannon of Internal Medicine Lingsu (Spiritual Pivot), Chapter 16-Ying qi" states: 'Another branch ascends to reach the forehead, runs along the centre of the top of head, descends to the neck, runs along the spinal column and enters into the sacral bone where the Du Channel passes' [7, p. 596].

"Neijing-Lingshu Chapter 33-Discourse of Sea" states: "Brain is the sea of Marrow, its transport (Openings) is in the upper region at the top of the skull and below the Fengfu DU-16 (opening)" [8, p. 345]. This statement has become one of the major principles of understanding the Brain physiological functions and possible treatment with scalp acupuncture and Du Mai points.

Above statements from classic TCM texts have clearly indicate that Du Mai (Governor Vessel) has a close relationship with the Brain.

3.2 The Modern Research on the Du Mai (Governor Vessel) and the Brain

With the development of TCM Brain theory, particularly the new understanding of the relationship of Brain and Du Mai (Governor Vessel, GV), there are increasing applications of Du Mai for the Brain related conditions.

Many of the new acupuncture theories with the majority using Du Mai points to treat Brain related diseases, such as; "Dredging Governor Meridian and Regulating Shen" [4, 9, 10], "Du-regulating and Cerebrovascular-unblocking" [11–13], "Tongdu Tiaoshen" [14], were developed and widely applied. Some commonly used Du Mai points, such as DU-24 Shenting, DU-20 Baihui, DU-16 Fengfu, DU-14 Dazhui, have the indications of regulating Shen, awaking the Brain. Due to Du Mai connect the Brain and the Heart, work together of dredging Du Mai to regulate the Brain, harmony Zangfu and Qi and Blood, nourish Shen and Qi, and regulate Shen and the awaking of the Brain. It is a unique example of Shen regulating method.

There are many recently published studies about the Brain related diseases treatment using regulating Du Mai or dredging Du Mai. Below are some samples, DU and GV are the same of the name of the acupoint of Du Mai.

Wang et al. [14] reported that they treated post-stroke depression patients with Tongdu Tiaoshen (Dredging Du Mai and Regulating Shen). The main points were DU-20 Baihui, DU-24 Shenting, DU-16 Fengfu, DU-14 Dazhui, DU-4 Mingmen, DU-7 Zhiyang and DU-3 Yaoyangguan, and combined with auricular point pressure seeds. A control group of patients were given 20 mg of oral fluoxetine every day after a break for 4 consecutive weeks. The 24-items Hamilton Depression Scale (HAMD), Self-Rating Depression Scale (SDS), TCM syndrome score, and Barthel Index (BI) were used to assess clinical outcome in both groups. There was no significant difference between two groups. They concluded that Tongdu Tiaoshen acupuncture technique combined with auricular point pressing seeds has a good clinical effect in the treatment of post stroke depression and can significantly improve the patient's symptoms and quality of life, with few adverse events. Guo et al. [11] reported how the group Du Regulating and Cerebrovascular Unblocking acupuncture therapy (DRCU) treated the patients with depression after cerebral infarction, compared with a control group of patients who admitted oral Escitalopram oxalate tablets. They also reposted the resulted of relief depression symptoms on both groups of patients. The main points of DRCU were DU-20, DU-24, DU-15 Yamen and plus other points. On the improvement of promoting the recovery of neural function and enhancing the quality of life, the treatment group was much better than the control group. Cheng et al. [9] observed Dredging Governor Meridian and Regulating Shen acupuncture therapy (DGRS), with main points were GV-24, GV-20, GV-16, GV-14, GV-11, GV-7, GV-4 and GV-3, in the treatment of vascular cognition impairment. Compared with oxiracetam only, the DGRS group had significantly better results with TCM core symptoms scales and the level of insulin-like growth factors 1 (IGF-1). They concluded that the patient's activities of daily living, cognitive function, and manifestation can be effectively improved by DGRS treatment. Jiang et al. [13] found that Tongdu Tiaoshen (Dredging Du Mai and Regulating Shen technique) combined with rehabilitation technology can significantly improve the neurological deficit, activities of daily living ability and motor function of limbs in patients with flaccid paralysis after stroke, with good long-term results. Sun et al. [10] compared Dredging Governor Meridian and Regulating Shen therapy (DGRS) with antidepressant Prozac for post-stroke depression (PSD). The main acupuncture points for DGRS were GV-20, GV-16, GV-24, GV-26 Shuigou, GV-14 and GV-11 Shendao. They found DGRS therapy could improve the PSD symptoms in patients and also recover neural function and improve daily life activities. These improvements were all prior to antidepressant. Huang et al. [12] also compared regulating Du meridian and dredging Brain acupuncture therapy on PSD with fluoxetine. Main points were GV-20, GV-24, Ex-Sishencong, CV-17 Tanzhong, LV-3 Taichong, KI-3 Taixi, HT-7 Shenmen, BL-19 Ganshu, BL-23 Shenshu. There were no significant differences between two groups. They concluded that regulating Du meridian and dredging Brain acupuncture therapy can effectively improve the symptoms of patients with PSD and nervous function defect, improve the quality of life, and had a curative effect in treatment of PSD. Chen et al. [4] used Dredging Governor Meridian and Regulating Shen therapy (DGRS) combined with fluoxetine to treat depression and compared that treatment with fluoxetine only. The main points were GV-16, GV-20, GV-24 and Ex-Yintang. The results indicated that DGRS plus antidepressants were much more effective than antidepressants only. Wang et al. [15] used the similar treatment protocol with Chen group [4] and reported similar results as well.

In summary of the short literature review above, Du Mai (Governor Vessel GV) points are increasing and more commonly used in clinical practice to treat Brain related conditions, particularly different types of depression and stroke. The commonly used main points are DU-20 Baihui, DU-16 Fengfu, DU-24 Shenting, DU-26 Shuigou, DU-14 Dazhui and DU-11 Shendao, et al.

Unfortunately, most of the above studies were done in China and published in Chinese with only few abstracts in English, excepted the last one [15].

In western English journal articles, Governor Vessel (Du Mai) is the channel of the Brain was first published in the EJOM 2015 [1]. The conclusion was based on the literature review of the TCM classic texts. The short review above was from the recent collection of clinical studies for the purpose of this research.

Twelve regular meridians have its affiliated Zang-fu organs and its name of the channels, such as hand Taiying Lung channel, shortly called Lung meridian, hand Shaoying Heart channel, called Heart meridian, foot Yangming Stomach channel, called Stomach meridian, and foot Jueying Liver channel, called Liver meridian, et al. It is clear that Du Mai is the channel of the Brian, can be called in short, the Brain channel (Nao Jing).

3.3   The Functions of the Du Mai (Governor Vessel)

Similar to other channels, main functions of Du Mai could be summarized as: contacting and communication, moving Qi and blood, induction and conduction, regulating balance.

3.3.1   Contacting and Communication

"Lingshu-Chapter 33 On the Four Seas" [7, p. 650] states: 'Since the twelve chan-nels connect the five solid and six hollow organs inside, and link the four extremities and joints outside.' The internal organs, the limbs, the five senses, the channels and collaterals, and the sinew, vessel, muscles and bones, each have different functions. However, they collectively carry out the overall functional activities of the internal organs. This kind of organic cooperation and communication of the organs is mainly achieved by the meridians. Twelve regular meridians and their branches criss-cross, into the inner and out the appearance, through the upper and reach the lower, affili-ated Zangfu organs. Eight extraordinary organs irrigate regulation and communica-tion with the 12 meridians, 12 sinews and tendons, 12 skins areas. It forms a unified whole of internal and external, surface, top, bottom, left and right, and mutual coordination.

The Du Mai (Governor Vessel), enters the Brain and is directly connected to the Brain with spine, uterus and perineum and connect other Zangfu organs through the three branches: Kidney, head, eyes, umbilicus, nose, throat and Heart. They are all connected to each other and complete the common physiological functions.

3.3.2   Moving Qi and Blood

"Lingshu-Chapter 47 Ben Zang (The Various Conditions of Internal Organs Relating to Different Diseases)" says: 'The functions of the channels are to promote the cir-culation of Blood and energy, to operate the *yin* and *yang*, to moisten the tendon and bone and to smooth the joints.' [7, p. 689]

The organs and tissues of the human body can maintain normal physiological functions and prevent pathological changes only if there is sufficient Qi and Blood. The visceral Blood must rely on the transmission of the meridians to reach the whole body and function.

Due to the communication between the Du Mai and the Brian, it can ensure the smooth flow of Blood in the Brain. After receive enough Blood nourish, and the normal physiological of the Brain can be fully exerted, and thus resist the evil spirits.

3.3.3   Response and Conducting Functions

"Lingshu-Chapter 1 The Nine Kinds of Needle and the Twelve Source Points" states 'The most important thing in acupuncture is to get the needling feeling' [7, p. 497]. It is pointed out that the key principle of acupuncture treatment is 'getting Qi', which is the function of response induction and conduction of the meridian system.

The physiological function or pathological changes of the internal visceral function can be influenced to the body surface through the meridians, which can be assisted through access of the function of the meridians and its points on the body surface. On the other hand, when the body surface is stimulated by acupuncture, moxibustion, et al., the stimulation will be transmitted along the meridians and other parts of the body surface or related organs, so that the function of that area or the organs can be changed to achieve the purpose of ventilating or circulating Blood and adjusting the function of the organs.

Du Mai (Governor Vessel), as the channel of the Brain, could have pathological reflections on it when the Brain related disorder happens, such as tenderness, soreness, depression or nodules. As an example, Zhang et al. [16] examined the Du Mai points of the hospitalized depression patients and found about 80% of the patients may have had tender points on the spinal of the governor vessel and most of them may have had 2–6 tender points. Their conclusion was that depression is closely related to the Du Mai and can be reflected at points on specific areas.

3.3.4   Regulating Balance

"Lingshu-Chapter 75 The Criterions of Pricking and the Difference Between Healthy Energy and the Evil Energy" says 'Purge when it having a surplus and in vigorous when it is insufficient, adjust the *yin* and *yang* to become normal' [7, p. 792].

When the human body has pathological conditions such as Qi and Blood disharmony or Yin and Yang disorders, it can be adjusted by acupuncture, massage and other external treatments to stimulate and adjust the balance of the meridians, so that the Yin and Yang are calm and the body is in harmony. Such adjustment is often two-way, which is to say, the original hyperactivity can be inhibited, and the original inhibitions can be excited. The Du Mai and most acupoints on it have the function of treating Brain-related diseases. Acupuncture, Tuina massage and other external therapies can treat stroke, convulsions, coma, depression, anxiety, and so on through regulating the balance of Du Mai and the Brain itself.

3.4   The Pathological Changes of Du Mai (Governor Vessel)

There are many statements about the Brain pathological changes in Huangdi Neijing, as Unschuld PU [5, VII p. 78–79] translated in "NJSW Chapter 60-Discourse on Bone Hollows" as 'When the supervisor vessel (Du Mai) causes a disease, [this causes] the spine to be stiff and to be bent backwards' and 'When it generates a disease, there is pain from the lower abdomen rushing upwards to the heart. [Patients] cannot [relieve nature] in front and behind. This causes the surging elevation illness.'

After that there are many descriptions in other classic TCM texts, such as "Nanjing-Chapter 19" 'when the Du Mai causes disease, the spine to be stiff and syncope'. "Yi Zong Jing Jian" explain that DU-26 Renzhong can treat 'stroke, stunned speech, the mouth closed and not open, the evil spirits and unconscious.'

In summary the pathological changes of Du Mai (Governor Vessel) are: spinal diseases, low back pain, especially middle line back pain, headache, neck pain, stroke and other Brain related disorders, the perineum area diseases, gynaecological diseases, male diseases, etc.

3.5   Clinical Application of the Theory Du Mai (Governor Vessel) Is the Channel of the Brain

Through the above analysis, it is not difficult to understand that Du Mai is the meridian of the Brain, referred as Brain channel. It has a broad guidance of clinical applications.

3.5.1   Clinical Diagnosis

Because of the inductive conduction the Du Mai can partially reflect the changes of Brain diseases. The search for the corresponding part of the Du Mai points can assist in the diagnosis of Brain related diseases. There have been some clinical reports [16], but further research is needed.

3.5.2   Du Mai Points Are the Key for Treating Brain Disease

In the above section, the modern research on the Du Mai (Governor Vessel) and the Bran, has reviewed some recent studies on using Du Mai points to treat Brain related disorders. There are several earlier sample studies. From early 1980', professor Hechun Luo and colleagues from mental health institute of Beijing medical university of China reported electro-acupuncture on DU-20 Baihui and DU-24 Shenting treatment for depression, results are better than controlled group with antidepressants, with less side-effects [17–19]. Professor Lingling Wang and colleagues from Nanjing University of Chinese medicine of China have treated hospitalised depression patients with a combination of acupuncture and antidepressant compared with antidepressants only, the main points were DU-20, DU-24, DU-14, DU-3 et al. Compared with antidepressants only, the treatment group had quicker response, from the first week, and with less side-effects, et al. [4, 15, 20]. The key point for the most commonly used treatment principle for stroke "Awake the Brain and Open Orifical" is DU-26 Renzhong [3, p. 112].

Du Mai (Governor vessel) enters the Brain at DU-16 Fengfu, which is the key pivot point to connect Du Mai and the Brain. As "Lingshu-Chapter 33 On the Four Seas" states: 'Brain is the sea of Marrow, its transport (Openings) are in the upper region at the top of the skull and below the Fengfu DU-16 (opening)' [7, p. 650]. DU-16 is also one of the 'Sun Simiao thirteen ghost points' [21, p. 548], also named as 'Ghost Pillow', which is one of the key points to treating mental illness.

3.5.3 Dao-Qi Acupuncture Technique Is Unique for Brain Conditions

Dao-qi technique was originally trace back to "Huangdi Neijing. Spiritual Pivot-34th The Five Disturbances": 'When one inserts and pulls out the needle slowly, it is called Dao-qi. When pricking without regular forms in invigorating and purging, it is called stabilizing the essence of life. It is because the evil energy that causes disturbances are falling into loggerheads and they must be dredged.' [7, p. 653]

After many clinical studies, it was concluded the manipulation of Dao-qi technique is: After achieving De-qi needling sensation, lifting-thrusting and rotating the needle with light and smooth stimulation. The amplitude was 1–2 mm; needle rotation angle <90° and frequency 60–100 times per minute for 1–2 min [15]. The main function of Dao-qi technique is guide the rebellious Qi to return to normal for treating Wuluan, or 'Five upheavals', including Heart, Lung, stomach and intestine, tibia arm and head. They are all involved the disturbance Qi of Zangfu or channels. Dao-qi on Du Mai, can directly affect the peace or the rebellion of the Brain, no matter if it is excess or deficient [22].

In the western literature, Dao-qi acupuncture technique and its detail manipulation was first published on the journal of Acupuncture in Medicine 2014 [15]. More detail of the Dao–qi technique will be seen in Chap. 6.

3.5.4 Guiding the Chinese Herbal Medicine Treatments of Brain Disorders

In the classic TCM texts, there were neither the Brain channel nor Brain patterns. There was almost no description about Chinese herbal medicine treatments for Brain conditions. After defining of that the Du Mai is the channel of the Brain, the herbs which related to the Du Mai can be used as the Brain guiding herbs. The sample Brain herbs, such as Gouqizi, Heshouwu, Nvzhenzi, Shudihuang, Shanzhuyu, et al., could be used to treating Du Mai and Brain related diseases, which still needs further research.

3.6 Common Patterns of the Brain and Their Points Selection

There is, so far, no text book that systematically explains the patterns of the Brain. Similar patterns were included and discussed within other Zangfu organs. Rossi [23, p. 171–215], in the book "Shen: Psycho-emotional aspect of Chinese Medicine" enumerated two emptiness-xu patterns, Emptiness of Heart and Spleen and Emptiness of Heart Yin with empty Fire, and five fullness, Shi patterns; they are stagnation of Liver Qi, Heart Fire, Liver Fire and Stomach Fire, obstruction by Phlegm-Tan and stasis of Blood-Xue, but no pattern of the Brain. Kaptchuk [24] and Liu et al. [25] did not mention the Brain.

> The only pathological pattern of the Brain discussed in Huangdi Neijing is in "Lingshu–Chapter 33 On the Sea"
> When the sea of bone marrow has an insufficiency, then the Brain revolves, and there are noises in the ears. The lower legs cramp, and vision is dimmed. The eyes see nothing. [Patients] are relaxed and sleep peacefully [8, p. 346].

Based on the review of classic TCM books and the understanding of its functions, the commonly clinical patterns of the Brain and its possible symptoms could be summarized as below, and they are on the way to further development.

3.6.1 Deficiency of Brain Marrow

Commonly seen signs and symptoms: Vertigo, tinnitus, dizziness, stress, depression, visual dim, insomnia or lethargy, infantile retardation of growth and closure of fontanel, physical stunting, amnesia and dull facial expression, light-colored or light red tongue, thin and deep pulse.

Points selection: DU-20 Baihui, DU-14 Dazhui, Ex-Bailaoxue, DU-4 Mingmen, KI-3 Taixi, GB-39 Xuanzhong/Juegu, and local area points. Techniques could include electric-acupuncture, scalp acupuncture, Dao-qi technique on Du Mai and Ren Mai points, et al.

3.6.2 Deficiency of Brain Yang Qi

Commonly seen signs and symptoms: Stress, mental depression, insomnia or lethargy, amnesia and dull facial expression, general cold sensation, cold limbs and body, dispirited, fatigue, whitish or pale tongue, weak and deep pulse.

Points selection: DU-20 Baihui, DU-16 Fengfu, DU-15 Yamen, DU-14 Dazhui, DU-9 Zhiyang, DU-4 Mingmen, DU-3 Yaoyangguan, REN-12 Zhongwan, REN-10 Xiawan, REN-6 Qihai, REN-4 Guanyuan, plus local suffered area points. Scalp acupuncture and Dao-qi technique may be included as well. Moxa could be applied.

3.6.3 Brain Yang Hyperactive

Commonly seen signs and symptoms: Anxiety, irritability, fever, distending headache, hallucinations or delusions, marked increase in energy, make impulsive decisions, instability; restlessness, restless sleep; blurred vision, dream disturbed, flushed face, red eyes, chatter, bitter taste in the mouth, tinnitus, thirst, dry throat, constipation, red tongue, yellow and scanty coat, fast and wiry pulse,

Points selection: DU-26 Renzhong, DU-24 Shenting, DU-20 Baihui, DU-16 Fengfu, DU-14 Dazhui, Ex-Yintang, REN-12 Zhongwan, REN-10 Xiawan, REN-6 Qihai, REN-4 Guanyuan, Ex- Shixuan, plus local suffered area points. Scalp acupuncture may be included. 1–2 key points may plus Dao-qi technique. Bleeding needling may apply for DU-14, Ex-Shixuan, et al.

3.6.4 Spine Marrow Stagnation

Commonly seen signs and symptoms: Stiffness and pain of neck and back, limited movement of spinal and limbs, spinal curvature straightened, segments skin and muscle pain, chronic flaccidity and weakness of the limbs with muscular atrophy; numbness of the limbs, blood vessels may be visible on the skin surface, dark-coloured skin. Purple or purple spots on tongue, wiry or unsmooth pulse.

Points selection: DU-20 Baihui, DU-16 Fengfu, DU-14 Dazhui, DU-9 Zhiyang, DU-8 Jinsuo, DU-7 Zhongshu, DU-3 Yaoyangguan, Ex-Shiqi Zhuixia, REN-11 Jianli, REN-10 Xiawan, REN-6 Qihai, REN-4 Guanyuan, plus local suffered area points. Dao-qi technique on selected Du Mai points. Scalp acupuncture may be included. Moxa or electric acupuncture could be applied.

3.6.5 Stagnation of Brain Collaterals

Commonly seen signs and symptoms: Hemiplegic, facial paralysis, aphasia, pain or numbness of one side limbs, headache, dizziness, anxiety, light-colored tongue with petechial or purple spots, wiry or taut pulse.

Brain acupuncture points selection: DU-20 Baihui, DU-16 Fengfu, DU-15 Yamen, DU-14 Dazhui, DU-9 Zhiyang, DU-3 Yaoyangguan, REN-12 Zhongwan plus, REN-10 Xiawan, REN-6 Qihai, plus local suffered area points. Scalp acupuncture and Dao-qi technique may be included. Moxa or electric acupuncture could be applied.

3.6.6 Disorder of Brain Shen

Commonly seen signs and symptoms: Mental depression, stress, anxiety, restlessness, insomnia or lethargy, delirium, murmuring, abnormal behavior, anorexia, polyphagia, dementia, drooling, schizophrenia, etc. light tongue with thin coating, wiry or slow pulse.

Brain acupuncture points selection: DU-24 Shenting, DU-20 Baihui, DU-16 Fengfu, DU-14 Dazhui, DU-26 Renzhong (Shuigou), Ex-Yintang, HT-7 Shenmen, plus local area points. Techniques could be selected through electric acupuncture, scalp acupuncture, Dao-qi techniques on Du Mai and Ren Mai, and so on.

3.6.7 Block of Brain Orifices

Commonly seen signs and symptoms: Sudden loss of consciousness, shock, coma with delirium, twitch or convulsion of limbs, epilepsy, grey or black tongue, rapid and weak pulse.

Brain acupuncture points selection: DU-26 Renzhong (Shuigou), DU-20 Baihui, DU-16 Fengfu, DU-14 Dazhui, REN-12 Zhongwan plus 1–4 needles, REN-6 Qihai, may add Ex-Shixuanxue with bleeding, KI-1 Yongquan. Scalp acupuncture, Dao-qi technique and electric acupuncture may be included.

3.7 Conclusion

With the development of TCM Brain theory, it is clear the Du Mai (Governor Vessel) is the channel of the Brain, in short the Brain meridian, which has positive and practical value for guiding the clinical practice of Chinese medicine, especially acupuncture. It would be an important clinical choice, that of acupuncture treatment for Brain related conditions, more focus on Du Mai points, plus Dao-qi technique.

References

1. Wang TJ. A new understanding of the brain and its clinical application. EJOM. 2015;8:28–31.
2. Wingate DS. Healing brain injury with Chinese medical approaches: integrative approaches for practitioners. London: Singing Dragon; 2018. eBook.
3. Shi XM. Stroke and awake the brain and open orifical acupuncture technique. Tianjin: Tianjin Science and Technology Press; 1998.
4. Chen L, Wang XJ, Wang LL. Clinical observation of dredging governor vessel and regulating Shen acupuncture method combined with fluoxetine treatment for 30 depression patients (in Chinese with English abstract). Jiangsu J Chin Med. 2011;12:57–9.
5. Unschuld PU, Tessenow H, Zheng JS. Huang Di Nei Jing Su Wen: an annotated translation of Huang Di's inner classic–basic questions. Berkeley: University of California Press; 2011. eBook.
6. Unschuld PU. Nan-Ching, the classic of difficult issues. Berkeley: University of California Press; 1986. eBook.
7. Wang B, Wu LS, Wu Q (Trans). Yellow emperors Cannon of internal medicine. Beijing: China Science & Technology Press; 1997.
8. Unschuld PU. Huang Di Nei Jing Ling Shu: the ancient classic on needle therapy. Berkeley: University of California Press; 2016. eBook.

 9. Cheng HL, Hu PJ, Zhang WD, et al. Clinical effect of dredging governor meridian and regulating Shen acupuncture method on the level of IGF-1 in the treatment of vascular cognition impairment. (Chinese with English abstract). World Chin Med. 2015;10(10):1586–9.
10. Sun PY, Chu HR, Li PF. Post-stroke depression treated with acupuncture therapy of dredging Governor Vessel and regulating mentality: a randomized controlled trial. (Chinese with English abstract). Chin Acupunct Moxibustion. 2013;1:3–7.
11. Guo XF, Lian LX, Wang YJ, et al. Clinical effect on Du regulating and cerebrovascular unblocking acupuncture therapy in the treatment of depression after cerebral infarction. World Chin Med. 2018;13(4):687–9.
12. Huang WX, Yu XM, Zhi QM. Curative effect of regulating Du Meridian and dredging brain acupuncture therapy on post—stroke depression (Chinese with English abstract). J Clin Acupunct Moxibustion. 2017;33(4):13–6.
13. Jiang TX, Wu WW, Li PF. Dredging governor Meridian and regulating Shen technique combined with rehabilitation technology for the patients with flaccid paralysis after stroke. (Chinese with English abstract). J Changchun Univ Chin Med. 2018;34(1):102–5.
14. Wang YL, Gao DH, Mu DZ, et al. Clinical effect of Tongdu Tiaoshen acupuncture combined with auricular point pressing seeds in treatment of post-stroke depression. J Anhui Chin Med. 2018;37(4):44–8.
15. Wang TJ, Wang LL, Tao WJ, et al. Acupuncture combined with an antidepressant for patients with depression in hospital: a pragmatic randomised controlled trial. Acupunct Med. 2014;32:308–12.
16. Zhang JB, Wang LL. Clinical study on the distribution of tender points in the spinal column of governor vessel of depression patients (in Chinese). Jiangsu J Chin Med. 2007;39(3):16–8.
17. Luo HC, Jia YK, Zhan L. Electro-acupuncture versus amitridtyline in the treatment of depressive states (in Chinese). J Trad Chin Med. 1985;5:3–8.
18. Luo HC, Jia YK, Wu XH, et al. Electro-acupuncture in the treatment of depressive psychosis. J Cliri Aorpririctirre. 1990;1:7–13.
19. Luo HC, Meng FQ, Jia YK, et al. Clinical research on the therapeutic effect of the electro-acupuncture treatment in patients with depression. Psychiatry Clin Neurosci. 1998;52:S338–40.
20. Wang J, Jiang JF, Wang LL. Clinical observation on governor vessel *Dao-qi* method for treatment of dyssomnia in the patient of depression (Chinese with English abstract). Chin Acupunct Moxibustion. 2006;26(5):328–30.
21. Deadman P, Al-Khafaji M, Baker K. A manual of acupuncture. 2nd ed. East Sussex: JCM; 2003.
22. Zhao JS. The study of Dao-qi acupuncture method on 'yellow emperors Cannon of internal medicine' (in Chinese). J Nanjing Univ Chin Med. 1993;9(2):49–50.
23. Rossi E. Shen: psycho-emotional aspects of Chinese medicine. Edinburgh: Churchill Livingstone; 2007.
24. Kaptchuk T. Chinese medicine, the web that has no weaver. London: Rider; 2000.
25. Liu ZW, Liu L. Essentials of Chinese medicine, vol. 3. London: Springer; 2009.

Chapter 4
Acupuncture Research for the Brain

4.1 Introduction

Huangdi Neijing, in short, Neijing, the bible of Chinese medicine [1, p. 25], in part two "Lingshu (Spiritual Pivot) chapter 73-Function and Competence" states: 'The laws date from the past. Their verification lies in the presence' [2, p. 624]. There are many theories and laws in Neijing and other classic of traditional Chinese medicine (TCM), that predates the currently held knowledge of physiology and pathology for millennia. Are they still practical and suitable for modern medical treatment after 2000 years?

Acupuncture, as part of TCM, has been practiced in China thousands of years and is expanding worldwide, due to its unique clinical effectiveness and minimal side-effects. Modern studies have found it often provides measureable improvements in patient's health outcome, particularly in the area of chronic pain. The national institutes of health (NIH) in the United States have recommended acupuncture as an alternative and complementary treatment for multiple health conditions [3]. However, the inner working of acupuncture mechanism and its practice remains unclear from the aspect of modern medicine. There are many positive results from controlled trials, as well as many negative controlled trials as well. These complicated and somewhat conflicting results necessitated a reconciliation to close the gulf between TCM and modern medicine.

Acupuncture is the insertion and stimulation of acupuncture needles at specific acupoints on the body to facilitate recovery of overall health. More recently with its public acceptance, increasing attentions has been given to the scientific explanations regarding the physiological mechanism of acupuncture.

Due to the complexities of the therapeutic mechanisms of acupuncture, research has increased of neural mechanism and has raised several methodological issues [4]. Lack of evidence from well-designed, randomized controlled trials that validate its efficacy and safety, as well as the lack of clear underlying mechanisms,

© Springer Nature Switzerland AG 2021   37
T. Wang, *Acupuncture for Brain*, https://doi.org/10.1007/978-3-030-54666-3_4

contribute to its limited application in clinical practice [5]. The exact physiological mechanism of acupuncture therapy remains unclear [6].

According to the traditional Chinese acupuncture theory as well as clinical practices, performance in specific acupoints can treat specific disorders. Acupuncture works mainly through the Brain [7]. More evidence has indicated one of the major mechanisms of acupuncture is the impact the Brain, through influence central neurotransmitters and/or remap the Brain.

4.2   Acupuncture Influence on Central Neurotransmitters

The major and most studied area of acupuncture for the Brain is, the neuro-humoral theory, which was introduced in the 1980s and the most well-known theory to describe mechanistic actions of acupuncture [8]. According to this theory, the analgesic effect of acupuncture is explained by production of endogenous, painkilling opiate substances, i.e. endorphins, enkephalins and dynorphins, and other neurotransmitters, serotonin and noradrenalin, which are released in the synapses, the connecting points of nerves [9].

Critics of acupuncture believe that if acupuncture works, it is merely a placebo effect. Many studies in human and in animals, however, show that this is not true. Additional research has found that the analgesic effect of acupuncture could be blocked by naloxon, an opiate antagonist, which implies that the action of acupuncture could be based partly on stimulating the endogenous painkilling substances. It could not be happening in the body if it were only a placebo effect [9].

One study for example, investigated the effect of acupuncture on acute pain. Reduction of pain was accomplished by needling the true acupuncture points, whereas needling inaccurate acupuncture points had observed a much weaker effect [10].

In past decades, multiple studies confirmed acupuncture on experimental animals, to show that acupuncture elicits therapeutic effect through modulating the neuroendocrine system [7]. Acupuncture can balance Brain functions through the regulation of central neurotransmitters/modulators, because all the acupuncture-influenced neurotransmitters/ modulators participate directly or indirectly to the neural regulation in almost all aspects [11]. The main neurotransmitters mechanisms for acupuncture include an increase in endogenous opioids and a decrease in substance P [12].

4.2.1   Increase Endogenous Opioids

Some neurotransmitters, including serotonin, opioid peptides, catecholamines, and amino acids in the Brain appear to participate or play a part in the modulation mechanism of acupuncture for certain autonomic nervous system (ANS) [13, 14].

A 2013 study determined that acupuncture can cause the Brain to release neuro-peptides molecules that allows neurons and effector cells to communicate with the central nervous system. In turn, this can help relieve pain and stimulate the body's self-healing process [4].

An increase in endogenous opioids in plasma or cerebrospinal fluid has been observed in humans who receive electro acupuncture [15]. Analgesic relief involves the activation of endogenous opioid systems and mu-opioid receptors (MOR) which have been shown in animal models [16–18]. Furthermore, part of the response to electro acupuncture is that if alienates the opioid receptor antagonist naloxone [19].

A 2003 study further deciphered that low-frequency (2 Hz) electro acupuncture (EA) induces the activation of delta-opioid receptors via the release of enkephalin, beta-endorphin, and endomorphs in supraspinal CNS regions, whereas the effects of high-frequency (100 Hz) electro acupuncture involve the actions of dynorphin on kappa opioid receptors in the spinal cord [20].

Studies have shown that acupuncture therapy evoked not only short-term increases in MOR binding potential, but also long-term increases in multiple pain and sensory processing regions of the Brain. These effects on MOR binding potentials were absent in the sham acupuncture group. The study showed acupuncture increased the binding availability of MOR in regions of the Brain that process and dampen pain signals–specifically the cingulate, insula, caudate, thalamus and amygdala [16].

EA was able to restore the impaired gastric motility and dysrhythmic slow waves by enhancing vagal activity, which was mediated via the opioid pathway [21, 22]. Ameliorating effects of EA at ST-36 Zusanli on gastric motility might activate the central opioids that, in turn, inhibit sympathetic outflow [23]. Although acupuncture produced significant heart rate decreases in pentobarbital anesthetized rats, this response is related to the activation of GABAergic neurons instead of opioid [24]. This opinion is proved by another study, which indicates that an opioid receptor-mediated transmission is not responsible for the present bradycardic response induced by acupuncture like stimulation [25]. These views suggest that acupuncture treatment on different diseases may be mediated by different neurotransmitters, which is in accordance with holistic view of acupuncture treatment in TCM theory.

EA activates enkephalinergic neurons in several Brain areas that regulate sympathetic outflow, including the arcuate nucleus, rostral ventrolateral medulla, raphe nuclei, amongst others [26, 27]. Consistent with this, a later study [28] found that EA at PC5 Jianshi-PC6 Neiguan transiently stimulates the production of enkephalin in a region of the Brain, which regulates sympathetic outflow. It is suggested that a single brief acupuncture treatment can increase the expression of this modulatory neuropeptide. The β-endorphin is a key mediator of changes in autonomic functions [29]. Acupuncture may hypothetically affect the hypothalamic-pituitary-adrenal (HPA) axis by decreasing cortisol concentrations and the hypothalamic pituitary-gonadal (HPG) axis by modulating central β-endorphin production and secretion [30]. Some reports have also shown that a negative perception of acupuncture might produce enhanced sympathetic activation to the acupuncture stimulus [31]. This may be mediated through endorphin pathways [32]. It is conceivable that a specific neuroendocrine-immune network is essential to acupuncture therapeutic effect. Further studies are required to reveal involved molecules and underlying mechanisms.

The term, endogenous opioid circuit (EOC) influences the hypothalamus and is one of the largest manufacturers of beta-endorphins. The endogenous poly-opioids reduce pain. Signals from needle insertion make their way to the hypothalamus. These opioid substances immediately travel to the periaqueductal grey to depress all pain signalling from the periphery. Serotonin is also released in the brainstem and stimulates further serotonin releases, along with norepinephrine within the dorsal horn. Both strongly inhibit pain signalling in both directions. Opioid release has been studied extensively in treatment of addiction disorders utilizing electro-acupuncture. Specific mill current frequencies have been shown to elicit greater releases of specific endorphins [33, p. 40–42].

Important new research about the effects of acupuncture on the Brain may provide an understanding of the complex mechanisms of acupuncture and could lead to wider acceptability of the treatment. The study indicates that acupuncture has a significant effect on specific neural structures. When a patient receives acupuncture treatment, a sensation called *de qi* can be obtained; scientific analysis shows that this deactivates areas within the Brain that are associated with the processing of pain [34].

These results provide objective scientific evidence that acupuncture has specific effects within the Brain which hopefully will lead to a better understanding of how acupuncture works. The results are fascinating. Whether such Brain deactivation constitute a mechanism which underlies or contributes to the therapeutic effect of acupuncture is an intriguing possibility which requires further research.

4.2.2 Decrease Substance P

Substance P (SP) exists in primary afferents that respond to painful stimuli and appear to transmit pain information into the central nervous system [35, 36].

Recent evidence has suggested that neuropeptides, and more specifically the substance P (SP), may play a critical role in the development of morphological injury and functional deficits following acute insults to the Brain. Those studies that have been reported suggest that SP is released following injury to the CNS and facilitates the increased permeability of the blood Brain barrier. They further reveal that the development of vasogenic oedema and the subsequent cell death and functional deficits are associated with these events. Inhibition of the SP activity, either through inhibition of the neuropeptide release or the use of SP receptor antagonists, have consistently resulted in profound decreases in oedema formation and marked improvements in functional outcome. The current review summarizes the role of SP in acute Brain injury, focusing on its properties as a neurotransmitter and the potential for SP to adversely affect outcome [36].

Several Brain-gut peptides, such as SP and vasoactive intestinal peptide (VIP), are involved in the regulation of gastrointestinal motor and sensory functions. SP and VIP are important Brain-gut peptides that are widely distributed in the central nervous system, gastrointestinal tract, and immune organs. These Brain-gut peptides can affect gastrointestinal movements through various systems; nervous, endocrine, immune, and by other means and may result in abdominal pain or discomfort, abnormal defecation, and other visceral hypersensitivity reactions [37, 38].

Electro Acupuncture (EA) and moxibustion (Mox) have been shown to down-regulate expressions of the abnormal increases in colonic mucosa-associated neuropeptide SP in patients with irritable bowel syndrome The study showed the effect that EA and Mox had on the primary gastrointestinal symptoms with irritable bowel syndrome (IBS) and assessed the expressions of colonic mucosa-associated neuropeptide SP and VIP. Both EA and Mox treatments were effective at relieving abdominal pain in IBS and concluded that both EA and Mox treatments are effective at ameliorating gastrointestinal symptoms by reducing SP and VIP expression in the colonic mucosa of IBS patients [39].

Immunofluorescence studies of SP in the spinal cord, and dorsal root ganglion tissues in rats also suggest a possible involvement of the primary SP-positive sensory neurons in the transmission of acupuncture stimulation signals [40].

4.2.3   Other Possible Neuropeptides Involved in Acupuncture's Mechanism of Action

Animal studies on the effect of acupuncture and moxibustion interventions in depression rats suggest an up-regulation response of 5-hydroxytryptamine (5-HT)/hydroxyindole acetic acid (5HIAA), and downregulation of tryptophan content in the frontal cortex [41]. Another mechanism by which acupuncture has been reported in the literature is through the upregulation of the Glutamate receptor 1 in the amygdala [42].

The mechanisms underlying the beneficial effects of acupuncture are associated with modulation of sympathetic outflow and possibly the endocrine system. The central action of EA may also affect the endocrine system and lead to a decrease in plasma renin, aldosterone, angiotensin II, norepinephrine, and serotonin [14].

In addition, there are some other neurotransmitters involved in the modulation mechanism of acupuncture for the Brain.

Amino acid sensors could regulate the activity of vagal afferent fibers. Amino acids are directly involved in signalling the vague nerve pathway in the Arcuate. Studies conducted so far on amino acids suggest that glutamate and gamma-aminobutyric acid (GABA) are involved in the mechanism of acupuncture for autonomic alteration [8].

The nerve growth factor (NGF) is a neurotrophin, which regulates the function and survival of peripheral sensory, sympathetic, and forebrain cholinergic neurons.

It could modulate sensory and autonomic activity as a mediator of acupuncture effects in the CNS. The therapeutic potential of EA could modulate the activity of the autonomic nervous system (ANS) by a long-lasting depression of the sympathetic branch, which is associated with a peripheral downregulation of NGF in organs. Although NGF in organs has been proved to be associated with the acupuncture effect on ANS, there is a lack of sufficient evidence to demonstrate the relationship between acupuncture effect and NGF in central autonomic nerve system [43].

Needling affects the cerebrospinal fluid (CSF) concentrations that naturally occur in opiate substances: dynorphin (acting at spinal level), endorphin (acting within the Brain), and encephalin (acting both in the Brain and at a spinal level). Endorphins and enkephalins are potent blockers or modulators of pain arising from the musculoskeletal system [8]. Neurotrophins are a subfamily of neurotrophic factors (NTFs) that regulate many aspects of neuronal development and functions, such as neurogenesis and differentiation, neurite outgrowth, synaptogenesis and synaptic plasticity, and circuit maintenance. The neurotrophins include brainderived NTF (BDNF), nerve growth factor, neurotrophin-3, and neurotrophin-4. In particular, BDNF is crucial for controlling normal adult Brain function and is the major activity-dependent modulator of neuronal and synaptic activity in the Brain [35]. Amongst of the neurotrophins, extensive studies have focused mainly on the association of BDNF and depression [44].

4.3   Acupuncture May Remap the Brain

In recent years, Brain imaging technologies, such as functional magnetic resonance imaging (fMRI) and positron emission tomography (PET), have been used to assess Brain responses to acupuncture in a dynamic, visual, and objective way. These techniques are frequently used to explore neurological mechanisms of responses to acupuncture and provide neuroimaging evidence as well as identifying the starting points to elucidate the possible mechanisms [5]. The study of the mechanism of acupuncture action was revolutionized by the use of fMRI, as it enabled in vivo investigation of Brain function and definition of additional Brain networks [7, 45] which opened a window into the neurobiological foundations of acupuncture [4].

4.3.1   Homeostatic Role

It is generally agreed that acupuncture plays a homeostatic role and may have a greater effect on patients with a pathological imbalance compared to healthy controls. Hence, imaging acupuncture and its effect on the Brain networks in patients may further help to elucidate the mechanisms by which acupuncture achieves its therapeutic effects [46].

An imaging study using fMRI showed that acupuncture could activate the median raphe nucleus, which is rich in serotonergic neurons. Previous research using fMRI showed that acupuncture stimulation could modulate the activity of the Brain limbic structures. These structures were deactivated during acupuncture and, more specifically, how the amygdala and hypothalamus responded the most to the treatment. This central effect of acupuncture results in suppressing the Hypothalamus-Pituitary-Adrenal (HPA) axis hyperactivity might underlie acupuncture's effects in ameliorating depressive symptoms [45].

The fMRI studies have shown that acupuncture stimulation, when associated with sensations comprising De-qi evokes deactivation of a limbic-paralimbic-neocortical network, which encompasses the limbic system, as well as activation of somatosensory Brain regions. Studies have also shown that the effect of acupuncture on the Brain is integrated at multiple levels, down to the brainstem and cerebellum. The studies support the hypothesis that the effect of acupuncture on the Brain goes for beyond the effect of attention on the default mode network or the somatosensory stimulation of acupuncture needling. These results suggest that acupuncture mobilizes the functionally anti-correlated networks of the Brain to mediate its actions, and that the effect is dependent on the psychophysical response [45].

Converging evidence focused on acute effects of acupuncture has revealed significant modulatory activities at widespread cerebrocerebellar Brain regions. Expectation in acupuncture treatment has a physiological effect on the Brain network, which may be heterogeneous from acupuncture mechanism. "De-qi" response, bearing clinical relevance and association with distinct nerve fibers, has the specific neurophysiology foundation reflected by neural responses to acupuncture stimuli [4].

4.3.2   Acupoints Specific Activities

Many studies have reported that different acupoints may have specific results activated in areas of the Brain [6, 7].

The study through fMRI conclude that acupuncture at LV-3 (Taichong) specifically activated contralateral middle occipital gyrus, ipsilateral medial frontal gyrus, superior parietal lobe, middle temporal gyrus, rostral anterior cingulate cortex (rACC), lentiform nucleus, insula, and contralateral thalamus. While stimulation at ST-44 (Neiting), which is close to LV-3, selectively activated ipsilateral secondary somatosensory area (SII), contralateral middle frontal gyrus, inferior frontal gyrus, lingual gyrus, lentiform nucleus, and bilateral posterior cingulate cortex (PCC). The conclusion was that acupuncture at adjacent acupoints elicits distinct cerebral activation patterns, and those specific patterns might be involved in the mechanism of the specific therapeutic effects of different acu-points [7].

Acupuncture at vision-related acupoints in the foot, activated the visual association cortex with fMRI imaging, at acupoints with strong analgesic effect, such as LI-4 (Hegu), ST-36 (Zusanli), and GB-36 (Waiqiu), can modulate the hypothalamus and limbic system which are pain-related neuromatrix. These results imply that the modulation effect of acupuncture might be related to the central nervous system. Moreover, acupuncture at specific acupoints could induce cerebral specific activation patterns [7].

A study [47] observed the relevant Brain areas activated by acupuncture at the Taichong acupoint (LV-3) and analysed the functional connectivity among Brain areas using the resting state fMRI to explore the acupoint specificity of the LV-3 Taichong acupoint. It is concluded that acupuncture at LV-3 mainly and more specifically activated the Brain functional network that participates in visual function, associative function, and emotion cognition, which are similar to the features on LV-3 in tradition Chinese medicine. These Brain areas constituted a neural network structure with specific functions that had specific reference values for the interpretation of the acupoint specificity of the LV-3 acupoint.

4.3.3 Clinical Treatment Study

The neuroscience techniques were not only used with health volunteers, but also introduced to the clinical treatment of patients.

A recently clinical study [48] used fMRI Brain scan to investigate the selected patients with carpal tunnel syndrome (CTS) and showed that when particular fingers were manipulated that would increase the pressure on the meridian nerve the Brain scans showed areas of the Brain as blurry. Eligible patients were enrolled and placed in randomized controlled trails, into two intervention groups: real electroacupuncture (EA) group, which included further subgroups, local points group and distal points group, and sham EA group. The real EA groups were superior to sham in producing improvements in neurophysiological outcomes, both local to the wrist and in the Brain. Moreover, greater improvement in second/third interdigital cortical separation distance following real acupuncture predicted sustained improvements in symptom severity at 3-month follow-up, while sham patients did not. In addition, compared to healthy adults, patients with CTS demonstrated increased fractional anisotropy in several regions and for these regions found that improvement in median nerve latency was associated with reduction of fractional anisotropy. Acupuncture at local versus distal sites may improve median nerve function at the wrist by somatopicapic arrangement, distinct neuroplasticity in the primary somatosensory cortex following therapy. The same part of the Brain was re-scanned following the acupuncture treatment and shows that the area re-mapping immediately following therapy was linked with better long-term symptom reduction. The study further suggests that improvements in primary somatosensory cortex somatotopy can predict long-term clinical outcomes for CTS.

There are now several trials showing that even when patients in acupuncture and placebo groups report similar drops in pain, the physical effects of treatment can be quick different [5].

A very recent review [5] summarizes the existing Brain imaging evidence that explains the effects of acupuncture for Alzheimer's disease (AD) and analyses Brain responses to acupuncture at cognitive-related acupoints Baihui (GV-20), Shenmen (HT-7), Zusanli (ST-36), Neiguan (PC-6), and Taixi (KI-3) from perspectives of acupoint specificity and acupoint combinations. Key issues and directions to consider in future studies are also put forward. This review should deepen our understanding of how Brain imaging studies can be used to explore the underlying mechanisms of acupuncture in AD.

Advances in functional neuroimaging have made it possible to study Brain responses to acupuncture. The study focus on the functional Brain responses that occur because of needle insertion into the body. An estimated study of the likelihood of meta-analysis was carried out to investigate common characteristics of Brain responses to acupuncture needle stimulation compared to tactile stimulation. A total of 28 functional magnetic resonance imaging studies, which consisted of 51 acupuncture and 10 tactile stimulation experiments, were selected for the meta analysis. Following acupuncture needle stimulation, activation in the sensorimotor cortical network, including the insula, thalamus, anterior cingulate cortex, and primary and secondary somatosensory cortices, and deactivation in the limbic-paralimbic neocortical network were assessed. Included were the medial prefrontal cortex, caudate, amygdala, posterior cingulate cortex, and parahippocampus, were detected and assessed. Following control tactile stimulation, weaker patterns of Brain responses were detected in areas similar to those stated above. The activation and deactivation patterns following acupuncture stimulation suggest that the hemodynamic responses in the Brain simultaneously reflect the sensory, cognitive, and affective dimensions of pain [49].

4.3.4   Resting-State Functional Magnetic Resonance Imaging

Resting-state functional magnetic resonance imaging (rs-fMRI) has a number of advantages, including precise positioning, the lack of radioactive injury, and the ability to combine functional and anatomic imaging. rs-fMRI can reflect spontaneous Brain activity and functional connectivity in vivo [50]. It is a highly promising and non-invasive imaging technique that was applied in the study of many neuropsychiatric diseases, including AD and other dementia. Existing rs-fMRI studies have demonstrated that the intrinsic Brain functional architecture can be modulated by acupuncture [47].

Accumulating neuroimaging studies in humans have shown that acupuncture can modulate a widely distributed Brain network in mild cognitive impairment (MCI) and Alzheimer's disease (AD) patients. Acupuncture at different acupoints could exert different modulatory effects on the Brain network. However, whether acupuncture at real or sham acupoints can produce different effects on the Brain network in MCI or AD patients remains unclear [46]. Using rs-fMRI, the study has reported that acupuncture induced amplitude of low-frequency fluctuation (ALFF) changes of different Brain regions in MCI patients from those shown in healthy controls. In MCI patients, acupuncture increased or decreased ALFF in the different regions from those activated by acupuncture in healthy controls. Acupuncture at the sham acupoint in MCI patients activated the different Brain regions from those in healthy controls. Therefore, the conclusion is acupuncture displays more significant effect on neuronal activities of the above Brain regions in MCI patients than that in healthy controls. Acupuncture exhibits different effects on the neuronal activities of the Brain regions from acupuncture at sham acupoint, although the difference is only shown at several regions due to the close distance between the above points [47].

Another more recent rs-fMRI study [51] indicated that connections between cognition-related regions such as the insula, dorsolateral prefrontal cortex, hippocampus, thalamus, inferior parietal lobule, and anterior cingulate cortex increased after acupuncture. The insula, dorsolateral prefrontal cortex, and hippocampus acted as central Brain hubs. In the sham acupoint acupuncture group, connections between Brain regions were dispersed. These results indicate that acupuncture can regulate Brain networks by increasing connectivity between cognition-related regions, thereby improving cognitive function in patients with mild cognitive impairment.

4.4 Possible Bias on Languish Publishing

Some researchers have pointed out the possible bias of some databases which was indexed as meta-analyses. As the literature review [52] found at least 288 articles from the MEDLINE/PubMed database indexed as meta-analyses of the efficacy of treatments for dementia. Among them, only 19 articles were studies from China. Many articles that were written in Chinese in other electronic databases were not included in previous research. This exclusion might have hindered the depth of the meta-analyses. On the other hand, a meta-analysis of randomized controlled trials of acupuncture for cerebral palsy by a Chinese researcher has indicated that most of the studies (on cerebral palsy) were conducted by Chinese researchers. Only one study was conducted by non-Chinese researchers. This may be related to the fact that acupuncture treatment originates from China [53].

4.5 Conclusion

There are two major parts of the acupuncture research for the Brain, one is the research on acupuncture mechanism through the Brain, the other one is the research of acupuncture treatment for Brain related conditions. This chapter focusd on the former. The latter one will be discussed in detail in the individual chapters of disease from Chaps. 7 to 18.

There are many different mechanisms on acupuncture research, while the central mechanism is the consensus by majority scholars. Acupuncture can impact the Brain, through influencing the central neurotransmitters and/or remapping the Brain.

The main neurotransmitters mechanisms for acupuncture include an increase in endogenous opioids and a decrease in substance P. Some other possible neuropeptides involved in acupuncture's mechanism are, 5-hydroxytryptamine (5-HT), Amino Acids, Nerve Growth Factor (NGF), Endorphins and enkephalins, neurotrophic factors (NTFs), et al.

Brain imaging technologies, such as functional magnetic resonance imaging (fMRI), resting-state functional magnetic resonance imaging (rs-fMRI) and positron emission tomography (PET), have been used to assess Brain responses to acupuncture in a dynamic, visual, and objective way. The neuroimaging researches have studied the mechanism of homeostatic role, acupoints specific activities and many clinical treatments for depression, Parkinson's disease, Alzheimer disease, etc.

References

1. Kaptchuk T. Chinese medicine, the web that has no weaver. London: Rider; 2000.
2. Unschuld PU. Huang Di Nei Jing Ling Shu: the ancient classic on needle therapy. Berkeley: University of California Press; 2016.
3. NIH. NIH consensus conference. Acupuncture. J Am Med Assoc. 1998;280(17):1518–24.
4. Bai LJ, Lao LX. Neurobiological foundations of acupuncture: the relevance and future prospect based on neuroimaging evidence. Evid Based Complement Alternat Med. 2013;812568:9 p. https://doi.org/10.1155/2013/812568.
5. Yu CC, Ma CY, Wang H, et al. Effects of acupuncture on Alzheimer's disease: evidence from neuroimaging studies. Chin J Integr Med. 2019;25(8):631–40.
6. Cho ZH, Chung SC, Wong EK, et al. Neural substrates, experimental evidences and functional hypothesis of acupuncture mechanisms. Acta Neurol Scand. 2006;113:370–7.
7. Liu H, Xu JY, Li L, et al. fMRI evidence of acupoints specificity in two adjacent acupoints. Evid Based Complement Alternat Med. 2013;932581:5 p.
8. Li QQ, Shi GX, Xu Q, et al. Acupuncture effect and central autonomic regulation. Evid Based Complement Alternat Med. 2013;267959
9. Cabýoglu MT, Ergene N, Tan U. The mechanism of acupuncture and clinical applications. Int J Neurosci. 2006;116(2):115–25.
10. Brockhaus A, Elger CE. Hypalgesic efficacy of acupuncture on experimental pain in man. Comparison of laser acupuncture and needle acupuncture. Pain. 1990;43(2):181–5.
11. Wen GQ, He XZ, Lu Y, et al. Effect of acupuncture on neurotransmitters/modulators. In: Xia Y, Cao X, Wu G, Cheng J, editors. Acupuncture therapy for neurological diseases. Berlin: Springer; 2010.
12. Malone M, Tsai. A review of the current acupuncture mechanisms of action from both an eastern and western perspective. SM group, Feb 2017. 7 p.
13. Li P, Longhurst JC. Neural mechanism of electroacupuncture's hypotensive effects. Auton Neurosci. 2010;57(12):24–30.
14. Zhou W, Longhurst JC. Neuroendocrine mechanisms of acupuncture in the treatment of hypertension. Evid Based Complement Alternat Med. 2012;878673:9 p.
15. Sjolund B, Terenius L, Ericsson M. Increased cerebrospinal fluid levels of endorphins after electro-acupuncture. Acta Physiol Scand. 1977;100:382–4.

16. Harris RE, Zubieta JK, Scott DJ, et al. Traditional Chinese acupuncture and placebo (sham) acupuncture are differentiated by their effects on μ-opioid receptors (MORs). J NeuroImage. 2009;47(3):1077–85.
17. Jiang Y, He X, Yin X, et al. Anti-inflammatory and synovial-opioid system effects of electroacupuncture intervention on chronic pain in arthritic rats (in Chinese with English abstract). Zhongguo Zhen Jiu. 2015;35:917–21.
18. Hsieh YL, Hong CZ, Liu SY, et al. Acupuncture at distant myofascial trigger spots enhances endogenous opioids in rabbits: a possible mechanism for managing myofascial pain. Acupunct Med. 2016;34:302–9.
19. Pomeranz B, Chiu D. Naloxone blockade of acupuncture analgesia: endorphin implicated. Life Sci. 1976;19:1757–62.
20. Han JS. Acupuncture: neuropeptide release produced by electrical stimulation of different frequencies. Trends Neurosci. 2003;26:17–22.
21. Chen J, Song GQ, Yin JY, et al. Electroacupuncture improves impaired gastric motility and slow waves induced by rectal distension in dogs. Am J Phys. 2008;295(3):G614–20.
22. Hui QY, Xing JH, Chen JDZ. Electroacupuncture restores impaired gastric accommodation in vagotomized dogs. Dig Dis Sci. 2004;49(9):1418–24.
23. Yin JY, Chen J, Chen JDZ. Ameliorating effects and mechanisms of electroacupuncture on gastric dysrhythmia, delayed emptying, and impaired accommodation in diabetic rats. Am J Phys. 2010;298(4):G563–70.
24. Uchida S, Kagitani F, Hotta H. Mechanism of the reflex inhibition of heart rate elicited by acupuncture-like stimulation in anesthetized rats. Auton Neurosci. 2008;143(1–2):12–9.
25. Uchida S, Kagitani F, Hotta H. Neural mechanisms of reflex inhibition of heart rate elicited by acupuncture-like stimulation in anesthetized rats. Auton Neurosci. 2010;157(1–2):18–23.
26. Guo ZL, Longhurst JC. Expression of c-Fos in arcuate nucleus induced by electroacupuncture: relations to neurons containing opioids and glutamate. Brain Res. 2007;1166(1):65–76.
27. Guo ZL, Moazzami AR, Tjen-A-Looi S, et al. Responses of opioid and serotonin containing-medullary raphe neurons to electroacupuncture. Brain Res. 2008;1229:125–36.
28. Li M, Tjen-A-Looi SC, Longhurst JC. Electroacupuncture enhances preproenkephalin mRNA expression in rostral ventrolateral medulla of rats. Neurosci Lett. 2010;477(2):61–5.
29. Boyadjieva N, Advis JP, Sarkar DK. Role of β-endorphin, corticotropin-releasing hormone, and autonomic nervous system in mediation of the effect of chronic ethanol on natural killer cell cytolytic activity. Alcohol Clin Exp Res. 2006;30(10):1761–7.
30. Harbach H, Moll B, Boedeker RH, et al. Minimal immunoreactive plasma β-endorphin and decrease of cortisol at standard analgesia or different acupuncture techniques. Eur J Anaesthesiol. 2007;24(4):370–6.
31. Chae Y, Kim SY, Park HS, et al. Experimentally manipulating perceptions regarding acupuncture elicits different responses to the identical acupuncture stimulation. Physiol Behav. 2008;95(3):515–20.
32. Amanzio M, Benedetti F. Neuropharmacological dissection of placebo analgesia: expectation-activated opioid systems versus conditioning-activated specific subsystems. J Neurosci. 1999;19(1):484–94.
33. Wingate DS. Healing brain injury with Chinese medical approaches: integrative approaches for practitioners. London: Singing Dragon; 2018. eBook.
34. Asghar AU, Green G, Lythgoe MF, et al. Acupuncture needling sensation: the neural correlates of deqi using fMRI. Brain Res. 2010;1315:111–8.
35. De Felipe C, Herrero JF, O'Brien JA, Doyle CA, et al. Altered nociception, analgesia and aggression in mice lacking the receptor for substance P. Nature. 1998;392:394–7.
36. Donkin JJ, Turner RJ, Hassan I, et al. Substance P in traumatic brain injury. Prog Brain Res. 2007;161:97–109.
37. Kusano M, Sekiguchi T, Kawamura O, et al. Further classification of dysmotility-like dyspepsia by interdigestive gastroduodenal manometry and plasma motilin level. Am J Gastroenterol. 1997;92(3):481–4.

38. Dong WZ, Zou DW, Li ZS, et al. Study of visceral hypersensitivity in irritable bowel syndrome. Chin J Dig Dis. 2004;5(3):103–9.
39. Lu ZZ, Yin XJ, Teng WJ, et al. Comparative effect of electroacupuncture and moxibustion on the expression of substance P and vasoactive intestinal peptide in patients with irritable bowel syndrome. J Tradit Chin Med. 2015;35:402–10.
40. Zhang K, Xu DS, Cui JJ, et al. The expression of substance P in sensory neurons and nerve fibers associated with "Sanyinjiao" (SP 6) region in the rat. Zhen Ci Yan Jiu. 2015;40:449–54.
41. Ding N, Li R, Tian HH. Effect of acupuncture and moxibustion interventions on ethological changes and 5-HT/5-HIAA levels in prefrontal cortex in depression rats. Zhen Ci Yan Jiu. 2016;41:45–50.
42. Yan YX, Feng XM, Wang JY, et al. Effect of electroacupuncture intervention on expression of pain sensory and affective processing-related μ-opioid receptor, etc. in the amygdala in chronic neuropathy pain rats. Zhen Ci Yan Jiu. 2016;41:3–10,22.
43. Manni L, Albanesi M, Guaragna M, et al. Neurotrophins and acupuncture. Auton Neurosci. 2010;157(1–2):9–17.
44. Park H, Poo MM. Neurotrophin regulation of neural circuit development and function. Nat Rev Neurosci. 2013;14(1):7–23.
45. Hui KKS, Marina O, Liu J, et al. Acupuncture, the limbic system, and the anticorrelated networks of the brain. Auton Neurosci. 2010;157(1–2):81–90.
46. Jia HB, Liu ZS, Min BQ, et al. The effects of acupuncture at real or sham acupoints on the intrinsic brain activity in mild cognitive impairment patients. Evid Based Complement Alternat Med. 2015;529675:9 p.
47. Zheng Y, Wang YY, Lan YJ, et al. Imaging of brain function based on the analysis of functional connectivity-imaging analysis of brain function by fMRI after acupuncture at LR3 in heal the individuals. Afr J Tradit Complement Altern Med. 2016;13(6):90–100.
48. Maeda Y, Kim H, Ketter N, et al. Rewiring the primary somatosensory cortex in carpal tunnel syndrome with acupuncture. Brain. 2017;140(4):914–27.
49. Chae Y, Chang DS, Lee SH, et al. Inserting needles into the body: a meta-analysis of brain activity associated with acupuncture needle stimulation. J Pain. 2013;14(3):215–22.
50. Wang ZQ, Liang PP, Zhao ZL, et al. Acupuncture modulates resting state hippocampal functional connectivity in Alzheimer disease. PLoS One. 2014;9(3):e91160.
51. Tan TT, Wang D, Huang JK, et al. Modulatory effects of acupuncture on brain networks in mild cognitive impairment patients. Neural Regen Res. 2017;12(2):250–8.
52. Perng CH, Chang YC, Tzang F. The treatment of cognitive dysfunction in dementia: a multiple treatments meta-analysis. Psychopharmacology. 2018;235:1571–80.
53. Li LX, Zhang MM, Zhang Y, et al. Acupuncture for cerebral palsy: a meta-analysis of randomized controlled trials. Neural Regen Res. 2018;13(6):1107–17.

Chapter 5
Scalp Acupuncture

5.1 TCM Brain Theory and Practice

As Chaps. 1–3 explained, TCM has its Brain theory from Huangdi Neijing time. There are many texts that explain the Brain functions, pathological changes, the channel of Brain, etc. This section will focus on the acupuncture needling treatment for the Brain, particularly on the head.

5.1.1 Channels on the Head from Huangdi Neijing

In Huangdi Neijing, most of the channels are described in "Lingshu Chapter 10-The Conduit Vessels" [1, p. 171–204]. Here we will focus on the main channels and the branches with points located on the head.

5.1.1.1 Hand Shaoyang (Minor Yang) Sanjiao (Triple Burner) Channel

The hand minor yang [conduit] vessels of the triple burner… Their branches originate from the chest center and appear at the broken basin. They ascend along the nape and connect with the back of the ear. From there they ascend straight and appear at the upper corner of the ear. They bend downward and descend to the cheeks, reaching the bulging bones below the eye. Further branches extend from the back of the ear into the ear and appear in front of the ear. They pass in front of the ke zhu ren [opening], cross the cheek and reach the pointed corner of the eye.

© Springer Nature Switzerland AG 2021
T. Wang, *Acupuncture for Brain*, https://doi.org/10.1007/978-3-030-54666-3_5

5.1.1.2 Foot Yangming (Yang Brilliance) Stomach Channel

The foot yang brilliance [conduit] vessels of the stomach: … Then they extend along the low joint of the jaws to above the ears and reach beyond the ke zhu ren [opening] following the borderline of the hair to eventually reach the forehead and the skull.

5.1.1.3 Foot Shaoyang (Minor Yang) Gall Bladder Channel

The foot minor yang [conduit] vessels of the gall bladder: They originate from the pointed corner of the eye. They ascend through the temples and descend to behind the ears. They extend through the neck in front of the hand minor yang [conduits]… Their branches extend from behind the ear into the centre of the ear, and appear in front of the ear, from where they extend to behind the pointed corner of the eye. Further branches diverge from the outer corner of the eye and descend to the *da ying* [opening]. They unite with the hand minor yang [conduit] and extend below the bulging bone below the eye.

5.1.1.4 Foot Taiyang (Major Yang) Bladder Channel

The foot major yang [conduit] vessels of the urinary bladder: They originate from the inner corner of the eye. They ascend at the forehead and cross on the skull. … Their branches extend from the top of the skull to the upper corner of the ears. Their straight courses extend from the top of the skull into [the head] and connect with the Brain. Then they turn around and appear.

5.1.1.5 Foot Jueyin (Ceasing Yin) Liver Channel

The ceasing yin [qi] conduits of the Liver: … They link up with the eye connection, appear above at the forehead and merge on the head with the supervisor [conduit].

5.1.1.6 Du Mai (Supervisor Vessel, or Governor Vessel)

Another channel, Du Mai or Governor Vessel was found in "Neijing Suwei chapter 60-Discourse on Bone hollows" states 'As for the supervisor vessel… emerge together with the major yang [conduit] from the inner canthi of the eyes, rise to the forehead, intersecting [with the major yang conduit] on the peak of the skull, enter and enclose the Brain.' [2, p. 78]

We can see there are six channels directly connected with head and even enter the Brain. They are Hand Shaoyang Sanjiao (Triple Burner) channel, Foot Yangming stomach channel, Foot Shaoyang Gallbladder channel, Foot Taiyang (major yang) Bladder Channel, Foot Jueyin Liver channel, and Du Mai (Governor vessel).

5.1.2 Channel Points on the Head

In Huangdi Neijing, there are 25 points on the head, as described in "Chapter 58-Discourse on Qi holes" 'five [conduit] lines on the head: [each] line has five [holes]; five [times] five is 25 holes' [2, p. 50].

Based on the locations described on the "A Manual of Acupuncture" [3, p. 123–557], in summary there are 38 channel points located on the skull head, they are ST-8 Touwei, BL-3 Meichong, BL-4 Qucha, BL-5 Wuchu, BL-6 Chengguang, BL-7 Tongtian, BL-8 Luoque, BL-9 Yuzhen, SJ-18 Chimai, SJ-19 Luxi, SJ-20 Jiaosun, SJ-22 Heliao, SJ-23 Sizhukong, GB-1 Tongziliao, GB-3 Shangguan, GB-4 Hanyan, GB-5 Xuanlu, GB-6 Xuanli, GB-7 Qubin, GB-8 Shuaigu, GB-9 Tianchong, GB-10 Fubai, GB-11 Touqiaoyin, GB-13 Benshen, GB-14 Yangbai, GB-15 Toulinqi, GB-16 Muchuang, GB-17 Zhengying, GB-18 Chengling, GB-19 Naokong, DU-17 Naohu, DU-18 Qiangjian, DU-19 Houding, DU-20 Baihui, DU-21 Qiangding, DU-22 Xinhui, DU-23 Shangxing, DU-24 Shenting.

There are many additional points located around the ear, on top of the neck and the face.

The indications of many above the head points included neurological and psychological disorders, such as headache, dizziness, dimness of vision, hemiplegia (ST-8) [3, p. 136], loss of consciousness (BL-7) [3, p. 261], epilepsy (SJ-19) [3, p. 409], loss of speech (GB-7) [3, p. 426], mania and spasm (DU-17) [3, p. 550], wind stroke, loss of consciousness, poor memory, mental problems (DU-20) [3, p. 552], et al.

5.1.3 Channel Diseases and Treatment on Head

In clinic practice, we choose points mainly on the channels to treat related conditions, including the local area symptoms. Above the channels where their points are located on the head; these are commonly used to treating head and Brain related conditions, some according to the channels and some just for the local area symptoms. As some sample indications of the channels in Neijing [1]

- The foot yang brilliance [conduit] vessels of the stomach… When [these vessels] are excited, then the resulting disease will be a shivering with cold, and a tendency to moan, with frequent yawning. The complexion is black.
- When the disease emerges, [patients] develop an aversion to other persons and fire. When they hear sounds of wood, they are cautious and fearful. The heart is about to move. Those alone close the door and the windows and prefer to stay at home. In serious cases [patients] are inclined to ascend to high places and to sing. They throw off their garments and run away. The intestines have noises and the abdomen is swollen…. These are diseases generated by the blood: Madness, malaria, excessive warmth, sweating…

- The hand major yang [conduit] vessels of the small intestine: These are diseases generated by the ye liquids: The ears are deaf. The eyes are yellow.
- The foot major yang [conduit] vessels of the urinary bladder: … When [these vessels] are excited, then the disease presses into the head and causes pain there. The eyes feel as if they were to fall out. The nape feels as if it were pulled… These are diseases generated by the sinews: Piles, malaria, madness, peak-illness, headache, nape pain, yellow eyes, tear flow, nasal flow and nosebleed.
- The hand minor yang [conduit] vessels of the triple burner… When [these vessels] are excited, then this will result in the patient's suffering from deafness of the ears with mental confusion. The esophagus is swollen; the throat is blocked. These are diseases generated by the qi: Sweating. The pointed corners of the eyes ache.
- The foot minor yang [conduit] vessels of the gall bladder: When [these vessels] are excited, then this will result in the patient's suffering from a bitter flavour in his mouth and a tendency to deep breathing. These are diseases generated by the bones: Headache, aching chin and pointed corners of the eyes.

'When the supervisor vessel (Du Mai) generates a disease, treat the supervisor vessel.' "Neijing-Discourse on Bone hollows" [2, p. 80]

Ancient Chinese doctor has already known the importance of the channels and acupoints on the head. There were many theories and statements about the needling on head, as a sample of the famous stories is the point Baihui (DU-20).

One of the most celebrated doctor in Chinese history, Bian Que., cured a special patient, the crown prince of Guo State during the Spring and Autumn period (770 BC–475 BC) with needling on Baihui (DU-20) from his false death. This story, Bian Que. Jian Qihuangong (Bian Que. meets Duke Huan of Qi State—a chapter from the first Century BC book Shiji (Historical Records)), remains a required reading in junior high school curriculum in China [4].

According to legend, Bian Que. travelled through the state of Guo and heard that the Prince had died for half a day. Bian Que. asked the details from the warlock in the palace and thought that the Prince was suffering from a "Corpse" disease that suddenly made him faint and become unconscious. He went to see the Prince himself and then asked his disciples to grind the stone needle, stab the Baihui (DU-20) point, and made the herb medicine that could be put into the body for five points. After mixing with the medicine, the prince actually sat up and was no different from ordinary people. He continued to adjust and nourish Yin and Yang, 2 days later, the Prince completely recovered.

5.2   Modern Development on Head Acupuncture

Not like other TCM theory developments, the Brain theory and the related needling therapy was not thoroughly developed.

The most rapid development of head acupuncture was from 1950s after "new China" was founded. Inspired by some micro-acupuncture systems, such as ear acupuncture, nose acupuncture and eye acupuncture, some acupuncture experts began to practice needling on the head to treat diseases on other parts of the body. For example, Yunpeng Fang in Shanxi province at the end of 1950s and Yansong Tang in Shanghai at the end of 1960s began to apply head acupuncture for treating diseases, and gradually improved this therapy [5].

In the early 1970s, influenced by neurological knowledge, head acupuncture was mainly separated from traditional acupuncture system, i.e. no need guidance of channel, acupoints and classic TCM theory. In 1971, Dr. Shunfa Jiao from Shanxi province in China first published this modern acupuncture technique, which was combined with traditional acupuncture needling and the knowledge of modern physiology and anatomy of the nervous system and in 1972 it was systematically summarized and named of "Tou Zhen (head acupuncture or in translation in English scalp acupuncture SA)" [6, p. 7] Later, Yunpeng Fang's style scalp acupuncture was published in 1976. The other styles of scalp acupuncture are Mingjiu Zhang, Xuejian Lin, and so on. Each of them proposed different diagrams and groupings of scalp acupuncture points. For example, some divided the scalp into zones or regions, while some focus on points or lines [5, 7]. Dr. Mingqing Zhu began developing Zhu's style scalp acupuncture later in the 1980s and began to practice and educate many about his style of scalp acupuncture in American in 1991. His book "Zhu's Scalp Acupuncture" was published in 1992 [8]. In Japan, another style scalp acupuncture was published in 1973 by Dr. Toshikatsu Yamamoto, which is known as Yamamoto New Scalp Acupuncture (YNSA). His book with the same name published in 1998 [9, 10]. There were some papers which introduce scalp acupuncture in the treatment of Brain disease and were published in English journals from 1970's onward [11–13].

From the 1970s scalp acupuncture was widely used in China, with its clinical effectiveness and that was easy to follow. In the 1980s Jiao's style was covered in the higher education of acupuncture courses in most Chinese medicine universities and colleges in China [14, p. 81–84].

With the development of scalp acupuncture, many different styles were added which generated a level of confusion. Therefore, it was urgently required that standardization of the names of the acupoints or stimulation areas be established. In 1984 China Acupuncture Association prepared a protocol of Standard Nomenclature of Scalp Acupuncture lines, which was entrusted by the World Health Organization (WHO). After several years of discussion and research, in 1991, WHO published the scheme Standard International Acupuncture Nomenclature: 3.6 Scalp acupuncture lines [15]. Soon after the International Standard Scalp Acupuncture (ISSA) was incorporated into the higher education of acupuncture courses in almost all Chinese medicine universities and colleges in China, which replaced Jiao's style SA, in the early 1990s [16].

Compared with ISSA, Jiao's SA use the modern neurological language was easies to remember and practice, and more convenient to communicate with western practitioner and patients. In addition, the second edition of Jiao's Scalp Acupuncture (in Chinese) had updated several new stimulation areas, particularly the Spirit-Emotion Area, and the Maness-Control Area [17, p. 42–44]. These two updated areas are encouraging for the treatment of psychological conditions. Furthermore, the book "Chinese Scalp Acupuncture" published by famous neuro-acupuncturists Mr. and Mrs. Hao in USA in 2011, used Jiao's style as well [18]. This book, Acupuncture for Brain, will based on the second edition of Jiao's Scalp Acupuncture and embedding some useful materials from ISSA.

5.3   Chinese Scalp Acupuncture Stimulate Areas and Indications

If without specified, Chinese scalp acupuncture (CSA) in this book refers to Jiao's style [17, p. 41–45]. There are some revised on their locations and indications based my clinical experiences and researches. The relevant ISAA lines [15] are added after the areas in brackets.

5.3.1   Motor Area (MTA), (ISSA-MS6, dingniè qiánxiéxiàn)

Location: A line connecting 2 points called the upper and lower points of the Motor Area. The upper point is situated on the antero-posterior midline, 0.5 cm behind its midpoint. The lower point is the point in the temporal region where the supercilio-occipital line intersects the anterior hairline. The whole area line is divided into five equal parts, and grouped with three sections, upper one-fifth, middle two-fifths and lower two-fifths (see Figs. 5.1, 5.23 and 5.24).

Indications: Generally, for motor paralysis of the contralateral side.

- Upper one-fifth: Paralysis of the contralateral lower limb, trunk, spine and neck.
- Middle two-fifths: Paralysis of the contralateral upper limb
- Lower two-fifths: Central facial paralysis of the contralateral side, motor aphasia, dripping of saliva, disturbance of phonation, etc. (Also called First Speech Area, FSA)

5.3.2   Sensory Area (SSA), (ISSA-MS7 dingniè hòuxiéxiàn)

Location: A line parallel to and 1.5 cm posterior to the Motor Area. The whole area line is divided into five equal parts, and grouped with three sections, upper one-fifth, middle two-fifths and lower two-fifths.

(see Figs. 5.2, 5.23 and 5.24)

Indications: Generally, for the sensory disorders of the contralateral side.

Fig. 5.1 MTA:
Motor Area. MP:
Midpoint; APM:
Anterior Posterior
Midline; FSA:
First Speech Area

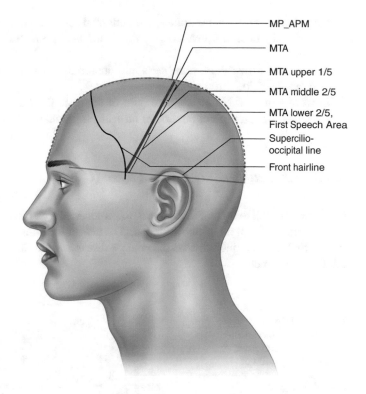

MP_APM

MTA

MTA upper 1/5

MTA middle 2/5

MTA lower 2/5,
First Speech Area

Supercilio-
occipital line

Front hairline

Fig. 5.2 SSA:
Sensory Area. MAT:
Motor Area;
MP-APM: Midpoint
of Anterior
Posterior Midline

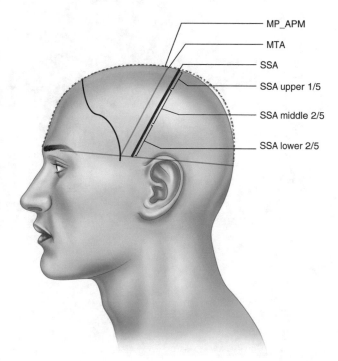

MP_APM

MTA

SSA

SSA upper 1/5

SSA middle 2/5

SSA lower 2/5

- Upper one-fifth: Pain, numbness and abnormal sensation of the contralateral side in the back, occipital headache, pain of the neck, and tinnitus, phantom low limb pain.
- Middle two-fifths: Pain, numbness and abnormal sensation of the contralateral arm, phantom low limb pain.
- Lower two-fifths: Numbness and pain of the contralateral side in the head and face, migraine, temporomandibular arthritis, trigeminal neuralgia, etc.

5.3.3 Chorea-Tremor Control Area (CTCA)

Location: Parallel to and 1.5 cm anterior to Motor Area (see Figs. 5.3, 5.23 and 5.24).

Indications: Involuntary movement and tremor of the contralateral side head and limbs, Sydenham's chorea, Parkinsonism's disease, tremors, essential tremor and related syndromes.

Fig. 5.3 CTCA: Chorea-Tremor Control Area. MAT: Motor Area; MP-APM: Midpoint of Anterior Posterior Midline

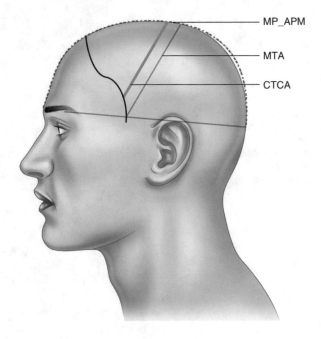

Fig. 5.4 VMA:
Vasomotor Area.
MAT: Motor Area;
MP-APM:
Midpoint of
Anterior
Posterior Midline

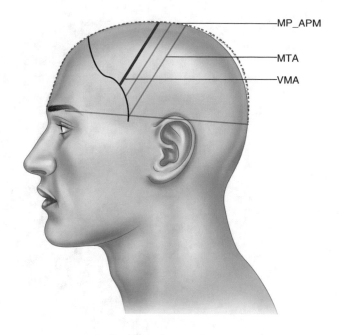

5.3.4   Vasomotor Area (VMA)

Location: Parallel to and 1.5 cm anterior to Chorea-Tremor Control Area (see Figs. 5.4, 5.23 and 5.24).

Indication: Cortical superficial oedema, essential hypertension, chronic pain, Alzheimer's disease, dementia, Brain injuries, etc.

5.3.5   Foot-Motor Sensory Area (FMSA)
(ISSA-MS5 dingzhongxiàn)

Location: Parallel to and 1 cm lateral to the anterior-posterior line. The line is 3 cm long and starts 1 cm posterior to the line representing the sensory area. Or, 1 cm lateral to the midpoint of the midline, draw a 3 cm long line to the posterior (see Figs. 5.5, 5.22 and 5.24).

Indication: Paralysis, pain or numbness of contralateral lower limb, pain of the back and neck, nocturnal enuresis, frequent urination, prolapsed uterus, poor memory, etc.

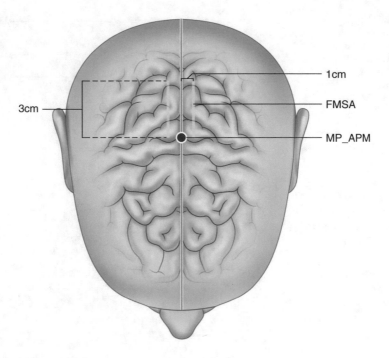

Fig. 5.5 FMSA: Foot-Motor Sensory Area. MP-APM: Midpoint of Anterior Posterior Midline

5.3.6 Dizziness and Auditory Area (DAA), (ISSA-MS11 nièhòuxiàn)

Location: A horizontal line 4 cm long, its midpoint 1.5 cm above the apex of the ear (see Figs. 5.6 and 5.23).

    Indication: Ipsilateral dizziness, deafness, tinnitus, auditory vertigo, Meniere's syndrome, etc.

5.3.7 First Speech Area (FSA)

Location: Lower two-fifths of the Motor area (see Figs. 5.7 and 5.23).

    Indications: Motor aphasia, dripping of saliva, disturbance of phonation, etc.

Fig. 5.6 DAA:
Dizziness and
Auditory Area

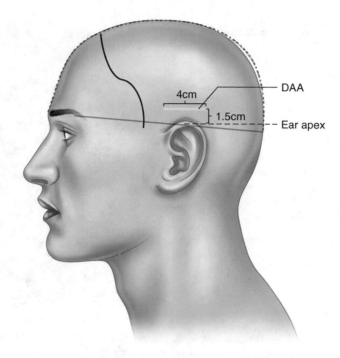

Fig. 5.7 FSA: First
Speech Area. MP:
Midpoint; APM:
Anterior
Posterior Midline

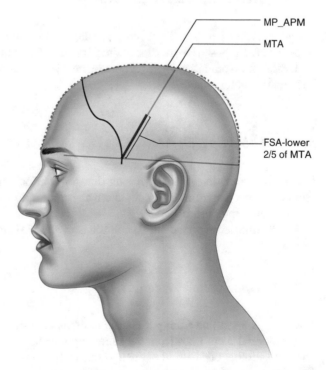

Fig. 5.8 SCSA:
Second Speech Area

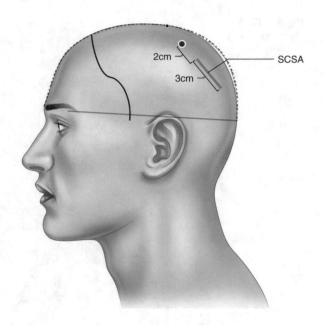

5.3.8   Second Speech Area (SCSA)

Location: A vertical line 3 cm long, parallel to the anterior-posterior midline, its upper end 2 cm posterior-inferior to the parietal tubercle (see Figs. 5.8 and 5.23).

   Indication: Nominal aphasia (cannot express the words who want to say, particularly nouns such as name).

5.3.9   Third Speech Area (TSA)

Location: A horizontal line 4 cm long drawn posteriorly from the midpoint of the Auditory Area. Or: from the point 1.5 cm above the apex of the ear draw a horizontal line 4 cm long posterior.

   Indication: Sensory (receptive) aphasia (see Figs. 5.9 and 5.23).

5.3.10   Application Area (APA)

Location: A 3 cm line from parietal tuber to the center of the mastoid process and two additional 3 cm lines from the same origin of the first line at the tuber, one in front and another one behind of the first line with an angle of 45-degree between the first line and each of the latter lines (see Fig. 5.10).

   Indication: Apraxia, difficulty on fine movement.

Fig. 5.9 TSA: Third
Speech Area

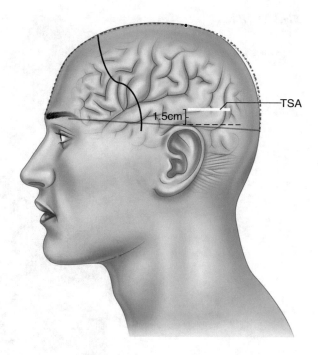

Fig. 5.10 APA: Application Area

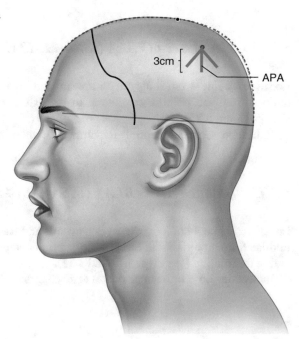

Fig. 5.11 VSA:
Visual Area

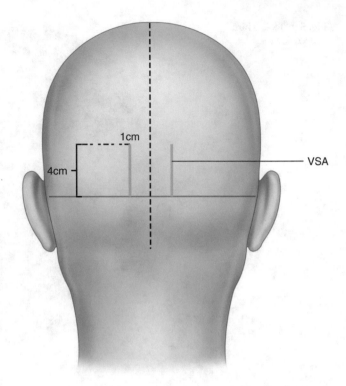

5.3.11   Visual Area (VSA), (ISSA-MS13 zhenshàng pángxiàn)

Location: A line 4 cm long drawn upwards and parallel to the anterior-posterior
midline from the point 1 cm lateral to the external occipital protuberance (see
Figs. 5.11 and 5.25).

Indication: Cortical (central) impairment of vision and cataract.

5.3.12   Balance Area (BLA), (ISSA-MS14 zhenxià pángxiàn)

Location: A line 4 cm long drawn downwards and parallel to the anterior-posterior
midline from a point at the level of the external occipital protuberance, 3.5 cm lateral to the midline (see Figs. 5.12 and 5.25).

Indication: Loss of balance due to cerebellar disorders, Brain atrophy, et al.

Fig. 5.12 BLA:
Balance Area

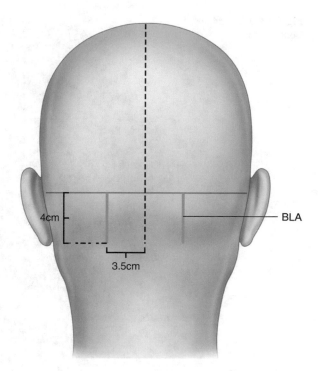

5.3.13   *Mania Control Area (MCA), (ISSA-MS12 zhenshàng zhèngzhongxiàn)*

Location: On the anterior-posterior midline, from the tip of external occipital protu-berance, draw a line 4 cm long drawn downwards on the midline (see Figs. 5.13 and 5.25).

Indication: Mania, anxiety, medulla and brainstem injuries.

5.3.14   *Stomach Area (STA), (ISSA-MS3 épángxiàn II)*

Stomach Area: A line 2 cm long drawn directly backwards and parallel to the anterior-posterior midline from a point on the anterior hairline vertically above the pupil of the eye (see Figs. 5.14 and 5.26).

Indication: Disorders of the upper abdomen and general malaise, gastritis, stom-ach pain, poor appetite, esophageal reflux, and TCM Spleen and Stomach conditions.

Fig. 5.13 MCA: Mania
Control Area

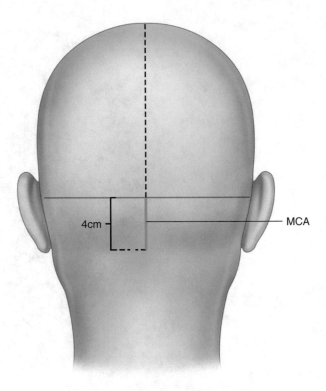

Fig. 5.14 STA:
Stomach Area

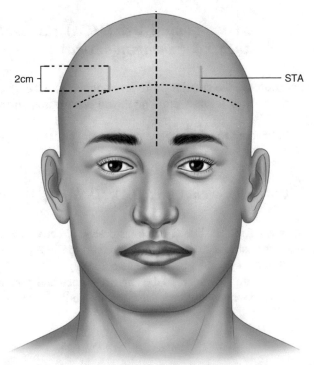

Fig. 5.15 LGA:
Liver and
Gallbladder Area
(or Hepatic
Area). STA:
Stomach Area

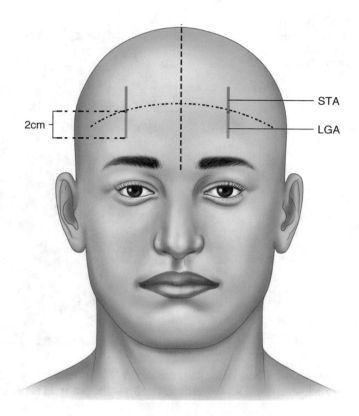

5.3.15   Liver and Gallbladder Area (LGA) or Hepatic Area (HTA), (ISSA-MS3 (épángxiàn II)

Location: A line 2 cm long extending anteriorly from the Stomach area (see Figs. 5.15 and 5.26).

Indication: Pain or discomfort in the epigastric and right hypochondriac, diseases of the Liver and gallbladder system, emotion disorders, general pain, and TCM Liver and Gallbladder conditions.

5.3.16   Thoracic Cavity Area (TCA) or Chest Area (CHA), (ISSA-MS2 épángxiàn I)

Location: A line 4 cm long, parallel to the anterior-posterior midline, with its midpoint at the anterior hairline, midway between the stomach area and the midline (see Figs. 5.16 and 5.26).

Fig. 5.16 TCA:
Thoracic Cavity
Area. STA:
Stomach Area

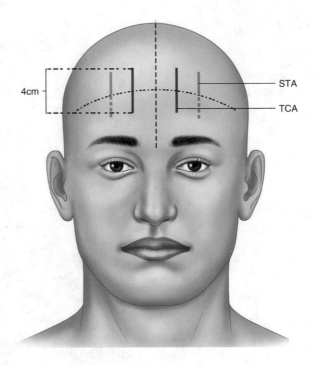

Indication: Chest pain, palpitation, stable angina, shortness of breath, bronchial asthma, paroxysmal supraventricular tachycardia, and TCM Heart and Lung conditions.

5.3.17   *Reproduction Area (RPA), (ISSA-MS4 épángxiàn III)*

Location: A 2 cm long line parallel from the frontal corner upward. Or a line 2 cm long, parallel to the anterior-posterior midline, drawn directly backwards from the anterior extremity of the Stomach Area at the same distance which separates the Stomach area from the Thoracic Cavity Area (see Figs. 5.17 and 5.26).

Indication: Impotence, ejaculation praecox, functional uterine bleeding, frequent urination, cystitis, prolapsed uterus, and TCM Kidney conditions.

5.3.18   *Intestine Area (ITA) (ISSA-MS4 épángxiàn III)*

Location: A 2 cm long line, extended from the reproduction area downward (see Figs. 5.18 and 5.26).

Indication: Large intestine and small intestine conditions, IBS, diarrheal, constipation, urinal track infection (UTI), and TCM Small Intestine and Large Intestine conditions.

Fig. 5.17
RPA:
Reproduction Area

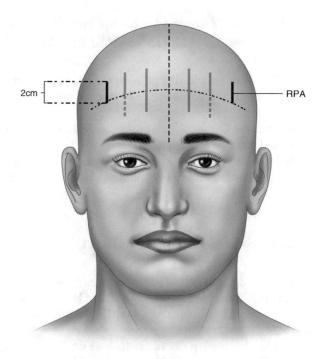

Fig. 5.18 ITA:
Intestine Area. RPA:
Reproduction Area

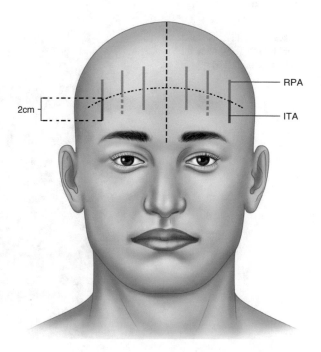

5.3.19   Nose Throat Mouth Tongue Area (NTMTA) or Head Area (HDA), (ISSA-MS1 ézhongxiàn)

Location: From the meeting point of the anterior-posterior midline with front hairline, draw a line 4 cm long, 2 cm upward and 2 cm down ward (see Figs. 5.19 and 5.26).

Indications: Centre of face problems, nose, throat, month, tongue related conditions; and emotion conditions.

Note: Nose Throat Mouth Tongue Area (NTMTA) and Head Area (HDA) are the same area. The later one was published in the book "Chinese Scalp Acupuncture" in 2011 [14, p. 57].

5.3.20   Spirit-Emotion Area (SEA)

Location: 2 cm side of the antero-posterior midline, a 4 cm line from Vasomotor Area to front (refer to Fig. 5.24). Or: 2 cm lateral to the point of 3.7 cm front of the middle point of mid line, draw a 4 cm line to front parallel to midline (see Figs. 5.20 and 5.24).

Indication: emotion disorders, such as depression, stress, anxiety, bipolar disorder, epilepsy, post-traumatic stress disorder (PTSD), insomnia and substance abuse, et al.

Fig. 5.19 NTMTA: Nose Throat Mouth Tong Area (or Head Area, HDA)

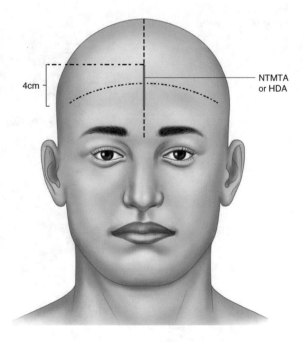

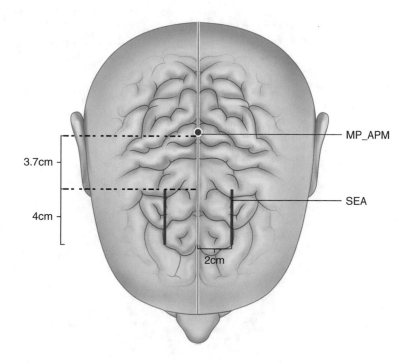

Fig. 5.20 SEA: Spirit-Emotion Area. MP-APM: Midpoint of Anterior Posterior Midline

5.3.21 Central Area (CTA) (ISSA-MS5 Dingzhongxian)

Location: On the anterior-posterior midline, a 3 cm line from the midpoint back ward (see Figs. 5.21 and 5.22).

Indication: Poor memory, emotion disorders, children stunting, frequency urination, infertility, prolapsed uterus, etc.

Note: This is the only area which is not listed on Jiao's books [13, p. 41–45]. It is major based on the ISSA-MS5 and personal clinical experiences.

There are two lines of ISSA have no similar areas with Jiao's style:

- MS9 dingpangxian II:

  - Location: lateral line 2 of vertex 2.25 cun lateral to middle line of vertex, 1.5 cun from GB-17 (Zhengying) backward along the meridian.
  - Indication: Pain, numbness and paralysis of the upper limb.

- MS10 nieqianxian:

  - Location: anterior temporal line from GB-4 (Hanyan) to GB-6 (Xuanli).
  - Indication: Migraine, headache, motor aphasia, trigeminal neuroglia, Bell's palsy, toothaches, etc.

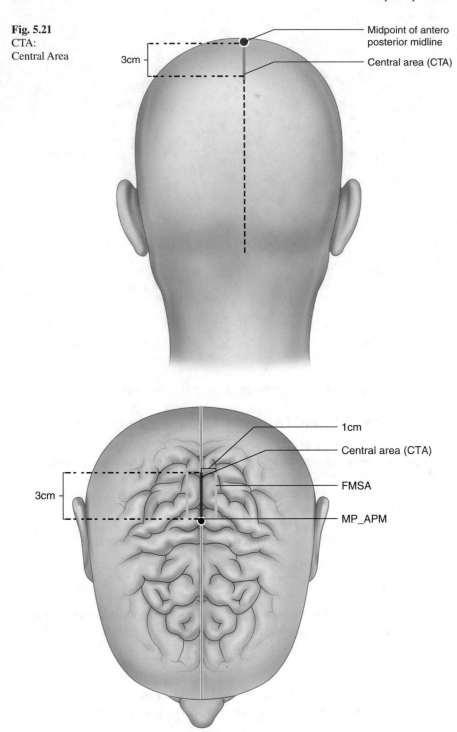

Fig. 5.21 CTA: Central Area

Midpoint of antero posterior midline

3cm

Central area (CTA)

1cm

Central area (CTA)

FMSA

3cm

MP_APM

Fig. 5.22 CTA and FMSA. MP-APM: Midpoint of Anterior Posterior Midline

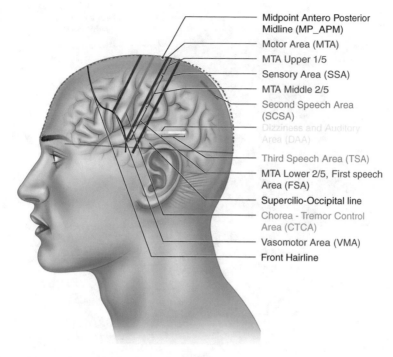

Midpoint Antero Posterior Midline (MP_APM)

Motor Area (MTA)

MTA Upper 1/5

Sensory Area (SSA)

MTA Middle 2/5

Second Speech Area (SCSA)

Dizziness and Auditory Area (DAA)

Third Speech Area (TSA)

MTA Lower 2/5, First speech Area (FSA)

Supercilio-Occipital line

Chorea - Tremor Control Area (CTCA)

Vasomotor Area (VMA)

Front Hairline

Fig. 5.23 Side view of scalp acupuncture areas

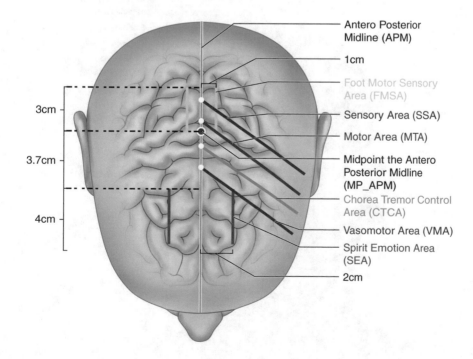

Antero Posterior Midline (APM)

1cm

Foot Motor Sensory Area (FMSA)

Sensory Area (SSA)

Motor Area (MTA)

Midpoint the Antero Posterior Midline (MP_APM)

Chorea Tremor Control Area (CTCA)

Vasomotor Area (VMA)

Spirit Emotion Area (SEA)

2cm

3cm

3.7cm

4cm

Fig. 5.24 Top view of areas

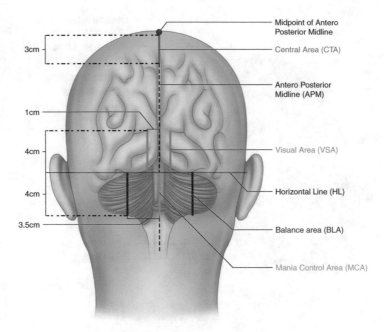

Fig. 5.25 Back view of areas

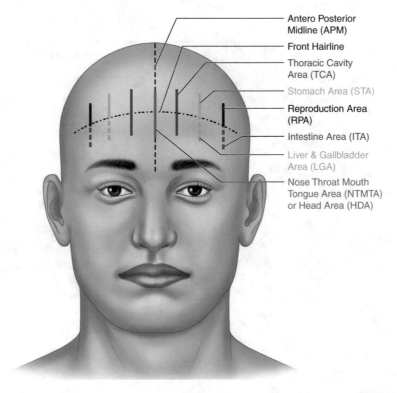

Fig. 5.26 Front view of areas

5.4 Scalp Acupuncture Needling Techniques

5.4.1 Needle Size

The commonly used needle sizes are 0.25 × 25 mm and 0.30 × 40 mm. Due to the first three layers of the scalp, skin, sense connective tissue and epicranial aponeurosis, are tightly bound together as a single unit. The stronger material of the needle body is more suitable for scalp insertion, as the scalp skin is thicker than general body skin.

5.4.2 Angle and Depth of Needling

The angle for inserting the needle is 20°–30°, according to the area of the skull, i.e., flat area lower angle (see Fig. 5.27). After rapid needle insertion, slightly down the angle to 10°–20°, push the needle to suitable depth according to the length of the stimulation area and the response of the patient. As a sample of Foot Motor-Sensory Area, which is 3 cm in length, then the needle depth should be better in 3 cm as well.

Fig. 5.27 Scalp acupuncture needling angle

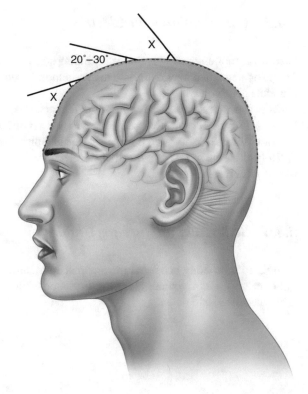

5.4.3   Needling Manipulation

After the needle is inserted in the scalp, if the patient has already gained considerable sensation, do not need more manipulation. If there is not much sensation, and the condition requests it, such as in severe cases or if there is not so much of a response for just needling, then further manipulation is needed. Different styles of scalp acupuncture suggest different manipulations. ISSA and Jiao's style request rapid rotation needling. The better frequency of rotation is 200 movements per minute.

5.4.4   Needle Removing

When SA needles are removed, should press the insertion point with a cotton ball or cotton stick after the needle is removed and press the pinhole several seconds to reduce the pain and avoid bleeding or subcutaneous hematoma. If bleeding occurs, should press longer 10–30 s. Occasionally there are 1–2 areas sore and with tension after needle removed. We can ask the patient to slightly press or massage the area, and warm the area after 12 h, if needed.

5.4.5   Combination with Electric

Electric acupuncture can generate continuing stimulation, through the needles to the points or areas, and may stimulate neuro-humoral regulation system to enhance the clinical effectiveness.

May choose two needles on the same line or areas, such as the upper 1/5 and the lower 2/5 of the Motor area. May choose the two different SA lines or areas, such as Foot Motor-Sensory area plus same side of Spirit-Emotion area.

Regarding the nature or pattern of the electro pulses, the frequency, timing, et al., please refer to relevant books.

5.4.6   Scalp Acupuncture for Children

Compared with body acupuncture, scalp acupuncture is more suitable for children patients as it is not visible, and mobility is possible during needling, play games while needling, and so on.

5.4.7   Combination with Other Techniques

Scalp acupuncture, whatever the style, can be combined with other acupuncture techniques, beside combination with electro acupuncture. The most combination is with SA in general body acupuncture, abdominal acupuncture, etc.

5.5   Notice and Cautions of Scalp Acupuncture

5.5.1   Scalp Layers

The scalp is the soft tissue envelope of the cranial vault. The scalp has five layers, they are the skin, the connective tissue, the epicranial aponeurosis, the loose areolar tissue, and the pericranium. The first three layers are bound together as a single unit. This single unit can move along the loose areolar tissue over the pericranium, which is adherent to the calvaria. Scalp acupuncture needling should pass through this single unit, and the needle tip and main body reaching the layer of loose areolar tissue, which is approximately 4–6 mm underneath the surface of scalp.

5.5.2   Careful Notice

- For stroke patients, waiting until the life factors stable including blood pressure, heartbeat and breathing, before scalp acupuncture is necessary.
- Not suitable for high temperature without known reason, or heart failure, etc.
- Should be more carefully that the needling does not cause the patient to faint due to strong stimulation.
- Compared with body acupuncture, scalp acupuncture there is more possibility of bleeding after removing the needle due to the countless number of arteries and veins. Careful attention is required for patients with hemophilia, or prescribed bleed thinning medicine. When removing the needles, should be pressure the needling points with cotton ball or stick for several seconds. If bleeding continues, more pressure should be given.
- It is inadvisable to apply scalp acupuncture on any scalp area where there is wound, infection, ulcer, tumour, big scar, a postoperative skull defect, or avoid inserting needle directly to the shunt.
- If the scalp skin is not clean enough or sweating, the needling points' area should be cleaned.

5.5.3 Scalp Acupuncture for Children and Women

- It is inadvisable to treat an infant whose fontanel has not yet closed, same as for other Brain delayed developments with exceptional care. If treatment is necessary, carefully avoid the fontanel.
- More attention is required for pregnant women. General principle to avoid applying scalp acupuncture for the first 3 months and last 2 months of pregnancy if they have a history of miscarriages or risks of miscarriage.

5.6 Summary

Acupuncture on head has a long history which we could trace back to almost 2000 years ago. Scalp acupuncture, as an independent acupuncture system, started in the early 1970s. There are many styles of scalp acupuncture, Jiao's style is the first published system and is widely practiced. The location of scalp acupuncture areas, indications and needling techniques in the book are mostly according to Jiao's style with some revisions which based on clinical experiences and additional research. The created design of colourful illustrations of scalp acupuncture areas highlight the stimulation zones with measurements which is easy to follow and practice.

References

1. Unschuld PU. Huang Di Nei Jing Ling Shu: the ancient classic on needle therapy. Berkeley: University of California Press; 2016. eBook.
2. Unschuld PU, Tessenow H, Zheng JS. Huang Di Nei Jing Su Wen: an annotated translation of Huang Di's inner classic – basic questions. Berkeley: University of California Press; 2011. eBook.
3. Deadman P, Al-Khafaji M, Baker K. A manual of acupuncture. 2nd ed. East Sussex: JCM; 2003.
4. Zhan M. A doctor of the highest calibre treats an illness before it happens. Med Anthropol. 2009;28(2):167.
5. Liu Z, Guan L, Wang Y, et al. History and mechanism for treatment of intracerebral haemorrhage with scalp acupuncture. Evid Based Complement Alternat Med. 2012;895032:9 p.
6. Jiao SF. Scalp acupuncture and clinical cases. Beijing: Foreign Languages Press; 1997.
7. Wang FC. Chinese alternative treatment methods-scalp acupuncture therapy (Chinese). 2nd ed. Beijing: People's Medical Publishing House; 2008.
8. Zhu MQ, Kong RQ, Peng ZY, etc. Chinese scalp acupuncture (in Chinese). Guagnzhou: Guangdong Science and Technology Press; 1993.
9. Yamamoto T. New scalp acupuncture. Acupunct Med. 1989;6(2):46–8.
10. Yamamoto T, Yamamoto H. Yamamoto new scalp acupuncture. 1st ed. Tokyo: Axel Springer Japan Publishing; 1998. eBook.
11. Liu TH, Sadove MS. Scalp needle therapy: acupuncture treatment for central nervous system disorders. Am J Chin Med. 1974;2(3):261–9.
12. Chiao SF. Scalp acupuncture in brain diseases. Chin Med J. 1977;3(5):325–8.

13. Wen W. Scalp acupuncture in China. Am J Chin Med. 1977;5(1):101–4.
14. Xi YJ, Situ L. Acupuncture and moxibustion techniques (Chinese). Shanghai: Shanghai Science and Technology Press; 1985.
15. WHO Scientific Group on International Acupuncture Nomenclature. A proposed standard international acupuncture nomenclature: report of a WHO scientific group. Geneva: World Health Organization; 1991.
16. Yang ZM. Acupuncture and moxibustion techniques (Chinese). Shanghai: Shanghai Science and Technology Press; 1996.
17. Jiao SF. Scalp acupuncture (Chinese). 2nd ed. Beijing: People's Health Press; 2009.
18. Hao JJ, Hao LL. Chinese scalp acupuncture. Boulder: Blue Poppy Press; 2011.

Chapter 6
Dao-qi Needling Technique with Du Mai and Ren Mai

6.1 Dao-qi Needling Technique, Origin and Development

The ancient texts were remarkably simple and concise, how to translate them into modern language is often confused even in Chinese itself. One can image the difficulty and possible misunderstanding in translation to other languages, including English. There are several translations of Huangdi Neijing, some by Western and some by Chinese people. For the comparing of Western and Eastern translations, two samples are both listed below for the Dao-qi in Neijing.

6.1.1 The Origin of Dao-qi Needling

Dao-qi (guiding the Qi) needling technique was original from Neijing. There are two chapters in Huangdi Neijing that reference Dao-qi (导气), Chapters 34 and 71.

6.1.1.1 Neijing-Lingshu-Chapter 34

黄帝曰:五乱者，刺之有道乎?…黄帝曰:补写奈何?歧伯曰:徐入徐出，谓之导气。补写无形，谓之同精。是非有馀不足也，乱气之相逆也。黄帝曰:允乎哉道, 明乎哉论, 请著之玉版, 命曰治乱也。 [1, p. 653].

Two Chinese doctors Mr. Wu and Son translated Neijing in 1997 which were published in Chinese and English "Yellow Emperors Cannon of Internal Medicine, Lingshu-Chapter 34—Wu Luan (The Five Disturbances)" [1, p. 653].

> Yellow Emperor asked: Is there any principle for treating the five kinds of disturbances stated above by pricking?……Yellow Emperor asked: How to invigorate or purge? Qibo said: When one inserts and pulls out the needle slowly, it is called the **inducement of the energy**. When pricking without regular forms in invigorating and purging, it is called stabilizing the essence of life, this is not for invigorating the insufficient energy nor purging the

surplus energy, it is because the evil energies that cause disturbances are falling into log-gerheads and they must be dredged.

Professor Paul Unschuld translated Neijing Suwen in 2011 and Neijing Lingshu in 2016, which are the most widely accepted works in western. In his "Huang Di Nei Jing Ling Shu: The Ancient Classic on Needle Therapy-Chapter 34—The Five Disturbances" [2, p. 354].

Huang Di: These five disturbances, is there a WAY of piercing them?
    Huang Di: How are they supplemented and drained?
    Qibo:
    Slow insertion and slow withdrawal, that is called "**guiding the qi**".
    Supplementation and drainage are directed at [qi] without physical appearance.
    This is called "gathering the essence".
    It is like this:
    [These treatments] are not directed at a surplus or an insufficiency. They are directed
    at disturbed qi engaged in movements contrary to the norms.

It is not so difficult to understand the meaning of Dao-qi, either inducence of the energy [1, p. 653] or guiding the qi [2, p. 354]. Its manipulation is also similarly described, inserts and pulls out the needle slowly [1, p. 653] or slow insertion and slow withdrawal [2, p. 354]. Its function is not reinforcing or reducing, or without regular forms in invigorating and purging by Wang [1, p. 653], or supplementation and drainage are directed at [qi] without physical appearance by Unschuld [2, p. 354]. Its main functions 'are directed at disturbed qi engaged in movements contrary to the norms' [2, p. 354].

Interestingly, here the translation of Dao-qi by above two are written in two different ways, inducence of the energy by Mr. Wu [1, p. 653] or guiding the Qi by Mr. Unschuld [2, p. 354]. In terms of the Qi (气), Chinese doctors used the word of 'energy', while western professor used the directly pinyin word of 'Qi'. Energy is one of the common translation of Qi, but more TCM masters from Western and Eastern prefer to use the origin pinyin word Qi, instead of the close English word 'energy', which is close but not cover some meaning of the Qi.

6.1.1.2   Neijing-Lingshu-Chapter 71

持针之道，欲端以正，安以静。先知虚实而行疾徐。左手执骨，右手循之。无与肉果。写欲端以正，补必闭肤。辅针导气，邪得淫泆，真气得居。 [1, p. 775].
    "Neijing-Lingshu Chapter 71-Xieke (Retention of the Evil)".

In the manipulation of pricking, one should be upright and calm. He should know the asthe-nia and sthenia of the disease first, and then, decide the speed of the needle insertion. In the insertion, hold the bone of the patient with the fingers of the left hand, and press the acu-point with the fingers of the right hand to avoid the tangle of the needle by fibre the muscle. In pricking, the needle must be kept straight, and insertion should be right forward; in invigorating, the needle hole on the skin must be sealed up, apply the manipulation of twist-ing the needle to guide the energy to keep it not run rashly, and in this way, the health energy can be stabilized. [1, p. 775]

Unschuld in "Evil Visitors Chapter 71" translated:

The WAY of handling the needles requires sincerity and a proper [attitude], peace and calmness.
  At first one must know whether it is a condition of depletion or repletion, and then.
  [the needle] is applied swiftly or slowly.
  One's left hand holds the bones; the right hand follows them.
  [The needle] must not get stuck in the flesh. To conduct a drainage, [the needle].
  must be held vertically.
  For supplementation the skin is to be closed [with the finger once the needle is.
  withdrawn]. One supports the needling [by a manual massage] to guide the qi.
  This way the evil [qi] are dissipated, and the true qi can settle down. [2, p. 607]

For this chapter, two translations are quite similar, except the Qi or energy. It is not difficult to understand; the translation of Dao-qi is a challenge. The translation phases, 'inducement of the energy' or 'gathering the essence', are not accurate to the original meaning of Dao-qi, which is more closely related to 'guiding the Qi'. Thus in this chapter of the book, and subsequent chapters, Dao-qi will be formally used and with not often explanation of the meaning similar of English translation 'guiding the Qi'.

6.1.2   Modern Development of Dao-qi Needling

Unfortunately, Neijing, and later texts, did not explain how to practice Dao-qi in detail, such as lifting and twisting, at which lever and with what duration, etc. During my PhD research with Professor Lingling Wang at Nanjing University of Chinese Medicine (NJUCM), my colleagues and me studied in detail the manipulations of Dao-qi needling technique and its clinical practice including the treatment for depression. There are many papers published on this technique and most of them are in Chinese [3–6]. In 2014, the detail explanation of Dao-qi needling technique was published in the journal *Acupuncture in Medicine* by the author Dr. Tianjun Wang. The paper, "Acupuncture combined with an antidepressant for patients with depression in hospital: a pragmatic randomised controlled trial" [7] explained the detail manipulations of Dao-qi technique, as stated in citation below. It is believed that this was the first published text on this subject in English text in the western world about Dao-qi acupuncture technique and its manipulations.

This manipulation (of Dao-qi needling technique) involved lifting-thrusting and rotating the needle with light and smooth stimulation. The amplitude was 1–2 mm; needle rotation angle <90° and frequency 60–100 times per minute for 1–2 min.

6.2   Process of Dao-qi Needling

6.2.1   Patient Selected and Indications of Dao-qi

As Neijing stated, Dao-qi techniques is used mainly for the Five Disturbances, which are the disturbances in the Heart, in the Lung, in the Stomach, in the upper arms and in the head [2, p. 352].

The fact is:
  The qi,
  when they are disturbed in the heart, then the heart is vexed with closure and silence.
  [Patients] lower the head and silently withdraw;
  when they are disturbed in the lung, [patients] may lower or raise [their head]. They
  pant and shout loudly. They press6 with their hands [the chest] to be able to breathe;
  when they are disturbed in the stomach and intestines, then that is cholera;
  when they are disturbed in the upper arms and lower legs, then this is associated.
  with recession in the four limbs;
  when they are disturbed in the head, then this is associated with recession and.
  counter flow. The head is heavy and [the patient] feels dizzy and falls to the ground.

In modern language, the conditions of Dao-qi technique indications are:

- Spirit and emotion diseases
- Shortness of breath
- Diarrheal
- Recession in the four limbs
- Headache and dizziness
- Other diseases which are not good response to conventional acupuncture
  treatments

6.2.2 Points Selected

In terms of the points of the five disturbances, in the same Neijing chapter there are
listed some points on the relevant channels, which are still used from day-to-day in
clinic. With the development of TCM Brain theory and the understanding that Du
Mai is the Brain channel, more practice and studies are focus on Du Mai points, and
Ren Mai points which will be explained detail in Sect. 6 of this chapter.

6.2.3 De-qi First

De-qi, or Qi arrive, is the essential application of classic acupuncture. This is the
principle of acupuncture. 'The curative effect is so reliable as the blue appearing
when the clouds are blown away by the wind' [1, p. 496].

- "Spiritual Pivot—first Nine Needles and the Twelve Source Points" says 'The
  most important thing in acupuncture is to get the de qi sensation, when it appears,
  the curative effect will appear in the wake of it, and the curative effect is so reliable as the blue appearing when the clouds are blown away by the wind. This is
  the principle of acupuncture.'

The Nine Needles and the Twelve Origin [Openings] [2, p. 33].

As for the needles,
> for each there is an appropriate usage; each has a different shape.
> Each fulfills its specific function. That is the essence of piercing.
> When the qi arrive, then this shows the effect. The effects, they are as reliable as the
> wind that blows away clouds; they are as clear as the appearance of a blue sky. This
> is all there is to the WAY of piercing.

After De-qi sensation, Dao-qi technique can apply for the relative points and patients.

6.2.4   Dao-qi Sensation of Practitioner

After de-qi sensation, the needle may thrust into further deeper, according to the location of points and therapeutic plan. The practitioner should very carefully feel the changes on the tip of the needle, and the level of the needle's touch. When the needle has a certain degree of tension, it can be freely inserted and twisted, indicating that is the right level of Dao-qi. At this ideal state, the resistance of the lifting and thrusting of the needle should be equal, and the resistance of the left and right turns of the needle should be the same. If there is a feeling of inequality, the uncoordinated resistance of the upper and lower sides should be corrected by proper manipulation.

6.2.5   Dao-qi Sensation of the Patient

After De-qi sensation, with agreement of the patient, needle should go further to deep level. When Dao-qi technique is applied, the patient may get the feeling of soft, comfortable, long-lasting, and the feeling may spread over a certain area or to a certain direction. Most of times, the feeling will go to the area or the direction of the body that is suffering parts of the body. The Qi is clever, may moving to the area of weakness or stagnation to generate positive response. After Dao-qi, the spread feeling may change or disappear in specific sections of the suffered area of a certain distance, which is called 'QiZhiBingSuo (Qi extending affected parts)'.

The Dao-qi sensation for the majority is soft and gentle, most patients can tolerate and enjoy it. Most times it is a comfortable feeling with happy mood. This enjoyable needling feeling can provide the patients a state of complete relaxation and positive mind set, which benefit all the clinical results.

6.3   Shen During Dao-qi Needling

"Lingshu-chapter 8–To Consider the Spirit as the Foundation" says 'All norms of piercing [require one] to first of all consider the spirit as the foundation.' [2, p. 145]

The essence of the Dao-qi technique is to adjust the Shen (spirit). The spirit in TCM is the general term of all kinds of the vitality phenomena of the human body, and the external manifestation of all activates.

In order to ensure the success of the Dao-qi needling, it is necessary to pay attention to the following issues:

6.3.1 Setting the Shen Before Dao-qi

The acupuncturist and the patient should adjust their mind state together before needling, adjust their breathing rhythm and stabilize their concentration.

6.3.2 Comfort the Shen During Dao-qi

Based on the patient's psychological changes, find the roots of their emotional state of mind, conduct speech counselling to comfort the patient.

6.3.3 Governing Shen of Practitioners

Own concentration, mastering the patients mental state and Qi changes.

6.3.4 Keeping Shen from Patients

Including the cooperation with the practitioner, the experience and perception of the needling and the response of the Dao-qi needling, etc.

6.3.5 Detail Methods for Shen Keeping

6.3.5.1 Quiet Environment

A quiet and good environment is a necessary condition for the partition to eliminate interference, concentrate on the Shen, and focus on the needling. The quiet environment is not only conducive to the practitioner's special mind, but also to the patient's concentration. In order to better follow the practitioner's requirements, and to easily accept the suggestion and help improve the efficacy.

6.3.5.2 Stabilize the Patient

The acupuncturist's serious and focused operation attitude will consciously and unconsciously affect the patient, making it easier for the patient to calm down when receiving treatment and focus on the needle. Suitable position could benefit to stabilize the patient, such as seating down with higher chair back better for Dao-qi on DU-16 Fengfu.

6.3.5.3 Condense on the Needle

The practitioners are highly concentrated, carefully operating and understanding the feelings and changes under the needle.

6.3.5.4 Check Its Response

According to the operation requirements of the Dao-qi needling, the acupuncturist wholeheartedly puts into the operation of acupuncture, eliminates all external disturbances, and concentrates on the needle with high concentration. At this time, the local reaction of the acupuncture point and the patient cannot escape the acupuncturist. The practitioner is keen to observe the response of the needling feeling and any response from the patient including body languages.

6.4 Precaution and Notice of Dao-qi Needling

In addition to the requirements of the above mentioned Dao-qi needling operation, in order to produce a soft, comfortable and long-lasting feeling of the needle, it is also necessary to pay attention to the following notice points:

6.4.1 Explanation First

A comprehensive understanding of the patient's condition and a correct diagnosis of the patient's pattern of physical and pathological situation, based on the knowledge of TCM and western medicine. Different types of diseases, under the same practice, may have different acupuncture induction. There should be a direction prediction and judgment for this kind of induction. If there is any possibility of discomfort, the patient should be reminded not to be nervous beforehand. Different patients of different constitution types have different degrees of time for generating acupuncture induction, and the amount of the manipulation should be adjusted within a certain range. In addition, different patient may have different response to the needling. All above explanation should discussion with the patient before the Dao-qi needling start.

6.4.2   Select the Appropriate Acupoints

The manipulation of the Dao-qi needling is specifically implemented on the acupoints. Therefore, it is very important to choose suitable acupoints. Different acupoints can produce different needling reaction. As example if that of Jing-well points, which are very shallow and generally painful feeling, so they are not suitable for Dao-qi needling.

6.4.3   Maintain a Comfortable Position

The position is the posture of the patient during acupuncture treatment. The different parts and different therapeutic plan require different position. For sample, the points on the posterior head or neck such as DU-16 Fengfu, are better used in the siting position and relax the head. Clinical experience suggests that a higher chair back with a small soft pillow against the forehead can stabilize the patient's head and neck and make it easier to perform the Dao-qi needling on these points. The points on the back and particularly on Du Mai channel, need a prone position and is often better with a soft pillow under the chest or abdomen to relax the whole body. The supine position is better for the acupoints in front of the body, and so on.

6.5   Commonly Used Dao-qi Points

For the easier understanding for the western readers, all acupoints' number, pinyin name, locations and some indications in this chapter are cited mainly from the book "A Manual of Acupuncture" [8, p. 495–560] with some revisions. This book is widely used in western countries, particularly in European countries.

6.5.1   Du Mai Points

As previous statement in Chap. 3, Du Mai (Governor Vessel) is the channel of the Brain. Du Mai points are commonly used to treat Brain related conditions. Besides the normal acupuncture techniques, Dao-qi needling is mainly used for these Brain conditions, particularly for severe patients and do not respond to routine needling techniques.

Commonly used Du Mai points for Brain related conditions and their Dao-qi needling techniques are listed as below:

DU-2 Yaoshu

- Location: On the midline, in the sacro-coccygeal hiatus.
- Dao-qi needling: Oblique superior insertion 1 to 1.2 cun.
- Dao-qi feeling: Sensation deep in the sacral hiatus and expending around.
- Dao-qi indications: Severe local pain with cold, female and male conditions, such as irregular menstruation, haemorrhoids, etc.

DU-3 Yaoyangguan

- Location: On the midline of the lower back, in the depression below the spinous process of the fourth lumbar vertebra.
- Dao-qi needling: Perpendicular insertion 1 to 1.5 cun.
- Dao-qi feeling: Sensation deep to the spine, one side or both sides of the hip and leg, may spread to the front lower abdomen.
- Dao-qi indications: Severe lower back and lower limb pain with cold, female and male conditions, such as impotence, irregular menstruation, etc.

DU-4 Mingmen

- Location: On the midline of the lower back, in the depression below the spinous process of the second lumbar vertebra.
- Dao-qi needling: Perpendicular insertion 1 to 1.5 cun.
- Dao-qi feeling: Sensation deep to the spine, one side or both sides of the lower back and hip, may spread to the front lower abdomen.
- Dao-qi indications: Severe lower back pain may with cold, tinnitus, headache, female and male conditions, such as impotence, irregular menstruation, fertility, etc.

DU-6 Jizhong

- Location: On the midline of the back, in the depression below the spinous process of the eleventh thoracic vertebra.
- Dao-qi needling: Perpendicular-oblique superior insertion 1 to 1.5 cun.
- Dao-qi feeling: Sensation deep to the spine, may radiate up and down alone spine, one side or both sides of the middle back or side of the ribs, may spread to the front middle abdomen.
- Dao-qi indications: Severe back pain on the middle spine, spinal cord injuries, chronic and severe spleen and stomach problems, etc.

DU-7 Zhongshu

- Location: On the midline of the back, in the depression below the spinous process of the tenth thoracic vertebra.

- Dao-qi needling: oblique superior insertion 1 to 1.5 cun.
- Dao-qi feeling: Sensation deep to the spine, may radiate up and down alone spine, one side or both sides of the middle back or side of the ribs, may spread to the front middle abdomen.
- Dao-qi indications: Severe back pain on the middle spine, spinal cord injuries, chronic and severe spleen and stomach problems, etc.

DU-8 Jinsuo

- Location: On the midline of the back, in the depression below the spinous process of the ninth thoracic vertebra.
- Dao-qi needling: Oblique superior insertion 1 to 1.5 cun.
- Dao-qi feeling: Sensation deep to the spine, may radiate up and down alone spine, one side or both sides of the middle back or side of the ribs, may spread to the front middle abdomen.
- Dao-qi indications: Severe back pain on the middle spine, spinal cord injuries, general tendon injuries, chronic or severe spleen and stomach problems, etc.

DU-9 Zhiyang

- Location: On the midline of the back, in the depression below the spinous process of the seventh thoracic vertebra.
- Dao-qi needling: Oblique superior insertion 1 to 1.5 cun.
- Dao-qi feeling: Sensation deep to the spine, may radiate up and down alone spine, one side or both sides of the chest or side of the ribs, may spread to the front chest.
- Dao-qi indications: Severe up back pain with particularly cold pain on the middle spine, spinal cord injuries, chronic or severe chest pain or chronic mild heart attack, etc.

DU-10 Lingtai

- Location: On the midline of the back, in the depression below the spinous process of the sixth thoracic vertebra.
- Dao-qi needling: Oblique superior insertion 1 to 1.5 cun.
- Dao-qi feeling: Sensation deep to the spine, may radiate up and down alone spine, one side or both sides of the chest or side of the ribs, may spread to the front chest.
- Dao-qi indications: Severe up back pain on the middle spine, spinal cord injuries, chronic chest pain or chronic mild heart attack, stress, depression, anxiety, etc.

DU-11 Shendao

- Location: On the midline of the back, in the depression below the spinous process of the fifth thoracic vertebra.

- Dao-qi needling: oblique superior insertion 1 to 1.5 cun.
- Dao-qi feeling: Sensation deep to the spine, may radiate up and down alone spine, one side or both sides of the chest or side of the ribs, may spread to the front chest.
- Dao-qi indications: Severe up back pain on the middle spine, spinal cord injuries, chronic chest pain or chronic mild heart attack, stress, depression, anxiety, insomnia etc.

DU-12 Shenzhu

- Location: On the midline of the back, in the depression below the spinous process of the third thoracic vertebra.
- Dao-qi needling: Oblique superior insertion 1 to 1.5 cun.
- Dao-qi feeling: Sensation deep to the spine, may radiate up and down alone spine, one side or both sides of the chest or side of the ribs, may spread to the front chest.
- Dao-qi indications: Severe up back pain on the middle spine or sides, spinal cord injuries, chronic chest pain, etc.

DU-13 Taodao

- Location: On the midline of the back, in the depression below the spinous process of the first thoracic vertebra.
- Dao-qi needling: Oblique superior insertion 1 to 1.5 cun.
- Dao-qi feeling: Sensation deep to the spine, may radiate up and down alone spine, one side or both sides of the chest or side of the ribs, may spread to the front chest.
- Dao-qi indications: Severe back pain on the middle spine, spinal cord injuries, chronic or severe chest pain with cold, cough, etc.

DU-14 Dazhui

- Location: On the midline at the base of the neck, in the depression below the spinous process of the seventh cervical vertebra.
- Dao-qi needling: Perpendicular or slightly oblique superior insertion 1 to 1.5 cun.
- Dao-qi feeling: Sensation deep to the spine, may radiate up and down alone spine, one side or both sides of the neck and chest, may spread to the shoulder and arm.
- Dao-qi indications: Severe neck or up back pain on the middle spine, whiplash injury, spinal cord injuries, chronic or severe chest pain with cold, cough, thyroid diseases, depression, anxiety, headache, etc.

DU-15 Yamen

- Location: On the midline at the nape of the neck, in the depression 0.5 cun inferior to DU-16 Fengfu, below the spinous process of the first cervical vertebra (impalpable).

- Dao-qi needling: Perpendicular insertion 1 to 1.3 cun, direction to the mouth (this needling not suitable for acupuncturists without supervised training).
- Dao-qi feeling: Sensation deep to the spine, may radiate up and down alone spine, one side or both sides of the neck, may spread to the mouth or tongue.
- Dao-qi indications: Aphasia due to stroke or other Brain injuries, severe neck pain on the middle spine, whiplash injury, stress, back headache, etc.
- Notes: According to many reference, the safety and effectively depth of needling of DU-15 Yamen is 25–33 mm (1 to 1.3 cun), according to the size of the neck.

DU-16 Fengfu

- Location: On the midline at the nape of the neck, in the depression immediately below the external occipital protuberance.
- Dao-qi needling: Perpendicular insertion 1 to 1.3 cun, direction to the tip on nose.
- Dao-qi feeling: Sensation deep to the spine, may radiate up and down alone spine, one side or both sides of the neck or ear, may spread to the mouth or nose, may upward to the top or frontal of the head (this needling not suitable for acupuncturists without supervised training).
- Dao-qi indications: Depression, anxiety, aphasia, stroke, Parkinson's disease, dementia, multiple sclerosis (MS), Brain injuries, severe back headache, etc.
- Notes: According to many references, the safety and effectively depth of needling of DU-16 Fengfu is 25–33 mm (1 to 1.3 cun), according to the size of the neck.

DU-17 Naohu

- Location: At the back of the head on the midline, 1.5 cun directly above DU-16 Fengfu, in the depression directly superior to the external occipital protuberance.
- Dao-qi needling: Transverse insertion superiorly 0.7 to 1.2 cun.
- Dao-qi feeling: Sensation may radiate upward to the top or frontal of the head, or spread to the sides of the head.
- Dao-qi indications: Anxiety, stress, dimness of vision, mania, epilepsy, back headache, etc.

DU-20 Baihui

- Location: At the vertex on the midline, in the depression 5 cun posterior to the anterior hairline and 7 un superior to the posterior hairline. More practically with straight head level, directly from the ear apex and meeting with midline.
- Dao-qi needling: Transverse insertion forward or backward 0.7 to 1.3 cun.
- Dao-qi feeling: Sensation may radiate upward to frontal or backward of the head, or spread to the sides of the head.
- Dao-qi indications: Anxiety, stress, mania, epilepsy, top headache, dementia, Parkinson's disease, prolapse of uterus, frequency urination, etc.

DU-23 Shangxing

- Location: At the top of the head on the midline, 1 cun posterior to the anterior hairline.
- Dao-qi needling: Transverse insertion forward 0.7 to 1.2 cun.
- Dao-qi feeling: Sensation may forward to the frontal of the head or nose, or spread to the sides of the forehead.
- Dao-qi indications: Rhinitis, nasal obstruction and discharge, frontal headache, nasal polyps; eye problems, stress, anxiety, etc.

DU-24 Shenting

- Location: At the top of the head on the midline, 0.5 cun posterior to the anterior hairline.
- Dao-qi needling: Transverse insertion forward 0.5 to 1 cun or backward 0.7–1.3 cun.
- Dao-qi feeling: Sensation may radiate forward to the frontal of the head or nose, or spread to the sides of the forehead or the top head.
- Dao-qi indications: Depression, stress, anxiety, epilepsy, insomnia; rhinitis, nasal obstruction, lose of smell, frontal headache, eye problems, etc.

DU-26 Shuigou (Renzhong)

- Location: Above the upper lip on the midline, at the junction of the upper third and lower two thirds of the philtrum.
- Dao-qi needling: Oblique insertion upward 0.5 to 1 cun to the root of the nasal septum.
- Dao-qi feeling: Strong sensation may radiate directly to the nose, or spread to the forehead, eyes and face. To restore consciousness, should wait for the tears out of the eyes or watery of eyes.
- Dao-qi indications: Sudden loss of consciousness, coma, mania, clinic depression, epilepsy, unexpected laughter and crying, severe stiffness and pain of the spine, sprain and pain of the lumbar spine, etc.

6.5.2 Ren Mai Points

6.5.2.1 Ren Mai with Brain

Du Mai is the channel of the Brain. In addition, perhaps Ren Mai (Conception Vessel) is also affiliated, or at least closely related to the Brain [9]. As the Su Wen pointed out: 'Ren Mai …. enters the eyes'. ("Plain Questions, Chapter 60—Discourse on Bone Hollows") [10, p. 77]. Many Ren Mai points have the indications for Brain problems. Below are some sample Ren Mai points' indications [8, p. 495–525]:

> REN-4 Guanyuan: Insomnia, dizziness, wind dizziness, headache. Sudden turmoil disorder, wind stroke, heaviness of the body like a mountain, tremor of the hands.
> REN-6 Qihai: Loss of consciousness from wind stroke.
> REN-12 Zhongwan: Injury by worry, anxiety and overthinking, chronic and acute childhood fright wind, loss of consciousness, mania-depression, epilepsy, tongue thrusting.
> REN-13 Shangwan: Wind epilepsy, visual dizziness.
> REN-17 Shanzhong (Danzhong): Loss of consciousness.
> REN-24 Chengjiang: Mania-depression.

6.5.2.2 Second Brain

Dr. Michael Gerson proposed the theory of 'Second Brain' or 'Gut Brain' in 1998 [11]. From the modern medicine aspect, during early fetal development, both the "gut" (esophagus, stomach, small intestine and colon) and the Brain start to develop from the same clump of embryonic tissue. When that piece of tissue is divided, one piece grows into the central nervous system (Brain and cranial nerves); the other section becomes the enteric nervous system. During later stages of fetal development, these two "Brains" become connected via the vagus nerve. The vagus nerve creates a direct connection between the Brain and the gut [12, p. 249–251].

6.5.2.3 Commonly Used Ren Mai Points with Dao-qi Needling Technique

REN-2 Qugu

- Location: On the midline of the lower abdomen, at the superior border of the pubic symphysis, 5 cun below the umbilicus.
- Dao-qi needling: Perpendicular insertion 0.7 to 1.3 cun, or transverse insertion downward 1 to 1.3 cun. Bladder should be empty before Dao-qi needling.
- Dao-qi feeling: Sensation may radiate deep to the lower abdomen or spread to the private area.
- Dao-qi indications: Difficult or frequency urination, urinary tract infection (UTI), impotence, seminal emission, itching of the scrotum, contraction of the penis, dryness and pain of the genitals, infertility, low ovarian function, etc.

REN-3 Zhongji

- Location: On the midline of the lower abdomen, 4 cun inferior to the umbilicus and 1 cun superior to the pubic symphysis.
- Dao-qi needling: Perpendicular insertion 0.7 to 1.3 cun, or oblique or transverse insertion downward 1 to 1.3 cun. Bladder should be empty before Dao-qi needling.

- Dao-qi feeling: Sensation may radiate deep to the lower abdomen, or spread downward to the private area.
- Dao-qi indications: Difficult or frequency urination, urinary tract infection (UTI), impotence, seminal emission, contraction of the penis, dryness and pain of the genitals, infertility, Low ovarian function, irregular menstruation, amenorrhoea, menorrhagia, etc.

REN-4 Guanyuan

- Location: On the midline of the lower abdomen, 3 cun inferior to the umbilicus and 2 cun superior to the pubic symphysis.
- Dao-qi needling: Perpendicular insertion 0.7 to 1.3 cun, or oblique or transverse insertion downward 1 to 1.5 cun. Bladder should be empty before Dao-qi needling.
- Dao-qi feeling: Sensation may radiate deep to the lower abdomen, or spread downward to the private area.
- Dao-qi indications: Impotence, seminal emission, contraction of the penis, dryness and pain of the genitals, infertility, difficult or frequency urination, urinary tract infection (UTI), irregular bowel syndrome (IBS), low ovarian function, irregular menstruation, amenorrhoea, menorrhagia, wind-stroke, heaviness of the body, etc.

REN-6 Qihai

- Location: On the midline of the lower abdomen, 1.5 cun inferior to the umbilicus and 3.5 cun superior to the pubic symphysis.
- Dao-qi needling: Perpendicular insertion 0.7 to 1.3 cun, or oblique or transverse insertion downward 1 to 1.5 cun. Bladder should be empty before Dao-qi needling.
- Dao-qi feeling: Sensation may radiate deep to the lower abdomen or spread downward to the private area.
- Dao-qi indications: Impotence, seminal emission, prolapse of the uterus, prolapse of the rectum; cold and pain on lower abdominal, limbs; chronic diarrhoea, dryness and pain of the genitals, infertility, difficult or frequency urination, urinary tract infection (UTI), IBS, low ovarian function, irregular menstruation, amenorrhoea, menorrhagia, wind-stroke, heaviness of the body, etc.

REN-9 Shuifen

- Location: On the midline of the upper abdomen, 1 cun above the umbilicus and 7 cun below the sternocostal angle.
- Dao-qi needling: Perpendicular insertion 0.7 to 1.3 cun.
- Dao-qi feeling: Sensation may radiate deep to the upper abdomen, or spread downward or sides.

- Dao-qi indications: Oedema, IBS, abdomen swollen, pain or cramp, chest pain, etc.

REN-10 Xiawan

- Location: On the midline of the upper abdomen, 2 cun above the umbilicus and 6 cun below the sternocostal angle.
- Dao-qi needling: Perpendicular insertion 0.7 to 1.3 cun.
- Dao-qi feeling: Sensation may radiate deep to the upper abdomen, or spread downward or sides.
- Dao-qi indications: Abdominal fullness, epigastric pain, nausea and vomiting after eating, focal distention, IBS, no pleasure in eating; pain around lower neck; thyroid problems, hypothyroidism, hyperthyroidism, thyroid nodules, etc.

REN-11 Jianli

- Location: On the midline of the abdomen, 3 cun above the umbilicus and 5 cun below the sternocostal angle.
- Dao-qi needling: Perpendicular insertion 0.7 to 1.3 cun.
- Dao-qi feeling: Sensation may radiate deep to the upper abdomen, or spread up or downward, or sides.
- Dao-qi indications: Abdominal distention, epigastric pain, nausea and vomiting after eating, focal distention, IBS, no pleasure in eating, front and back neck pain, pharyngitis, sore throat, hoarse voice, etc.

REN-12 Zhongwan

- Location: On the midline of the abdomen, 4 cun above the umbilicus and midway between the umbilicus and the sternocostal angle.
- Dao-qi needling: Perpendicular insertion 0.7 to 1.3 cun. May plus 2–4 needles around it with 0.5–1 cm distance, to enhance the functions.
- Dao-qi feeling: Sensation may radiate deep to the upper abdomen, or spread up or downward, or sides.
- Dao-qi indications: Abdominal distention or pain, nausea and vomiting, poor appetite, diarrhoea, IBS, heart pain, shortness of breath; dizziness, headache; neurological and psychological conditions, such as stroke, Parkinson's disease, dementia, poor memory, depression, anxiety and overthinking, bipolar, epilepsy, autism, etc.

REN-17 Danzhong (Shanzhong)

- Location: On the midline of the sternum, in a depression level with the junction of the fourth intercostal space and the sternum.
- Dao-qi needling: transverse insertion 0.8 to 1.3 cun.
- Dao-qi feeling: Sensation spread up or downward, or sides of chest.

- Dao-qi indications: Shortness of breath, cough, asthma, fullness and oppression of the chest and diaphragm, obstruction of the chest, pain of the chest and heart; difficult ingestion, acid regurgitation, oesophageal constriction, vomiting; goitre, wind painful obstruction, loss of consciousness, etc.

REN-22 Tiantu

- Location: On the midline, in the centre of the suprasternal fossa, 0.5 cun superior to the suprasternal notch.
- Dao-qi needling: needle first perpendicularly 0.2 to 0.3 cun, then direct the needle inferiorly along the posterior border of the manubrium of the sternum 0.5 to 1 cun (this needling not suitable for acupuncturists without supervised training).
- Dao-qi feeling: Sensation spread to the middle and side of chest.
- Dao-qi indications: Severe obstruction in the chest, fullness of the chest, obstruction of qi with Heart pain, pain of the heart and back, rebellious qi with cough, asthma, sudden dyspnoea, inability to breathe; severe rattling sound in the throat, accumulation of phlegm in the throat, plum-stone sensation (Meiheqi); sudden loss of voice, inability to speak, swelling of the neck, goitre, etc.

REN-23 Lianquan

- Location: On the anterior midline of the neck, in the depression above the hyoid bone.
- Dao-qi needling: Oblique insertion in the direction of tongue root, 0.8 to 1.5 cun.
- Dao-qi feeling: Sensation may spread to the tongue root and throat.
- Dao-qi indications: Swelling below the tongue with difficulty speaking, sudden loss of voice, loss of speech after wind-stroke, contraction of the root of the tongue; hard to swallow, etc.

REN-24 Chengjiang

- Location: Above the chin, in the depression in the centre of the mentolabial groove.
- Dao-qi needling: Oblique insertion upward, 0.5 to 1.0 cun.
- Dao-qi feeling: Sensation may spread to the mouth and sides.
- Dao-qi indications: Hemiplegia, deviation of the mouth, epilepsy, mania-depression; pain and numbness of the face, swelling of the face, pain of the teeth and gums, purple lips, excessive production of watery saliva, dry mouth, wasting and thirsting disorder with great desire to drink; dark urine or frequent urination, sweating, impotence, abdominal masses in women, uterine fibroids, infertility, face beauty, etc.

Above listed Du Mai and Ren Mai points are just some sample of commonly used Dao-qi needling points, which are mostly used to treating Brain related conditions. Of cause, there are lots of other points are suitable and commonly used for Dao-qi needling as well.

In summary, Dao-qi needling technique original from Huangdi Neijing, which is characterized by gentle and smooth manipulation and widely applied. Its main functions are regulating the reverse chaos and regulating the Qi of channels and internal organs, coordinated balance. Adjusting the Shen is the basic requirement of the Dao-qi technique, which require the coopetition of the practitioner and the patient. The successful application of the Dao-qi needling method needs to be a combination of biological and psychological effects. Commonly used Dao-qi point for Brain related conditions are Du Mai and Ren Mai points.

References

1. Wang B, Wu LS, Wu Q (Trans). Yellow Emperors cannon of internal medicine. Beijing: China Science & Technology Press, 1997.
2. Unschuld PU. Huang Di Nei Jing Ling Shu: the ancient classic on needle therapy. University of California Press, California, USA, 2016. eBook.
3. Wang J, Jiang JF, Wang LL. Clinical observation on governor vessel Dao-qi method for treatment of dyssomnia in the patient of depression (Chinese with English abstract). Chin Acupunct Moxibustion. 2006;26(5):328–30.
4. Jiang JF, Liu LY, Wang J, et al. Influence of combined acupuncture and medication on HAMD factors in depression patients (Chinese with English abstract). Shanghai J Acu-Mox. 2007;26)6:3–5.
5. Wang TJ, Wang LL, Tao WJ, et al. Dynamic observation of retained needles on HAMD factors scales in depression (Chinese with English Abstract). J Jiangsu Chin Med. 2008;40:192–4.
6. Wang TJ, Wang LL, Tao WJ, et al. Clinical study on combined needle-embedding and dedication for depressive sleep disorder. J Acupunct Tuina Sci. 2009;7:210–2.
7. Wang TJ, Wang LL, Tao W, et al. Acupuncture combined with an antidepressant for patients with depression in hospital: a pragmatic randomised controlled trial. Acupunct Med. 2014;32:308–12.
8. Deadman P, Al-Khafaji M, Baker K. A manual of acupuncture. 2nd ed. East Sussex: JCM Publications; 2003.
9. Wang TJ. A new understanding of the Brain and its clinical application. EJOM. 2015;8:28–31.
10. Unschuld PU, Tessenow H, Zheng JS. Huang Di Nei Jing Su Wen: an annotated translation of Huang Di's Inner Classic – basic questions. University of California Press, California, 2011. Volume II. eBook.
11. Gershon MD. The second brain. New York: Harper Collins; 1998.
12. Maciocia G. The psyche in Chinese medicine-treatment of emotional and mental disharmonies with acupuncture and Chinese berbs. Edinburgh: Churchill Livingstone; 2009.

Part II
Acupunture Treatment for the Diseases of the Brain

Chapter 7
Stroke

7.1 General Information

Acupuncture has been used in stroke and particularly on post stroke rehabilitation in China for over 3000 years, and still widely used as a part of the treatment for post stroke patients in almost all the hospitals in China. However, it is not part of the conventional treatment in most of the western countries.

7.1.1 Basic Background of Stroke

Stroke is defined by the World Health Organization (WHO): "rapidly developing clinical signs of focal (or global) disturbance of cerebral function, with symptoms lasting 24 h or longer or leading to death, with no apparent cause other than of vascular origin" [1]. It is an acute focal injury of the central nervous system (CNS) arising from a vascular cause such as cerebral infarction, intracerebral haemorrhage, or subarachnoid haemorrhage. Stroke is an ongoing global health problem. In 2016, stroke was the second-leading global cause of death after ischemic heart disease, representing 11.8% of total deaths worldwide. In some countries, such as China, stroke has been the leading cause of death with incidence increasing by 8.7% per annum. There were 5.53 million people who suffered from stroke worldwide. Stroke was also the second most common cause of premature mortality and secondary disability [2–4].

The worldwide burden of ischemic and haemorrhagic stroke increased significantly. Of the two major classes of stroke, ischemic (~80% of strokes) and haemorrhagic (~20% of strokes), the burden has increased in terms of the absolute number of people with incident ischaemic and haemorrhagic stroke (37% and 47% increase, resp.), number of deaths (21% and 20% increase), and Disability Adjusted of Life Years (DALYs) lost (18% and 14% increase) [4–6].

© Springer Nature Switzerland AG 2021
T. Wang, *Acupuncture for Brain*, https://doi.org/10.1007/978-3-030-54666-3_7

The symptoms caused by stroke, such as hemiplegia, cognitive disorder, aphasia, and dysphagia, greatly affect the ability of patients to perform activities of daily living (ADL), as well as social participation, imposing a great burden on families and communities. Stroke became an important public health-care and social issue because of its high prevalence, unsatisfactory treatment options, large medical burden, and serious reduction in quality of life (QoL). Hence, both patients and practitioners desire effective alternative therapies.

There is a special type of stroke, transient ischemic attack (TIA), also called mimic stroke-like symptoms. It is defined as an acute loss of focal cerebral or ocular function with symptoms lasting less than 24 h and which is thought to be Due to inadequate cerebral or ocular blood supply as a result of low blood flow, thrombosis or embolism associated with diseases of the blood vessels, heart, or blood [7].

7.1.2 The Aetiology and Pathogenesis

Stroke can be caused by ischemia or haemorrhage. Thrombosis, embolus and haemorrhage are causations of the damage to the Brain tissue, which lead to hemiplegia or some form of hemiparesis. Prognosis depends on the extensiveness of the stroke, type of stroke and the patient's general health condition. The prognosis is depended on how quickly a patient is able to get treatment after the onset.

The impact factors for stroke are mixed, external risk factor are geographic location, altitude, weather, etc. Internal risk factors are listed below:

- Age: The death cases over 45 years old, stroke is the first. The age group of prevalence rate of stroke is 60–74.
- Sex: The prevalence rate of stroke in man is almost double than women.
- High blood pressure: The most common risk factor for stroke, it is 2 to 7 times higher than non-high blood pressure.
- Other risks: Diabetes: TIA, previous stroke history, heart attack history, obesity, smoke, et al.
- Predisposing factor: any factor which may increase blood pressure which may induce stroke, such as sudden change in climate, diet disorders, severe diarrhoea, excessive drinking or drunkenness, over think, anxiety, excessive force, over tired, constipation, over sex, et al.

7.1.3 Typical Clinical Symptoms

7.1.3.1 FAST

Due to different part of body are controlled by different part the Brain, the symptoms vary and depend on the affected Brain. Below are some commonly seen signs and symptoms of urgent stroke, which could be abbreviated as FAST [8].

Face—the face may have dropped on 1 side, the person may not be able to smile, or their mouth or eye may have drooped.

Arms—the person with suspected stroke may not be able to lift both arms and keep them there because of weakness or numbness in one arm.

Speech—their speech may be slurred or garbled, or the person may not be able to talk at all despite appearing to be awake; they may also have problems understanding what you're saying to them.

Time—it's time to dial 999 immediately if you notice any of these signs or symptoms.

Other commonly seen symptoms for stroke we summarize as Five suddenly:

- Suddenly confusion or trouble speaking or understanding. Sometimes weakness in the muscles of the face can cause drooling.
- Suddenly trouble seeing in one or both eyes
- Suddenly trouble walking, dizziness, loss of balance or coordination
- Suddenly, severe headache with no known cause

7.1.3.2 Commonly Seen Problems After a Stroke or Sequel of Stroke

The commonly seen symptoms or sequel of stroke can be divided by two main categories, physical symptoms and mental problems. Most of these symptoms could be improved with time and particularly with rehabilitations [9]. Acupuncture is one of the effective and valuable methods for stroke rehabilitation.

Physical Symptoms

Paralysis mostly on one side (hemiplegia), weakness, balance or coordination problems.
Pain, numbness, burning or tingling sensations.
Fatigue, urinary or bowel incontinence, constipation.
Aphasia, unclear speech, or difficulty understanding speech, reading or writing.
Difficulty swallowing (dysphagia).
Visual problem, double vision, Partial blindness.

Mental Symptoms

Poor memory, difficulty making decision or poor concentration.
Post stroke depression or anxiety.

7.1.4 Examination and Diagnosis

With the developments of the modern medicine, the diagnosis of stroke has been much quicker and accurate. As the samples of widely applied of computerized tomography (CT) scan and magnetic resonance imaging (MRI) are usable achievement for early identify of haemorrhagic stroke from Ischemic stroke.

Other examinations, such as normal physical examination and neurological examination are still useful to understanding what the individual has suffered and help to establish the treatment methods and rehabilitation strategy.

7.1.5   The Treatment of Stroke with Modern Medicine

The treatment of stroke usually includes acute treatment, subacute care, spontaneous recovery, rehabilitation, and the return to community life. Acute treatment for stroke depends on what kind of stroke, ischemic stroke or haemorrhagic stroke.

The most effective therapy for acute ischemic stroke, the most common kind of stroke, is administration of recombinant tissue plasminogen activator (rtPA) within 3 h of stroke onset. Antithrombotic treatment includes antiplatelet use of aspirin within 48 h of stroke onset, which reduces the risk of recurrence and mortality [10]. The sooner the better. Quick treatment not only improve the chance of survival but also may reduce complications they may have. Unfortunately, rtPA must be administered within 4.5 h of stroke onset to be effective, and it often results in intracranial haemorrhage [11]. These two factors largely restrict the clinical use of rtPA [12].

The Emergency treatment of haemorrhagic stroke focuses on controlling the bleeding and reducing pressure in the Brain. Surgery may be needed to reduce future risk.

There is much debate about the amount and frequency of therapy that is needed for stroke rehabilitation, and each person with stroke should be assessed individually and reassessed regularly. Rehabilitation is an adaptive process, and practice and repetition are likely to be key components with optimal recovery often requiring many months of treatment [13, p. 51].

For promote a patient-centred approach, the updated fifth National Clinical Guideline for Stroke has structured by problems with Recommendations, as listed below:

- Activities of daily living
- Arm function
- Cognition (Apraxia, Attention and concentration, Executive function, Memory, Perception, Spatial awareness)
- Communication (Aphasia, Dysarthria, Apraxia of speech)
- Continence
- Fatigue
- Hydration and nutrition
- Mental capacity
- Mobility (Weakness and ataxia, Balance, Falls and fear of falling, Walking)
- Mood and well-being (Anxiety, depression and psychological distress, Emotionalism)

- Mouth care
- Pain (Neuropathic pain, central post-stroke pain), Musculoskeletal pain, Shoulder pain and subluxation,
- Sensation
- Sex
- Spasticity and contractures
- Swallowing
- Vision
  Implications of recommendations

7.2 TCM Understanding

Stroke in TCM theory could belong to "Wind-Stroke/ Attack (Zhong Feng)", "Hemiplegia (Pian Ku)" or Hemiparalysis (Ban Shen Bu Sui) [14]. The aetiology is complex, could be summarized as internal deficiency as the root, and Wind, cold, summer wet, humid dryness and fire are the branches. Overexertion, deficiency after disease or injury, weakness due to aging, imbalance of yin and yang, emotional distress or too much alcohol, et al. are commonly recognised reasons.

Stoke can be divided into internal Zangfu degree and Channel degree, or mild and severe degree. The mild or channel degree stroke affects the meridians and are related to symptoms such as hemiplegia, numbness, deviation of eyes and mouth, difficulty of speech. When the disease goes further into the inner organs and meridians, then severe degree stroke happens with aphasia, loss of consciousness, coma, aside of paralysis, numbness on side of the body [15, p. 1214–17].

7.3 General Acupuncture Treatment

Acupuncture is a kind of classical traditional Chinese medicine (TCM) that has been used for patients with stroke and post-stroke rehabilitation for thousands of years. WHO has listed stroke as the Diseases, symptoms or conditions for which acupuncture has been proved—through controlled trials—to be an effective treatment on its review in 2002 [16, p. 24]. Clinical trial and meta-analysis findings have demonstrated the efficacy of acupuncture in improving balance function, reducing spasticity, and increasing muscle strength and general well-being post-stroke (see Sect. 7.5 on this chapter). The mechanisms underlying the beneficial effects of acupuncture in stroke rehabilitation remain unclear.

According to the TCM theory about stroke classifications, the principle of general acupuncture treatment would be followed the pattern identification as well.

7.3.1 Mild Degree (Channel Degree)

7.3.1.1 Channel Blockage by Wind and Phlegm

Signs and Symptoms (SS): Hemiplegia, deviation of mouth and tongue, speech difficulty or Aphasia, feeling reduced or lost on limbs, dizziness and vertigo, lots of phlegm, dark tongue with white coat, wiry and slippery pulse.

Points selection: DU-20 Baihui, DU-16 Fengfu, GB-20 Fengchi, ST-40 Fenglong, ST-36 Zusanli, SP-10 Xuehai, REN-12 Zhongwan.

7.3.1.2 Wind and Fire Upper Disturbance

SS: Hemiplegia, deviation of mouth and tongue, speech difficulty or Aphasia, vertigo and headache, red face and eyes, bitter mouth and dry throat, upset and irritable, yellow urine and dry stool. Red tongue with yellow and dry coat, wiry and fast pulse.

Points selection: DU-20 Baihui, Ex-Sishencong, LI-11 Quchi, GB-34 Yanglingquan, LV-2 Xingjiang, LV-3 Taichong. SJ-6 Zhigou.

7.3.1.3 Hot Phlegm and Excess Fu

SS: Hemiplegia, deviation of mouth and tongue, speech difficulty or Aphasia, feeling reduced or lost on limbs, bloating and constipation, headache and vertigo, lots of phlegm, dark and red tongue with yellow and greasy coat, wiry and slippery pulse.

Points selection: DU-20 Baihui, GB-20 Fengchi, ST-36 Zusanli, LI-11 Quchi, ST-40 Fenglong, ST-44 Neiting, SJ-6 Zhigou, REN-12 Zhongwan, ST-25 Tianshu.

7.3.1.4 Qi Deficiency and Blood Stagnation

SS: Hemiplegia, deviation of mouth and tongue, speech difficulty or Aphasia, feeling reduced or lost on limbs, light face, short of breath and fatigue, sweating, palpitation, loose stool, swollen hand and feet. Light colour tongue with white and thick coat with teeth marks on sides, deep and thin pulse.

Points selection: REN-12 Zhongwan, REN-10 Xiawan, REN-6 Qihai, REN-4 Guanyuan, ST-36 Zusanli, SP-10 Xuehai, BL-17 Geshu,

7.3.1.5 Yin Deficiency with Internal Wind

SS: Hemiplegia, deviation of mouth and tongue, speech difficulty or Aphasia, feeling reduced or lost on limbs, vertigo and tinnitus, dry mouth and throat. Thin tongue body with less coat or no coat, wiry, thin or fast pulse.

Points selection: DU-20 Baihui, GB-20 Fengchi, ST-36 Zusanli, GB-39 Xuanzhong, SP-6 Sanyinjiao, KI-3 Taixi,

7.3.2   Severe Degree (Zangfu Degree)

7.3.2.1   Phlegm Heat Block the Brain

SS: Suddenly onset, loss of consciousness or coma, snoring and phlegm, Hemiplegia, deviation of mouth and tongue, limbs convulsion or spasm, stiff neck, fever, smelling mouth, disturbing, even cold hands and feet, frequently spasm, perhaps vomiting blood. Dark red tongue with dry yellow coat, wiry slippery fast pulse.

Points selection: 12-Jin-well points with bleeding, or 10-Xuan points with bleeding, DU-26 Renzhong (Shuigou), LI-11 Quchi, ST-40 Fenglong, LI-4 Hegu, LV-3 Taichong, Ex-Yintang.

7.3.2.2   Phlegm and Blood Stasis Blockage Heart Shen

SS: Suddenly onset, loss of consciousness or coma, snoring and phlegm, Hemiplegia, deviation of mouth and tongue, phlegm in throat, light face with purple lip, urine and stool incontinence, all body cold and wet, purple tongue with white and greasy coat, deep slippery slow pulse.

Points selection: 12-Jin-well points with bleeding, or 10-Xuan points with bleeding, DU-26 Renzhong (Shuigou), REN-12 Zhongwan, ST-36 Zusanli, ST-40 Fenglong, PC-6 Neiguan, SP-4 Gongsun, PC-8 Laogong.

Above pattern identifications may be separate used with general needling, or better combined with below unique Brain acupuncture techniques.

7.4   Unique Acupuncture Techniques for Stroke

Traditionally, acupuncture treatment for stroke are focused mainly on Yangming channels, i.e. Hand Yangming Large Intestine meridian and Foot Yangming Stomach meridian, which original from "Huangdi Neijing-Su Wen (Plain Questions) Chapter 44—Wei lun (on Flaccidity)" 'it is stated in the ancient books that when treating the flaccidity, it should treat the Yangming Channel alone' [14, p. 215]. This treatment principle has been guiding the acupuncture treatment for stroke over two thousand years and is still applied by many acupuncturists, particularly for sequel of stroke, followed by most of classic TCM textbooks.

Recently, with the development of TCM Brain theory, it is believed that TCM Brain has played a unique role of stroke, on its ethology, pathology, treatment strategy and recovery. It is believed that the internal and external pathological factors, cause Brain channels blockage or bleeding from Brain vessel, which may lead to damage of Brain marrow and result of stroke. The major organ location of stroke is no doubt in the Brain, and involve other Zang organs such as Heart, Liver, Spleen and Kidney, et al. Most stroke patients are deficient of root and excess on branches. One of the typical sample of this developments is Xing Nao Kai Qiao (Awake the Brain and Open Orificios) [17].

Due to the Brain marrow and Shen disorder, its ability of regulating other Zangfu organs has been decreased or lost, which lead several other Zangfu organs disorders. Stroke, with such complex clinical manifestation, hemiplegia, facial paralysis, speech difficulty, et al., there are definitely more than two organs involved.

In terms of the unique acupuncture treatment, Brain is the main location of disease and Du Mai is the channel of the Brain. The treatment principle will be more focused on the rebalance of the Brain and regulating Du Mai. Thus scalp acupuncture and Du Mai Dao-qi technique are mostly used in acupuncture practice.

7.4.1   Scalp Acupuncture for Treating Stroke (Detail of Scalp Acupuncture, Location and Needling, Please see Chap. 5)

- Hemiplegia: Opposite upper 1/5 and 2/5 Motor Area and Foot-Motor Sensory Area. During the needling, patients should move or helped to move their suffered limbs.
- Hemi-sensory disorder: Opposite upper 1/5 and 2/5 Sensory Area and Foot-Motor Sensory Area
- Hemianopia: Visual Area
- Motor aphasia: first Speech Area
- Anomic aphasia: second Speech Area
- Sensory aphasia: third Speech Area
- Dizziness: Vertigo and Auditory Area
- Ataxia: Balance Area
- Constipation: Intestine Area
- Frequently urination: Foot-Motor Sensory Area

7.4.2   Du Mai Dao-qi Technique (Detail of Dao-qi Technique on Du Mai, Points Location and Needling, Please see Chap. 6)

- DU-26 Renzhong (Shuigou): Dao-qi technique: request the patient with tear or watery in eyes.
- DU-16 Fengfu, DU-15 Yamen, DU-14 Dazhui, DU-9 Zhiyang, DU-4 Mingmen, DU-3 Yaoyangguan

7.4.3 Ren Mai Dao-qi Technique (Detail of Dao-qi Technique on Ren Mai, Points Location and Needling, Please see Chap. 6)

- REN-12 Zhongwan plus 2–4 needles around it with 0.5–1 cm distance, REN-10 Xiawan, REN-6 Qihai, REN-4 Guanyuan, REN-17 Danzhong (Shanzhong).

Above unique Brain acupuncture techniques can be combined with syndrome differentiation treatment.

7.4.4 Brain Pattern Differentiation

The common clinical Brain patterns of stroke and its possible symptoms could be summarized as below and are currently being developed and not perfected at the moment.

7.4.4.1 Deficiency of Brain Yang Qi

Signs and Symptoms (SS): Hemiplegia, deviation of mouth and tongue, speech difficulty or aphasia, feeling reduced or lost on limbs, light face, short of breath and fatigue, sweating, palpitation, loose stool, swollen hand and feet, cold on suffered side. Light colour tongue with white and thick coat with teeth marks on sides, deep and thin pulse.

Brain acupuncture treatment:

Scalp acupuncture on related areas as above 7.4.1.

Brain acupuncture points selection: DU-20 Baihui, DU-16 Fengfu, DU-15 Yamen, DU-14 Dazhui, DU- 9 Zhiyang, DU-4 Mingmen, DU-3 Yaoyangguan, REN-12 Zhongwan, REN-10 Xiawan, REN-6 Qihai, REN-4 Guanyuan, plus local suffered area points. Moxa could be applied, and Dao-qi technique may be added.

7.4.4.2 Stagnation of Brain Collaterals

SS: Hemiplegia, deviation of mouth and tongue, speech difficulty or aphasia, loss of balance, vague or double vision, feeling reduced or lost on limbs, pain on shoulder, arm and leg, swollen and purple on hand and feet. Purple with light coat, wiry pulse.

Brain acupuncture treatment:

Scalp acupuncture on related areas as above 7.4.1 plus Vasomotor Area.

Brain acupuncture points selection: DU-20 Baihui, DU-16 Fengfu, DU-15 Yamen, DU-14 Dazhui, DU-9 Zhiyang, DU-3 Yaoyangguan, REN-12 Zhongwan, REN-10 Xiawan, REN-6 Qihai, plus local suffered area points. Moxa could be applied, and Dao-qi technique may be added.

7.4.4.3   Disorder of Brain Shen

SS: Several weeks or months after stroke, hemiplegia, deviation of mouth and tongue, speech difficulty or aphasia, feeling reduced or lost on limbs; mental depression, stress, anxiety, insomnia or lethargy, delirium, murmuring, abnormal behavior, anorexia, polyphagia, dementia, drooling, etc. light tongue with thin coating, wiry or slow pulse.

Brain acupuncture treatment:

Scalp acupuncture on related areas as above 7.4.1.

Brain acupuncture points selection: DU-24 Shenting, DU-20 Baihui, DU-16 Fengfu, DU-14 Dazhui, Ex-Yintang, HT-7 Shenmen, plus local area points. Techniques could be selected through electric acupuncture, Dao-qi techniques, et al.

7.4.4.4   Blockage of Brain Orifical

SS: Suddenly onset, loss of consciousness or coma, hemiplegia, deviation of mouth and tongue, phlegm in throat, light face with purple lip, urine and stool incontinence, all body cold and wet, purple tongue with white and greasy coat, deep slippery slow pulse.

Brain acupuncture treatment:

Scalp acupuncture on related areas as above 7.4.1.

Brain acupuncture points selection: DU-26 Renzhong, DU-20 Baihui, DU-16 Fengfu, DU-14 Dazhui, REN-12 Zhongwan plus 2–4 needles, REN-6 Qihai, 10-Xuan points with bleeding. Techniques could be selected through electric acupuncture, Dao-qi techniques, et al.

Notes
- Treatment should be given as soon as possible for the best results. The acute stoke, particularly haemorrhagic stroke, should be waiting until the life figures, breathing, heartbeat, and blood pressure, are stable. The integrate with western medicine emergency care should be considered in acute stage.
- The treatment frequency: in the early stage, the more often the better. In western countries, suggest 2–3 times per week, then with time, move slow down to once per week followed by one in 2–4 weeks for maintenance and prevention. If in China, possible every day or even twice per day in early stage.
- Acupuncture can be combined with routine rehabilitations such as physiotherapy, speech therapy, etc.
- Above Brain related patterns for stroke can be identified separately for severe patients, and combined with classic TCM pattern identifications.

7.5   Research

Countless clinical trials have indicated acupuncture can enhance the muscles strength functions [18], improve balance function [19] and reduce spasticity [20] in stroke patients. A review conducted in 2016 has summarized that acupuncture is a prospective therapy targeting neurogenesis for ischemic stroke [12].

Positron emission tomography (PET), as it is a non-invasive method of central nervous system, has been used to explore mechanism of acupuncture treatment. One study [21] has demonstrated that electric acupuncture (EA) at head points, DU-20 Baihui and GB-7 Qubin could activate the cerebral structures related to motor function on the bilateral hemispheres, and concluded that EA was very helpful for the cerebral motor plasticity after the ischemic stroke.

One study [22] conducted 10 sessions of placebo or active low-frequency electrical stimulation (2/100 Hz) using subcutaneous acupuncture needles over the scalp at corresponding functional areas of the cerebral cortex. The finding suggested that the active group had a larger functional improvement.

Post stroke depression (PSD) is the most frequent and important neuropsychiatric consequence of stroke. It contributes to a variety of adverse health outcomes, including increased disability, morbidity, and mortality. Qian's study [23] concluded that body acupuncture was effective in reducing stroke patients' depressive symptoms and had fewer side-effects. It should be considered as an option for neuropsychiatric sequelae of stroke.

A systematic review and meta-analysis about eye acupuncture for stroke [24] indicated that when eye acupuncture was combined with conventional treatment, such as western medicine or rehabilitation, compared to conventional treatment alone, there was a significant difference in the areas of mental state, swallow function, and neurological function deficit scale (NDS), et al.

The recently Cochrane system review in 2018 indicates that the effects of acupuncture in reducing death or dependency or improving neurological and movement scores in trials is better than compared control [25].

Another literature review, conducted by Chavez et al. in 2017 [26] summarized the current known mechanisms in ischemic stroke rehabilitation through acupuncture and electro acupuncture (EA) therapy. The evidence in this review indicates that five major different mechanisms are involved in the beneficial effects of acupuncture/EA on ischemic stroke rehabilitation: (1) Promotion of neurogenesis and cell proliferation in the central nervous system (CNS); (2) Regulation of cerebral blood flow in the ischemic area; (3) Anti-apoptosis in the ischemic area; (4) Regulation of neurochemicals; and, (5) Improvement of impaired long-term potentiation (LTP) and memory after stroke. Their findings show that acupuncture exerts a beneficial effect on ischemic stroke through modulation of different mechanisms originating in the CNS.

7.6   Conclusion

Stroke is the second global leading cause of death, even the first cause in some developing countries such as China. The conventional medicine has played the mainstream role in the early interventions and then in recovery and rehabilitation. It has been developed very rapidly thus every four years the National Guidance should be updated.

Acupuncture has been used for patients with stroke and post-stroke rehabilitation for thousands of years. Acupuncture for stroke has been listed as the Diseases, symptoms or conditions for which acupuncture has been proved—through controlled trials—to be an effective treatment on WHO review in 2002.

Clinical trial and meta-analysis findings have demonstrated the efficacy of acupuncture in improving balance function, reducing spasticity, and increasing muscle strength and general well-being post-stroke, although the mechanisms underlying the beneficial effects of acupuncture in stroke rehabilitation remain unclear.

According to the TCM theory about stroke classifications, the principle of general acupuncture treatment would be followed by the pattern identification. With the development of TCM Brain theory, more clinical practice and researches focus on the Brain related acupuncture techniques such as scalp acupuncture and Du Mai Dao-qi technique. These special techniques can be used alone or combined with traditional acupuncture as well.

References

1. WHO MONICA Project Investigators. The World Health Organization MONICA project (Monitoring trends and determinants in cardiovascular disease). J Clin Epidemiol. 1988;41:105–14.
2. Stroke control project committee of national health and family planning commission of the People's Republic of China. Report on the Chinese stroke prevention (2015). 1st edn. Beijing: China Pecking Union Medical College Press, 2015.
3. GBD 2016 Causes of Death Collaborators. Global, regional, and national age-sex specific mortality for 264 causes of death, 1980–2016: a systematic analysis for the Global Burden of Disease Study 2016. Lancet. 2017;390:1151–210.
4. Truelsen T, Begg S, Mathers C. The global burden of cerebrovascular disease. https://www.who.int/healthinfo/statistics/bod_cerebrovasculardiseasestroke.pdf. Accessed on 26/04/2020.
5. Writing Group Members, Mozaffarian, D, Benjamin EJ, Go AS, et al. Heart disease and stroke statistics—2016 update: a report from the American heart association. Circulation. 2016;133:e38–e360.
6. Krishnamurthi RV, Feigin VL, Forouzanfar MH, et al. Global and regional burden of first-ever ischaemic and haemorrhagic stroke during 1990–2010: findings from the global burden of disease study 2010. Lancet Glob Health. 2013;1:e259–81.
7. Hankey GJ, Warlow C. Transient ischaemic attacks of the brain and eye. London: Saunders; 1994.
8. NHS, Symptoms of stroke. https://www.nhs.uk/conditions/stroke/symptoms/. Accessed 26/04/2020.
9. UPMC, Problems that occur after a stroke. https://www.upmc.com/services/rehab/rehab-institute/conditions/stroke/after-stroke. Accessed on 26/04/2020.
10. Smith WS, Johnston SC, Hemphill JC. Cerebrovascular diseases. In: Kasper D, Fauci A, Hauser S, et al., editors. Harrison's principles of internal medicine, vol. 2. 19th ed. New York, NY: McGraw Hill Education; 2014.
11. Powers WJ, Rabinstein AA, Ackerson T, et al. Guidelines for the early management of patients with acute ischemic stroke: a guideline for healthcare professionals from the American Heart Association/American Stroke association. Stroke. 2018;49(3):e46–e110.

12. Lin L, Zhong L, Bian ZX. Acupuncture for neurogenesis in experimental ischemic stroke: a systematic review and meta-analysis. Sci Rep. 2016;6:19521. https://doi.org/10.1038/srep19521.
13. Intercollegiate Stroke Working Party. National clinical guideline for stroke. 5th ed. London: Royal College of Physicians; 2016.
14. Wang B, Wu LS and Wu Q (Trans). Yellow Emperors cannon of internal medicine. Beijing: China Science & Technology Press. 1997.
15. Maciocia G. The practice of Chinese medicine, the treatment of diseases with acupuncture and Chinese herbs, 2nd edn. Edinburgh: Churchill Livingstone. 2007. eBook.
16. WHO. Acupuncture: review and analysis of reports on controlled clinical trials. World Health Organisation Geneva, 2002.
17. Bai XY, Jiang GL. Comparative analysis of therapeutic effects of apoplexy treated by Xingnao Kaiqiao acupuncture method and western medicine. World J Acupunct Moxibust. 1996;6(1):25–8.
18. Yan T, Hui-Chan CW. Transcutaneous electrical stimulation on acupuncture points improves muscle function in subjects after acute stroke: a randomized controlled trial. J Rehabil Med. 2009;41:312–6.
19. Liu S, Hsieh CL, Wei TS, et al. Acupuncture stimulation improves balance function in stroke patients: a single-blinded controlled, randomized study. Am J Chin Med. 2009;37:483–94.
20. Zhao JG, Cao CH, Liu CZ, et al. Effect of acupuncture treatment on spastic states of stroke patients. J Neurol Sci. 2009;276:143–7.
21. Fang Z, Ning J, Xiong C, et al. Effects of electro acupuncture at head points on the function of cerebral motor areas in stroke patients: a PET study. Evid Based Complement Alternat Med. 2012. Article ID 902413, 9 pages. https://doi.org/10.1155/2012/902413
22. Hsing WT, Imamura M, Weaver K. Clinical effects of scalp electrical acupuncture in stroke: a sham-controlled randomized clinical trial. J Altern Complement Med. 2012;18(4):341–6.
23. Qian XL, Zhou X, You YL. Traditional Chinese acupuncture for post stroke depression: a single-blind double-simulated randomized controlled trial. J Altern Complement Med. 2015;21:748–53.
24. Bai ZH, Zhang ZX, Li CR, et al. Eye acupuncture treatment for stroke: a systematic review and meta-analysis. Evid Based Complement Alternat Med. 2015. ID 871327, 11 pages. https://doi.org/10.1155/2015/871327.
25. Xu MM, Li D, Zhang SH. Acupuncture for acute stroke. Cochrane database of systematic reviews 2018, Issue 3. Art. No.: CD003317. https://doi.org/10.1002/14651858.CD003317.pub3
26. Chavez LM, Huang SS, MacDonald I, et al. Mechanisms of acupuncture therapy in ischemic stroke rehabilitation: a literature review of basic studies. Int J Mol Sci. 2017;18:2270–83.

Chapter 8
Parkinson's Disease

8.1 General Information

8.1.1 Basic Background of Parkinson's Disease

Parkinson's disease (PD), first reported by James Parkinson in 1817 in the UK, is an age-related and the second most common progressive neurodegenerative disorder. It is insidious onset and characterized by the presence of predominantly motor symptomatology such as bradykinesia, rest tremor, rigidity and postural disturbances, which is classified as the second most common neurodegenerative disease following the Alzheimer's disease (AD) [1, p. 140]. This disease affects about 3% of the elderly above 65, and the percentage is higher for males [2]. Although both genetic and environmental factors are implicated in the development of PD, the cause of disease is still unclear [3].

The majority of studies reporting overall crude prevalence (including males and females across the entire age range) fall between 100 and 200 per 100,000 persons, or one-two per thousand [1, p. 141]. This disease affects about 3% of the elderly above 65, and the percentage is higher for males [2].

8.1.2 The Aetiology and Pathogenesis

PD is caused by the selective loss of dopaminergic neurons in the substantia nigra (SN) and the depletion of striatal dopamine (DA) [4], which leads to a decrease in dopamine and then results in the loss of the basal ganglia's activities and the onset of neurodegenerative problems, result in an inability to control voluntary movement [1, p. 141]. It is well known that several factors including aging, inflammation, and oxidative stress can trigger PD, but the mechanism remains unclear [5].

© Springer Nature Switzerland AG 2021
T. Wang, *Acupuncture for Brain*, https://doi.org/10.1007/978-3-030-54666-3_8

Dopaminergic system dysfunction is implicated in a wide variety of neurological disorders, including Parkinson's disease. DA neurons play a central role in the control of motor functions and their loss causes behavioural dysfunctions. It is well known that several factors including aging, inflammation, and oxidative stress can trigger PD. Although both genetic and environmental factors are implicated in the development of PD, the cause of disease is still unclear [3].

Neurogenesis, which is the process by which neurons are generated from neural stem cells and progenitor cells, has been shown to occur in special zones of the adult Brain including the subventricular zone (SVZ) of the lateral ventricles and the dentate gyrus of the hippocampus. Interestingly, reduced proliferation of SVZ cells was observed in PD patients, suggesting that PD suppresses neurogenesis in the Brain. Promotion of neurogenesis and replacement of dead DA neurons with new ones in the Brains of PD patients would help alleviate PD symptoms. Therefore, adult neurogenesis has recently been considered a new therapeutic paradigm of PD. When neurogenesis occurs, several types of progenitor cells are observed. Type A cells are proliferating neuroblasts that form chains to migrate, while type B cells are similar to astrocytes morphologically. Doublecortin (DCX), a Brain-specific microtubule-associated protein, is considered a marker of type A migratory neuroblasts, while glial fibrillary acid protein (GFAP) is a marker of type B astrocytic cells [6].

8.1.3 Typical Clinical Symptoms

During the early years of the disease, motor disability may not be significant as symptoms are usually gentle and mild. If left untreated, after several years it causes significant motor deterioration with loss of independence and ambulation. As the disease progresses, the increasing motor disability affects the activities of daily living [1, p. 140].

The symptoms of PD can be variable in patients. Early signs may be mild and go unnoticed. The typical symptoms for PD are predominantly motor disorders, including bradykinesia, rest tremor, rigidity, postural disturbances and speech or writing changes. These symptoms often begin on one side of the body. It is also associated with diversity of non-motor symptoms, such as hyposmia, rapid eye movements, sleep behaviour disorder, personality changes, pain, paraesthesia and depression may be present and may even manifest before the motor symptoms. Urinary disturbances, orthostatic hypotension and neuropsychiatric disturbances (dementia, hallucinations and delirium) usually become evident and troublesome after several years in the course of the disease [1, 7, 8].

The typical clinical symptoms could be summary as below:

- Motor symptoms: bradykinesia, rest tremor, rigidity, postural disturbances and speech or writing changes
- Non-motor symptoms: hyposmia, rapid eye movements, sleep behaviour disorder, personality changes, pain, paraesthesia and depression.

8.1.4   Examination and Diagnosis

As there are no definitive biological or imaging markers, diagnosis is at present made through the use of stringent clinical criteria such as those developed by the Brain Bank of the Parkinson's Disease Society in the United Kingdom [9]. These criteria are used worldwide and provide for a definite diagnosis with a high degree of accuracy. Clinic pathological studies based on Brain bank material from Canada and the United Kingdom have shown that clinicians diagnose the disease incorrectly in about 25% of patients. In these studies, the most common reasons for misdiagnosis were presence of essential tremor, vascular parkinsonism and atypical parkinsonian syndromes [10].

Although the diagnosis is made exclusively on a clinical basis, there are new diagnostic tools that can be used to confirm the presence of dopaminergic denervation at the striatal level, thus lending support to the clinical diagnosis. These include fluorodopa positron emission tomography (FDOPA-PET) and dopamine transporter imaging with radionuclide tracers by means of single photon emission tomography (DAT-SPECT). Both methods are still used as investigational tools and not for the routine diagnosis of PD [1, p. 141].

8.1.5   The Treatment of PD with Modern Medicine

At present, there is no satisfactory therapy for PD [11, p. 216]. The available conventional treatment options include medical and surgical therapies [2]. The most commonly used medications include levodopa and anticholinergic drugs. However, its effectiveness decreases as the duration of treatment is prolonged. About 90% of patients show good response to levodopa, but 30%, 50%, and 70–80% of patients had adverse reactions after taking levodopa for 3 years, 5 years, and 10 years, respectively. Unfortunately, they are only symptomatic relief with limited effect, but has many adverse effects. Motor fluctuations and dyskinesia are the most common side effects of using levodopa and anticholinergic drugs in treating PD patients. More and more PD patients are actively looking for other methods of treatment, such as complementary and alternative medicine (CAM), such as acupuncture.

8.2   TCM Understanding

Traditional Chinese Medicine (TCM) regards PD as tremor paralysis or a trembling symptom in the book of "Huangdi Neijing (Yellow Emperor's Internal Classic)" for 2000 years ago, which results from pathological changes in internal organs with the majority of Kidney, Spleen, and Liver. Disorders in the Kidneys lead to inactivity. Deficiency of the Qi in the Spleen leads to muscular dystrophy and fatigue. 'Liver wind' leads to tremors, as stated below in "Huandi Neijing-Suwen Chapter 74-Zhizhengyao Dalunpian (Comprehensive Discourse on the Essentials of the Most Reliable)" [12, p. 626–8].

> All [diseases with] wind [causing] swaying and dizziness, without exception they are associated with the Liver.
> All [diseases with] cold [causing] contracting and pulling in, without exception they are associated with the Kidneys.
> All [cases of] tetany and stiff nape, without exception they are associated with dampness.

Based on the pattern identification and treatment, the symptoms can be divided into patterns of Liver and Kidney deficiencies, Qi and Blood deficiency, wind phlegm, Qi stagnation and Blood blockage, and Spleen deficiency with damp. TCM doctors usually use Chinese herbal formulas and acupuncture therapy to treating the PD patients according to above patterns.

8.3 General Acupuncture Treatment

Acupuncture, one of the therapies of TCM, has been used for more than 2000 years for PD or similar disorders in the China and east Asia. Due to the fact it is a very safe, has less side-effects and well-accepted treatment acupuncture has been expanding for hundreds of years and getting popular in the past a few decades, including PD. Many patients with PD are reported to using acupuncture as an alternative treatment at some point in their life. Indeed, it has been estimated that 7–49% of the PD patients have used acupuncture as an alternative therapy. Many patients with PD experienced an improvement of their conditions after acupuncture [3]. Many studies have been performed to prove the efficacy of this treatment and additional studies have reported that acupuncture treatment leads to significant improvements in patients with PD [13].

According to the TCM theory about Parkinson's disease classifications, the principle of general acupuncture treatment would to follow the pattern identification as well. As usual below patterns, symptoms and signs, and the points selection, are just sample suggestions. Clinic practice should follow each individual patient.

8.3.1 Deficiency of Qi and Blood

Signs and Symptoms (SS): Limb tremor or shaking his head for a long time, dump, pale complex, back stiffness, limb cramps, reduced activities, walking instability, shortness of breath, tired, dizziness, sweat, especially when moving, drool, big tongue with teeth marks, dull, thin coat, thin and weak pulse or deep.

Points selection: REN-12 Zhongwan, REN-6 Qihai, ST-36 Zusanli, SP-9 Yinlingquan, SP-6 Sanyinjiao, LU-5 Chize, LI-4 Hegu, GB-39 Juegu.

8.3.2 Deficiency of Kidney and Liver

SS: Severe limb tremor or shaking his head for a long time, dump and clumsy, back stiffness, limb cramps, reduced activities, walking instability, dizziness, tinnitus, insomnia and dreams, back pain and soft knee, limb numbness, poor memory, small or thin tongue with dark and red colour, less coat, thin and fast pulse.

Points selection: LV-3 Taichong, LV-8 Ququan, KI-3 Taixi, KI-10 Yingu, SP-6 Sanyinjiao, HT-7 Shenmen, PC-6 Neiguan, BL-18 Ganshu, BL-23 Shenshu, DU-20 Baihui, Ex-Sishencong.

8.3.3 Kidney and Spleen Yang Deficiency

SS: Limb tremor or shaking his head for a long time, dump and clumsy, pale face, cold limbs, back pain and soft knee, dizziness and tinnitus, long and cold urination, loose stool, swollen tongue with light colour, white and slippery coat, deep and slow pulse.

Points selection: BL-23 Shenshu, BL-20 Pishu, DU-3 Yaoyangguan, DU-4 Mingmen, KI-7 Fuliu, REN-6 Qihai, REN-4 Guanyuan, DU-20 Baihui.

8.3.4 Wind Due to Phlegm Heat

SS: Limb tremor or shaking of the head for a long time, smaller amplitude, light and heavy, self-control, may combine with chest tightness, head heavy and dizziness, cough with phlegm, thirsty, yellowish tongue coating, wiry and slippery pulse.

Points selection: GB-20 Fengchi, LU-5 Chize, LI-4 Hegu, ST-40 Fenglong, GB-34 Yanglingquan, LV-3 Taichong.

8.3.5 Stagnation of Internal Blood

SS: Limb tremor or shaking of the head for a long time, back stiffness, limb cramps, reduced activities, may be pain and heavy, purple tongue with spots, underneath blue vein, wiry and unsmooth pulse.

Points selection: LV-3 Taichong, LI-4 Hegu, SP-10 Xuehai, ST-36 Zusanli, REN-6 Qihai, GB-20 Fengchi.

Above pattern identifications may be separate used with general needling, or better combined with below unique Brain acupuncture techniques.

8.4   Unique Acupuncture Techniques for Parkinson's Disease

Above traditionally acupuncture treatment or similar for PD has been practiced for thousands of years and still often practiced in most acupuncture clinics. In the last a few decades, with the development of TCM Brain theory, it is believed that TCM Brain has played a unique role of PD, on its ethology, pathology, and treatment strategy. It is believed that the internal and external pathological factors, cause Brain channels stagnation, Brain Yin and Yang imbalance, may lead to damage of Brain marrow and result of PD. The major organ location of PD is no doubt in the Brain, and involved other Zangfu organs such as Liver, Spleen and Kidney, et al. Most PD patients are deficiency of root (Ben Xu) and excess on branches (Biao Shi).

In terms of the unique acupuncture treatment, due to the fact that the Brain is the main location of disease, the treatment principle will be more focused on the rebalance of the Brain and regulating Du Mai. Thus scalp acupuncture and Du Mai Dao-qi technique are mostly used in acupuncture practice.

8.4.1   Scalp Acupuncture for Treating PD (Detail of Scalp Acupuncture, Location and Needling, Please see Chap. 5)

- Limb tremor or shaking, back stiffness, limb cramps: Chorea-Tremor Control area
- Dizziness: Vertigo and Auditory Area
- Ataxia or walking instability: Balance Area
- Constipation: Intestine Area
- Frequently urination: Foot-Motor Sensory Area
- Depression: Spirit-Emotion Area

8.4.2   Du Mai Dao-qi Technique (Detail of Dao-qi Technique on Du Mai, Points Location and Needling, Please see Chap. 6)

- DU-16 Fengfu, DU-15 Yamen, DU-14 Dazhui, DU-9 Zhiyang, DU-4 Mingmen, DU-3 Yaoyangguan

8.4.3   Ren Mai Dao-qi Technique (Detail of Dao-qi Technique on Ren Mai, Points Location and Needling, Please see Chap. 6)

- REN-12 Zhongwan plus 2–4 needles around it with 0.5–1 cm distance, REN-10 Xiawan, REN-6 Qihai, REN-4 Guanyuan, REN-17 Danzhong (Shanzhong)

Above unique Brain acupuncture techniques can be combined with syndrome differentiation treatment.

8.4.4   Brain Pattern Differentiation

The commonly clinical Brain patterns of PD and its possible symptoms could be summarized as below and they are on the way for developing and not perfect at the moment.

8.4.4.1   Deficiency of Brain Marrow

SS: Severe and chronic limb tremor or shaking, back stiffness, limb cramps, back pain or stiffness, amnesia and dull facial expression, light-colored or light red tongue, thin and deep pulse.

Brain acupuncture treatment:

Scalp acupuncture on related areas as above 8.4.1.

Points selection: DU-20 Baihui, DU-14 Dazhui, Ex-Bailaoxue, DU-4 Mingmen, KI-3 Taixi, GB-39 Xuanzhong (Juegu), and local area points. Techniques could choose electric-acupuncture, Dao-qi technique, etc.

8.4.4.2   Deficiency of Brain Yang Qi

SS: Limb tremor or shaking, back stiffness, limb cramps, light face, short of breath and fatigue, sweating, palpitation, loose stool, swollen hand and feet, genera cold particularly on suffered side. Light colour tongue with white and thick coat with teeth marks on sides, deep and thin pulse.

Brain acupuncture treatment:

Scalp acupuncture on related areas as above 8.4.1 plus Central Area.

Points selection: DU-20 Baihui, DU-16 Fengfu, DU-14 Dazhui, DU-9 Zhiyang, DU-4 Mingmen, DU-3 Yaoyangguan, REN-12 Zhongwan, REN-10 Xiawan, REN-6 Qihai, REN-4 Guanyuan, plus local suffered area points. Moxa could be applied, with Dao-qi technique on 1–2 key points.

8.4.4.3   Stagnation of Brain Collaterals

SS: Limb tremor or shaking, back stiffness, limb cramps, back pain or stiffness, swollen and purple on hand and feet. Purple with light coat, wiry pulse.

Brain acupuncture treatment:

Scalp acupuncture on related areas as above 8.4.1 plus Vasomotore Area.

Brain acupuncture points selection: DU-20 Baihui, DU-16 Fengfu, DU-15 Yamen, DU-14 Dazhui, DU-9 Zhiyang, DU-3 Yaoyangguan, REN-12 Zhongwan, REN-10 Xiawan, REN-6 Qihai, plus local suffered area points. Moxa could be applied, with Dao-qi technique.

8.4.4.4 Disorder of Brain Shen

SS: Limb tremor or shaking, back stiffness, limb cramps, mental depression, stress, anxiety, insomnia or lethargy, poor memory, drooling, etc. light tongue with thin coating, wiry or slow pulse.

Brain acupuncture treatment:

Scalp acupuncture on related areas as above 8.4.1.

Brain acupuncture points selection: DU-24 Shenting, DU-20 Baihui, DU-16 Fengfu, DU-14 Dazhui, Ex-Yintang, HT-7 Shenmen, plus local area points. Techniques could be selected through electric acupuncture, Dao-qi techniques, etc.

Notes
- For treatment PD, the earlier involved the better the results.
- The treatment frequency: in the early stage, is the often the better. In western countries, suggest twice per week, then with time, move slow down to once per week followed by once every 2–4 weeks for maintenance. If in some areas, possibly start with every day.
- Acupuncture can be combined with routine therapy such as physiotherapy, speech therapy, etc.
- Above Brain related patterns for PD can be identified separately for severe PD, and combined with classic TCM pattern identifications.

8.5 Research

In the last two decades there are increasing number of clinical studies of acupuncture treatment in Parkinson's disease (PD). Acupuncture therapy, either manual or electro-acupuncture stimulation at specific acupoints, relieved some motor symptoms in patients with PD and markedly improved many non-motor symptoms such as psychiatric disorders, sleep problems, and gastrointestinal symptoms. When it was used as an adjunct for levodopa, acupuncture improved therapeutic efficacy and reduced dosage and the occurrence of side effects of levodopa [3].

A very recent study in China indicates that Scalp acupuncture by retaining lone time combined with exercise therapy can improve the motor function and activities of daily living of patients with early PD [14]. Another recent RCT study [15] indicates that compared head acupuncture points and scalp acupuncture plus levodopa with levodopa only, and found head acupuncture treatment improved PD related symptom scores, including tremor, movement and daily lift activities.

Most clinical studies are designed treatment group, manual acupuncture or electric acupuncture, scalp acupuncture or general body acupuncture, plus medication compared with medication only [16–18]. The commonly used monitor for motor function are UPDRS (Unified Parkinson's Disease Rating Scale) total scores and UPDRSIII scores. A study [16] combined electro-acupuncture at neck points and scalp with madopar on Parkinson's disease, compared with madopar only. After two period of treatment, the total effectiveness of treatment group showed an obvious increase, it was higher than control group. They concluded that the therapeutic effect of combined acupuncture and drug is more lasting and more prominent.

Gait disorder, a key contributor to fall and poor quality of life, represents a major therapeutic challenge in PD. A recently randomized pilot study [19], after three weekly electric acupuncture treatments showed significant improvement, prominently in gait speed.

There are increasing studies focused on the non-motor symptoms (NMS) of PD, ranges from autonomic dysfunction, neuropsychiatric disorders, sleep disturbance, sensory symptoms to gastrointestinal syndromes, fatigue, and many others and are often under-treated [8]. Non-motor aspects of PD had greater impact on quality of life and cause higher institutionalization rates and healthcare cost [20].

Recent reviews [3] has discovered that depression was the most reported symptom, followed by sleep disorder, constipation, and bladder dysfunction, and summarized that non-motor symptoms, such as psychiatric disorders, sleep disorders, gastrointestinal symptoms, autonomic symptoms, seems to be more beneficial from acupuncture treatment.

Patients with Parkinson's disease have focal cerebral perfusion reduction [21]. The transcranial doppler ultrasonography is effective in automatic monitoring of cerebral blood flow in Parkinson's disease [22]. Early study in China has indicated the choice of acupoints on the head for PD is fast and lasting for cerebral blood flow and may have a more direct therapeutic effect on the disease with Brain lesions as the main pathology [23]. Another China study found scalp acupuncture, combined with madopar, could improve the rigidity, tremor, dyskinesia and rCBT (Regional cerebral blood flow) in PD patients, which had close relationship with its effect on cerebral blood flow [24].

Basic studies indicated that acupuncture protected dopaminergic neurons against toxic insults and increase dopamine production in the Brain by inducing release of neurotrophic factor, enhancing antioxidant agents, and inhibit inflammatory [3].

Recently, many PD model studies suggest that stimulation at acupoints could enhance motor function and promote dopaminergic cells against toxic insults. Studies of fMRI on human subjects found that stimulation on GB34 activated motor-related Brain regions such as the putamen, caudate nucleus and thalamus and cerebellum [13].

Several reports have indicated that the mechanism of using acupuncture in treating PD is closely related to the neurological system. The messages can be integrated and pass through nerve pathways to the central nervous system when acupuncture points are stimulated, and consequently, the surrounding tissue is effected [2].

As a review [25] summarized that acupuncture stimulation in Parkinson's models had generated valuable mechanistic insight of Parkinson's and showed that acupuncture treatment is in fact a neuroprotective therapy that increases the release of various neuroprotective agents such as Brain-derived neurotrophic factor, glial cell line-derived neurotrophic factor, and cyclophilin A. In addition, acupuncture therapy slows cell death process and attenuates oxidative stress to dopaminergic neurons in the substantia nigra. Further, acupuncture therapy modulates neuronal activity of the basal ganglia output structures. These results suggest that early application of acupuncture therapy to Parkinson's patients may be helpful for the best efficacy of acupuncture treatment. It is hopeful that translation of achievement in acupuncture research in Parkinson's models will maximize the potentials of acupuncture treatment.

In acupuncture studies, functional magnetic resonance imaging (fMRI) is the most commonly applied method of functional neuroimaging, because it can indirectly measure Brain activity and functional changes of the Brain without harmful radiation and invasive procedures. In addition, acupuncture evoked different Brain activations in patients with Parkinson's disease than in healthy participants [26]. In their early study found acupuncture stimulation increased neural responses in regions including the substantia nigra, caudate, thalamus, and putamen, which are impaired caused by PD [13].

A very recent China fMRI study showed that real acupuncture had specific effects on Brain regions involved in the motor and cognitive management of movement, including the cerebellum, thalamus and motor cortex [15].

Adult neurogenesis has recently been considered a new therapeutic paradigm of Parkinson's disease. A study [6] indicate that acupuncture stimulation restores neurogenesis impairment. An early China study [27] to probe the mechanism of electro-scalp acupuncture in treatment of PD by single photon emission computer tomography (SPECT) and found electro-scalp acupuncture can decrease the loss of DAT (dopamine transporter) and improve the activities of DAT in the striatum of the patient of PD.

In summary, with the wide clinical practice on acupuncture for PD, particularly scalp and head acupuncture, increasing clinical studies has been published, mostly from China and Korea. The majority clinical trials are designed treatment group, manual acupuncture or electric acupuncture, scalp acupuncture or general body acupuncture, plus medication compared with medication only. Acupuncture has improved therapeutic efficacy and reduced dosage and the occurrence of side effects of medication. Except continuing study on motor function disorders, more interesting move on to the non-motor symptoms (NMS) of PD, ranges from autonomic dysfunction, neuropsychiatric disorders, sleep disturbance, sensory symptoms to gastrointestinal syndromes, fatigue, and many others. These NMS are even quicker and have a better response to acupuncture therapy.

The major possible mechanism of acupuncture treatment for PD are increase the release of various neuroprotective agents, protected dopaminergic neurons against toxic insults and to increase dopamine production in the Brain by inducing release of neurotrophic factor, enhancing antioxidant agents, and inhibit inflammatory, increased neural responses in regions including the substantia nigra, caudate, thalamus, and putamen, restores neurogenesis impairment, decrease the loss of DAT (dopamine transporter) and improve the activities of DAT, et al.

8.6 Conclusion

Parkinson's Disease (PD) is the second most common progressive neurodegenerative disorder worldwide. Although both genetic and environmental factors are implicated in the development of PD, the cause of disease and the mechanism remain still unclear. The most commonly used medications include levodopa and anticholinergic drugs. However, its effectiveness decreases as the duration of treatment is prolonged.

Chinese medicine and acupuncture has a long history of dealing with PD and similar symptoms, with rich clinical experiences. Some unique acupuncture techniques such as scalp acupuncture and Dao-qi technique, are more effective for PD related symptoms. Except traditional motor symptoms, non-motor symptoms are quick and have a better response to acupuncture treatment. Recent acupuncture studies indicate acupuncture protected dopaminergic neurons against toxic insults and increase dopamine production in the Brain by inducing release of neurotrophic factor, enhancing antioxidant agents, and inhibit inflammatory.

References

1. Baker M, Gershanik OS. Neurological disorders: public health challenges chapter 3.8 Parkinson's disease. WHO, Printed in Switzerland; 2006.
2. Chen FP, Chang CM, Shiu JH, et al. A clinical study of integrating acupuncture and western medicine in treating patients with Parkinson's disease. Am J Chin Med. 2015;43(3):407–23.
3. Zeng BY, Zhao KC. Effect of acupuncture on the motor and nonmotor symptoms in Parkinson's disease – a review of clinical studies. CNS Neurosci Ther. 2016;22:333–41.
4. Kim SN, Doo AR, Park JY, et al. Acupuncture enhances the synaptic dopamine availability to improve motor function in a mouse model of Parkinson's disease. PLoS One. 2011;6(11):e27566.
5. Hirsch EC, Hunot S. Neuroinflammation in Parkinson's disease: a target for neuroprotection? Lancet Neurol. 2009;8(4):382–97.
6. Jeon HJ, Sun R, Kin DS. Acupuncture stimulation at GB34 restores MPTP-induced neurogenesis impairment in the subventricular zone of mice. Evid Based Complement Alternat Med. 2017, ID 3971675, 9 pages.
7. Nutt JG, Wooten GF. Clinical practice. Diagnosis and initial management of Parkinson's disease. N Engl J Med. 2005;353:1021–7.
8. Chaudhuri KR, Yates L, Martinez-Martin P. The non-motor symptom complex of Parkinson's disease: a comprehensive assessment is essential. Curr Neurol Neurosci Rep. 2005;5:275–83.
9. Hughes AJ, Daniel SE, Lees AJ. Improved accuracy of clinical diagnosis of Lewy body Parkinson's disease. Neurology. 2001;57:1497–9.

10. Tolosa E, Wenning G, Poewe W. The diagnosis of Parkinson's disease. Lancet Neurol. 2006;5:75–86.
11. Asakawa T, Xia Y. Acupuncture treatment for Parkinson's disease. In: Xia Y, Ding G, Wu GC, editors. Current research in acupuncture. New York, NY: Springer; 2013.
12. Unschuld PU, Tessenow H, Zheng JS. Huang Di Nei Jing Su Wen: an annotated translation of Huang Di's inner classic – basic questions. University of California Press, California, 2011. V2 eBook.
13. Yeo SJ, Lim S, Choe IH, et al. Acupuncture stimulation on GB34 activates neural responses associated with Parkinson's disease. CNS Neurosci Ther. 2012;18:781–90.
14. Wang YS, Peng JD, Ruan SQ, et al. Effects of scalp acupuncture, by retaining long time combined with exercise therapy on motor function of patients with early Parkinson's disease. Shanxi J Chin Med. 2019;40(8):1124–30.
15. Li Z, Chen J, Cheng JB, et al. Acupuncture modulates the cerebello-thalamo-cortical circuit and cognitive brain regions in patients of Parkinson's disease with tremor. Front Aging Neurosci. 2018;5(10):206. 11 pages.
16. Suo QF, Wang LY, Pang MH. Clinical observation on 70 patients with Parkinson's disease treated by electro-acupuncture at neck points plus scalp acupuncture (in Chinese with English abstract). J Basic Chin Med 2015;21(7):860–61 and 83.
17. Chen YL, Feng WJ, Zhang XL. Parkinson's disease combined with overactive bladder syndrome treated with acupuncture and medication. Zhongguo Zhen Jiu. 2012;32:215–8.
18. Cho SY, Shim SR, Rhee HY, et al. Effectiveness of acupuncture and bee venom acupuncture in idiopathic Parkinson's disease. Parkinsonism Relat Disord. 2012;18:948–52.
19. Lei H, Toosizadeh N, Schwenk M, et al. A pilot clinical trial to objectively assess the efficacy of electro-acupuncture on gait in patients with Parkinson's disease using body worn sensors. PLoS One. 2016;11(5):e0155613.
20. Chaudhuri KR, Martinez-Martin P, Brown RG, et al. The metric properties of a novel nonmotor symptoms scale for Parkinson's disease: results from an international pilot study. Mov Disord. 2007;22:1901–11.
21. Yang JW, Hu ZP. The characteristics of cerebral blood flow perfusion in Parkinson's disease with accompanying depression and the influence of transcranial magnetic stimulation. ACTA Laser Biol Sinica. 2013;22(5):432–5.
22. Song HY. Clinical application value of transcranial Doppler ultrasonography in automatic monitoring of cerebral blood flow in Parkinson's disease (Chinese with English abstract). China's Rural Health. 2019;158(8):31.
23. Wang LL, He C, Zhao M, et al. Effect of acupuncture and moxibustion on brain blood flow status of Parkinson's disease (Chinese). Chin Acupunct Moxibustion. 1999;19(2):115–7.
24. Huang Y, Zhou Y, Jiang XM, et al. Effect of scalp acupuncture on regional cerebral blood flow in Parkinson's disease patients. China J Trad Chin Med. 2009;24(3):305–8.
25. Zeng BY, Salvage S, Jenner P. Current development of acupuncture research in Parkinson's disease. Int Rev Neurobiol. 2013;111:141–58.
26. Yeo SJ, Choe IH, van den Noort M, et al. Acupuncture on GB34 activates the precentral gyrus and prefrontal cortex in Parkinson's disease. BMC Complement Altern Med. 2014;14:336. 9 pages.
27. Jiang XM, Huang Y, Li DJ, et al. Effect of electro-scalp acupuncture on cerebral dopamine transporter in the striatum area of the patient of Parkinson's disease by means of single photon emission computer tomography. Chin Acupunct Moxibustion. 2006;26(6):427–30.

Chapter 9
Alzheimer's Disease and Other Dementias

9.1 General Information of Dementia

9.1.1 Basic Background of Dementia

Dementia is a common neurodegenerative disease of the central nervous system globally [1]. There are lots of diffcrent type of dementias. Alzheimer's disease (AD) is the most common cause of dementia, followed by vascular dementias (VaD) or mixed forms of AD and VaD. Other forms of neurodegenerative disorders or other type of dementias, such as Lewy body dementia, frontotemporal dementia, are accompanied with dementia as well [2]. AD, manifests with memory deficits and cognitive decline, is the most prevalent cause of neurodegenerative diseases characterized by progressive cognitive impairment and aging risk factor, with an insidious onset and a progressive impairment of cognitive function [3]. AD has been severe enough to impair activities of daily living, social function, and decreasing the Quality of Life (QoL) of both affected patients and their caregivers [4].

As the worldwide population ages, it is recognized that the disease burden worldwide will increase. According to the 2015 World Alzheimer Report, there were currently estimated to be 35.6 million people with dementia worldwide in 2012, which will double by 2030 and more than triple by 2050 [5]. This phenomenon will cause severe societal and economic burden to public health care due to the patients' cognitive disability and loss of independent function [6].

There is a special "predementia stage" which defined as Mild cognitive impairment (MCI). MCI refers to a cognitive state that is less than the expected level of cognitive function according to the individual's age or education level; it is not severe enough to interfere with activities of daily living (ADL) [7]. It is the primary target for early detection and management of dementia.

© Springer Nature Switzerland AG 2021
T. Wang, *Acupuncture for Brain*, https://doi.org/10.1007/978-3-030-54666-3_9

9.1.2   The Aetiology and Pathogenesis

The aetiology and pathology of dementia are still unclear. There are some hypotheses based on existing evidences. The amyloid cascade hypothesis has been central in drug development, however, other theories about AD have been postulated [2].

Several rs-fMRI (resting-state functional magnetic resonance imaging) studies have demonstrated that AD presents with disrupted functional characteristics at different levels, including in the amplitude of low-frequency fluctuations (ALFF), regional homogeneity and inter-regional functional connectivity [8].

9.1.3   Typical Clinical Symptoms

The symptoms of dementia include gradual memory loss and decline in thinking skills as well as problems concerning language, emotions, understanding, judgment, orientation, and walking [9].

Although Alzheimer disease (AD) is the most common type of dementia (accounting for approximately 60–70% of dementia cases), the underlying causes of AD remain unclear. The secondary type of dementia, vascular dementia (VaD), is mainly caused by stroke and accounts for approximately 25% of dementia cases.

Mild cognitive impairment (MCI) is the clinical stage of cognition impairment between normal aging and AD patients, with a diagnostic criterion of a symptomatic, predementia phase. It is important to find early and available interventions to delay the development from MCI to dementia [10].

Typical early symptoms of Alzheimer's may include [11]:

- Regularly forgetting recent events, names and faces.
- Becoming increasingly repetitive, e.g. repeating questions after a very short interval.
- Regularly misplacing items or putting them in odd places.
- Getting confused about the date or time of day.
- Being unsure of where you are or getting lost, especially in unfamiliar places.
- Having problems finding the right words.
- Having mood or behaviour problems such as loss of interest in daily activity, becoming easily upset or annoyed or losing confidence.

9.1.4   Examination and Diagnosis

Similar to many other neurological diseases, the diagnosis of dementia remains primarily clinical. First it is based on a careful history, obtained from the patient and their relatives and care givers. The history should demonstrate a typical progressive deterioration of cognitive and non-cognitive functions and some functional and behavioural consequences of this deterioration. Secondly at neurological and neuropsychological examination, there must be explicit impairments in memory and other cognitive domains, in the absence of developmental deficits. In addition, some Brain scans such as MRI may help to identify which kind of dementia and the level of suffer. As the biomarker field is evolving, the possibility to detect disease changes and progression in vivo, opens new regulatory scenarios including the possibility to intervene directly on the neuropathology before the appearance of symptoms [12].

In 2018, European Medicines Agency (EMA) [2] updated its Guideline on the clinical investigation of medicines for the treatment of Alzheimer's disease, with following criteria:

International Working Group (IWG) Criteria
(a) Prodromal AD

Predementia AD is represented by prodromal AD, with episodic memory impairment that is insufficient to disrupt the performance of accustomed instrumental activities of daily living (IADL).

(b) AD dementia

Indicates that episodic memory loss and other cognitive symptoms are sufficient to interfere with the usual performance of IADL

(c) Preclinical AD

Refers to the stage of AD that is not clinically expressed; that is, although the molecular pathology of AD is present in the Brain, symptoms are absent. The use of the preclinical AD definition signifies that this stage can only be detected by AD biomarkers, and not by currently available clinical methods. They are further subdivided in:

1. Asymptomatic at risk: cognitively normal individual with evidence of AD molecular pathology. It is not known whether progression to symptomatic AD will occur.
2. Presymptomatic AD: individuals with autosomal dominant gene mutations which almost certainly will develop the disease.

IWG-2 Criteria for Typical AD (A Plus B at Any Stage)
(A) Specific clinical phenotype

- Presence of an early and significant episodic memory impairment (isolated or associated with other cognitive or behavioural changes that are suggestive of a mild cognitive impairment or of a dementia syndrome) that includes the following features:

  - Gradual and progressive change in memory function reported by patient or informant over more than 6 months
  - Objective evidence of an amnestic syndrome of the hippocampal type, based on significantly impaired performance on an episodic memory test with established specificity for AD, such as cued recall with control of encoding test.

(B) In-vivo evidence of Alzheimer's pathology (one of the following)

- Decrease Aβ1–42 together with increased T-tau or P-tau in CSF
- Increased tracer retention on amyloid PET
- Alzheimer's disease Autosomal dominant mutation present (in PSEN1, PSEN2, or APP)

9.1.5   The Treatment of AD with Modern Medicine

Currently, there is no effective treatment for the disease, although some of the current treatments offer some symptomatic relief [8]. Drugs approved by the Food and Drug Administration (FDA) for AD treatment reported in mainstream medical articles were considered to have modest symptomatic effect, such as Cholinesterase-inhibitors (CIs) donepezil, rivastigmine, galantamine, and the glutamate receptor antagonist are recommended for clinical use [13].

The most effective intervention for dementia available is symptomatic treatment for vascular dementia. Antipsychotic treatment for dementia alleviates cognitive dysfunction less effectively than does symptomatic treatment. Alternative therapies are also effective at present [14].

There is now a consensus that treatment options should be evaluated in earlier disease stages before the full picture of dementia is reached. While the general approach for symptomatic drug development in mild to moderate and severe AD is still valid. The high efficacy of treatment of dementia depends on how early the treatment of individuals with dementia started [15]. Especially, reducing the risk of vascular dementia was reported to be a highly effective intervention [16].

According to literature review, the following types of treatment were reported effective: (1) antipsychotic drugs and cognitive enhancers, (2) symptomatic treatment drugs for VaD, (3) behavior therapy, (4) adjunctive therapy, and (5) other treatments [14].

However, no-medical treatment has been claimed to be able to stop or reverse the progression of AD or MCI [17]. Moreover, the inevitable adverse reactions are always related to [18].

9.2   TCM Understanding of Dementia

Traditional Chinese Medicine (TCM) believe that dementia caused by the Brain Shen damaged due to old age, essence and Qi deficiency, or toxicity, trauma, emotion disorder, insufficient endowment, etc. The pathological changes include deficiency of essence and Blood, Phlegm and stasis disturbed the Brain, or Brain marrow less nourish, Yuan Shen disorder. The basic principle is root deficient and superficial excessive. The main disease location is in the Brain [19].

There are some descriptions on classic TCM texts which ae similar to dementia. "Huangdi Neijing-Lingshu Chap. 54-Tiannian (Years Given by Heaven)" [20, p. 491].

> At the age of sixty, the heart qi begin to weaken, as if they were affected by grief. Blood and qi slowdown. Hence one is inclined to lie down.
> At the age of eighty the lung qi weaken. The *po* soul departs. Hence one tends to make false claims.

"The Chap. 33 Hailun-On the Four Sees in Yellow Emperors Cannon of Internal Medicine-Lingshu (Spirital Pivot)" [21, p. 651] stated 'When the sea of marrow is insufficient, one's Brain will feel like turning and he will have the syndromes of tinnitus, sore legs, dizziness, seeing nothing, slothful and sleepiness.' This statement about Brain pathological changes is quite similar with some symptoms of dementia.

"Yilin Gaicuo (Correcting the Errors in the Forest of Medicine Paperbook)—Naosuishuo (Discussion about Brain and Marrow)" states:

"Therefore, in children who do not have memory, the Brain marrow is not full. In older aged who do not have memory, the Brain marrow gradually emptying. Li Shi-zhen said: The Brain is the house of the Original spirit. Jin Zheng-xi said: The memory of men, it all is in the Brain" [22, p. 46].

9.3   General Acupuncture Treatment for Alzheimer's Disease

As a classic therapy in TCM, acupuncture has increasingly attracted attention for treating AD and other dementias. It is believed that acupuncture is effective in reducing the symptoms and slowing the progression of AD, although the neural mechanism underlying the effects is still not very clear at present [8].

More evidences indicated that acupuncture is more effective than medicine and could enhance the effects of drugs in terms of improving the cognitive function of AD patients and enhancing their ability to satisfy daily needs, with less adverse reactions and higher toleration. The safety of clinical acupuncture is verified and commonly recognised. Compared with medicine treatment, acupuncture also appeared to produce better outcomes in MCI patients [17].

According to the TCM theory about Alzheimer's Disease (AD) and other dementia classifications, the principle of general acupuncture treatment would follow the pattern identification as stated below.

9.3.1   Deficiency of Brain Marrow

Signs and Symptoms (SS): Memory and hearing decrease, dizziness and tinnitus, forgetfulness, insomnia, laziness and like lying, scorched teeth and withered hair, back pain and soft legs, unstable footsteps, pale tongue, white coating, with deep and weak pulses.

Points selection: DU-20 Baihui, Ex-Sishencong, BL-20 Pishu, BL-23 Shenshu, ST-36 Zusanli SP-6 Sanyinjiao, LV-3 Taichong, KI-3 Taixi, REN-12 Zhongwan, REN-4 Guanyuan.

9.3.2 Deficiency of Heart and Spleen

SS: Intelligence and memory decrease, dizziness, lacklustre complexion, body tiredness, sleeplessness, poor appetite, laziness, stress and easy crying, pale tongue and white coat, and weak pulse.

Points selection: DU-20 Baihui, Ex-Sishencong, BL-15 Xinshu, BL-20 Pishu, HT-3 Shaohai, HT-7 Shenmen, SP-9 Yinlingquan, SP-6 Sanyinjiao, REN-12 Zhongwan, REN-6 Qihai.

9.3.3 Liver and Kidney Yin Deficiency

SS: Memory decreasing, dull expression, silent words, difficult walking, thin body, dizziness, tinnitus, premature whiteness, loose teeth, soft back and legs, red face with night sweats, dim vision, red tongue and less coat, thin and wiry pulse.

Point selection: DU-20 Baihui, Ex-Sishencong, BL-18 Ganshu, BL-23 Shenshu, LV-8 Ququan, LV-Taichong, KI-10 Yingu, KI-3 Taixi.

9.3.4 Heart and Liver Heat

SS: Memory, cognition and judgment disorder, emotional irritability, anxiety, upset and insomnia, dizziness, headache, dry mouth, dry throat, dark urine, constipation, dry and red tongue, yellow coat, with thin and fast pulse.

Point selection: DU-20 Baihui, Ex-Sishencong, HT-8 Laogong, HT-7 Shenmen, PC-6 Neiguan, LV-2 Xingjiao, GB-20 Fengchi.

9.3.5 Stagnation of Phlegm and Stasis

SS: Intellectual and memory decline, abnormal thinking, dull expressions, speech-lessness, or erratic crying, phlegm in the throat, dizziness, headache and turbidity, numbness of the limbs, purple and dullness tongue, greasy coat, wiry, slippery or astringent pulses.

Point selection: DU-20 Baihui, Ex-Sishencong, ST-40 Fenglong ST-36 Zusanli, PC-6 Neiguan, REN-12 Zhongwan, LI-4 Hegu, LV-Taichong.

Above patterns, symptoms and signs, and the points selection, are just sample suggestions. Clinic practice should follow the real individual patient, with general needling, or combined with below unique Brain acupuncture techniques.

9.4   Unique Acupuncture Techniques for AD and Other Dementia

Traditionally TCM identification is more focus on five Zang and six Fu organs, similar with above general acupuncture pattern identification. With development of TCM Brain theory, more Chinese scholars generally believe that the disease major location of Alzheimer's disease and other dementia are in the Brain [19]. Their treatment principles, particularly for acupuncture, should be based on this development and choose relevant points and needling techniques. Scalp acupuncture and Dao-qi technique are mostly selected techniques for Brain related diseases, including dementia.

9.4.1   Scalp Acupuncture for Treating AD and Other Dementia (Detail of Scalp Acupuncture, Location and Needling, Please see Chap. 5)

- Intellectual, cognition, or memory decline, sleep disorders, depression, anxiety, et al.: Spirit-Emotion Area, Foot-Motor Sensory Area, Central Area
- Hearing problems, tinnitus, dizziness: Auditory Area
- Limb numbness: Sensory area and Foot-Motor Sensory Area

9.4.2   Du Mai Dao-qi Technique (Detail of Dao-qi Technique on Du Mai, Points Location and Needling, Please see Chap. 6)

- DU-26 Renzhong, DU-20 Baihui, DU-16 Fengfu, DU-15 Yamen, DU-14 Dazhui, DU-9 Zhiyang, DU-4 Mingmen, DU-3 Yaoyangguan

9.4.3   Ren Mai Dao-qi Technique: (Detail of Dao-qi Technique on Ren Mai, Points Location and Needling, Please see Chap. 6)

- REN-12 Zhongwan plus 2–4 needles around it with 0.5–1 cm distance, REN-10 Xiawan, REN-6 Qihai, REN-4 Guanyuan, REN-17 Danzhong (Shanzhong).

Above unique Brain acupuncture techniques can be combined with syndrome differentiation treatment.

9.4.4 Brain Pattern Differentiation

The commonly clinical Brain patterns of dementia and its possible symptoms could be summarized as below, which are currently in the development phase and soon to be confirmed.

9.4.4.1 Deficiency of Brain Marrow

SS: Memory and hearing decrease, dizziness and tinnitus, forgetfulness, insomnia, laziness and like lying, scorched teeth and withered hair, back pain and soft legs, unstable footsteps, pale tongue, white coating, with deep and weak pulses.

Scalp acupuncture: Spirit-Emotion Area, Foot-Motor Sensory Area, Auditory Area, Central Area.

Brain acupuncture points selection: DU-20 Baihui, DU-14 Dazhui, Ex-Bailaoxue, DU-4 Mingmen, REN-4 Guanyuan, KI-3 Taixi, GB-39 Xuanzhong, and local area points. Techniques could choose electric-acupuncture, scalp acupuncture, Dao-qi technique, etc.

9.4.4.2 Deficiency of Brain Yang Qi

SS: Intelligence and memory decrease, dizziness, lacklustre complexion, shortness of breath and body tiredness, sweating, sleeplessness, poor appetite, laziness, stress and easy crying, general cold, loose stool, pale tongue with white coat, and weak pulse.

Scalp acupuncture: Spirit-Emotion area, Foot-Motor Sensory Area, Auditory Area, Central Area.

Brain acupuncture points selection: DU-20 Baihui, DU-16 Fengfu, DU-14 Dazhui, DU-9 Zhiyang, DU-4 Mingmen, DU-3 Yaoyangguan, REN-12 Zhongwan, REN-10 Xiawan, REN-6 Qihai, REN-4 Guanyuan. Moxa could be applied, with Dao-qi technique on 1–2 key points.

9.4.4.3 Stagnation of Brain Collaterals

SS: Intellectual and memory decline, abnormal thinking, dull expressions, speech-lessness, or erratic crying, phlegm in the throat, dizziness, headache and turbidity, numbness of the limbs, purple and dullness tongue, thin coat, wiry or astringent pulses.

Scalp acupuncture: Spirit Emotion Area, Vasomotor Area, Sensory Area, Foot-Motor Sensory Area, Auditory Area, Central Area.

Brain acupuncture point selection: DU-20 Baihui, Ex-Sishencong, DU-16 Fengfu, DU-15 Yamen, DU-14 Dazhui, DU-9 Zhiyang, DU-3 Yaoyangguan, REN-12 Zhongwan, REN-10 Xiawan, REN-6 Qihai, plus local suffered area points. Moxa could be applied. Dao-qi technique may add for 1–2 key points.

9.4.4.4 Disorder of Brain Shen

SS: Memory, cognition and judgment disorder, emotional irritability, stress and anxiety, insomnia, dizziness or headache, drooling, light tongue, thin coat, with thin and uneven pulse.

Scalp acupuncture: Spirit-Emotion Area, Foot-Motor Sensory Area, Auditory Area, Central Area.

Brain acupuncture point selection: DU-26 Renzhong DU-24 Shenting, DU-20 Baihui, DU-16 Fengfu, DU-14 Dazhui, Ex-Yintang, REN-12 Zhongwan, HT-7 Shenmen, plus local area points. Techniques could be selected through electric acupuncture, Dao-qi techniques, etc.

Notes
- For treatment of Alzheimer's disease and other dementia, the early involved the better results.
- The treatment frequency: in the early stage, more often the better. In western countries, suggest twice per week, then with time, move slow down to once per week followed by once in 2–4 weeks for maintenance. If in some areas, possibly start with every day.
- Acupuncture can be combined with routine therapy such as cognition behaviour therapy (CBT), physiotherapy, speech therapy, etc.
- Above Brain related patterns for dementia can be combined with classic TCM pattern identifications.
- Due to the memory decreasing, patient missing is one of the major problems for the family and society. More attention should be paid for severe cases.

9.5 Research

The acupuncture research for Alzheimer's disease (AD) and other dementia has been over decades, majority focus on clinical efficacy verification and search the mechanism. A systematic review indicated that acupuncture was more effective than drugs and could enhance the effects of drugs in terms of improving the cognitive function of AD patients and enhancing their ability to satisfy daily needs [17]. Nevertheless, the underlying mechanism of acupuncture is still unclear. Some researchers found that acupuncture may lead to beneficial Brain changes in AD patients, such as ameliorating impaired cholinergic function, relieving amyloid neu-rotoxicity, and reducing hyperphosphorylated Tau protein and oxidative stress. However, these experimental clues were mostly controversial hypotheses, and few of them have been confirmed in vivo. Therefore, it is necessary to demonstrate the objective validation and therapeutic specificity of acupuncture before it is generally approved by clinical use [23].

Recent meta-analysis study investigated ten randomized controlled trials (RCTs) with AD treated by acupuncture [18]. Six trials showed that acupuncture was better than drugs on improving MMSE (Mini-Mental State Exam) scores. Furthermore, there were evidence of 3 trails indicating that acupuncture plus donepezil was more effective than donepezil alone at improving the MMSE scale score. As a conclusion, clinical practice on AD confirmed the effect of acupuncture, which was better than that of drugs, and acupuncture can enhance the effect of drugs for treating AD.

More studies have shown that acupuncture might be effective in improving the cognitive function of AD patients [24, 25]. A very recent study concluded that acu-puncture could induce significant regional alterations in AD patients, including increased and decreased spontaneous Brain activity, as well as enhanced hippocampal connectivity. These findings may be helpful for deeper insight into the mechanisms of acupuncture and may provide a new method for the treatment of AD in the future [8].

Accumulating neuroimaging studies in humans have shown that acupuncture can modulate a widely distributed Brain network in mild cognitive impairment (MCI) and Alzheimer's disease (AD) patients. Acupuncture at different acupoints could exert different modulatory effects on the Brain network [26].

Acupuncture could activate the temporal lobe (such as hippocampus, insula), some regions of the parietal lobe, and cerebellum in AD patients [27]. These regions are consistent with impaired Brain areas in AD patients, which are closely corre-lated with the cognitive function (memory, reason, language, executive, etc.). This study also provides the preliminary neurophysiological evidence for the potential effect of acupuncture on AD [28].

A study [17] indicate that compared with HC (Health Controls), AD and MCI (mild cognitive impairment) patients showed similar activations in cognitive-related Brain areas (inferior frontal gyrus, supramarginal gyrus, and rolandic operculum) as well as deactivations in cognitive-related areas, visual-related areas, basal ganglia, and cerebellum, which were not found in HC. Compared with sham acupuncture points, real acupuncture points produced more specific Brain changes with both activated and deactivated Brain activities in AD and MCI. The preliminary results in our study verified the objective evidence for neuronal specificity of acupuncture in AD and MCI patients.

Resting-state functional magnetic resonance imaging (rs-fMRI) is a highly promising noninvasive imaging technique that is applied in the study of many neu-ropsychiatric diseases, including AD and other dementia. Existing rs-fMRI studies have demonstrated that the intrinsic Brain functional architecture can be modulated by acupuncture [8].

Using resting-state fMRI, a study [26] reported that acupuncture induced ampli-tude of low-frequency fluctuation (ALFF) change of different Brain regions in MCI patients from those shown in the healthy controls. In MCI patients, acupuncture increased or decreased ALFF in the different regions from those activated by acupuncture in the healthy controls. Acupuncture at the sham acupoint in MCI patients activated the different Brain regions from those in healthy controls. Therefore, we concluded that acupuncture displays more significant effect on neuronal activities of the above Brain regions in MCI patients than that in healthy controls. Acupuncture exhibits different effects on the neuronal activities of the Brain regions from acupuncture at sham acupoint, although the difference is only shown at several regions due to the close distance between the above points.

9.6 Conclusion

Alzheimer's disease (AD) and other dementias are common neurodegenerative disease of the central nervous system, which has severe impact on the patient's daily activities. The aetiology and pathology of dementia are still unclear. Currently, there is no effective treatment for the disease.

Acupuncture has increasingly attracted attention for treating AD and other dementias. It is believed that acupuncture is effective in reducing the symptoms and slowing the progression of AD, although the neural mechanism underlying the effects is still not very clear at present. Some researchers found that acupuncture may lead to beneficial Brain changes in AD patients, such as ameliorating impaired cholinergic function, relieving amyloid neurotoxicity, and reducing hyperphosphorylated Tau protein and oxidative stress.

Alongside with the general acupuncture treatment for dementia, based on the development of TCM Brain theory, more practice and studies are focused on Brain acupuncture techniques such as scalp acupuncture, Dao-qi technique, Du Mai and Ren Mai points.

References

1. Ferri C, Prince M, Brayne C, et al. Alzheimer's disease international global prevalence of dementia: a Delphi consensus study. Lancet. 2005;366:2112–7.
2. European Medicines Agency. Guideline on the clinical investigation of medicines for the treatment of Alzheimer's disease. 2018. CPMP/EWP/553/95 Rev.2.
3. Prince M, Wimo A, Guerchet M, et al. The global impact of dementia: an analysis of prevalence, incidence, cost and trends in Alzheimer's Disease International, London, UK, 2015. http://www.alz.co.uk/research/statistics.htnril. Accessed on 26/04/2020.
4. Posadzki P, Ernst E, Lee MS. Complementary and alternative medicine for Alzheimer's disease: an overview of systematic reviews. Focus Altern Complement Ther. 2012;17(4):186–91.
5. WHO. World Health Organization and Alzheimer's disease international. dementia: a public health priority. Geneva. 2012:112. ISBN: 978 92 4 156445 8. http://www.who.int/mental_health/publications/dementia_report_2012/en/. Accessed on 26/04/2020.
6. Petrella JR. Neuroimaging and the search for a cure for Alzheimer disease. Radiology. 2013;269(3):671–91.
7. Petersen C, Smith GE, Waring SC, et al. Mild cognitive impairment: clinical characterization and outcome. JAMA Neurol. 1999;56(3):303–8.

8. Zheng WM, Su ZZ, Liu XY, et al. Modulation of functional activity and connectivity by acupuncture in patients with Alzheimer disease as measured by resting-state fMRI. PLoS One. 2018;13(5):e0196933. 14 pages. https://doi.org/10.1371/journal.pone.0196933.
9. Gehrman P, Gooneratne NS, Brewster GS, et al. Impact of Alzheimer disease patients' sleep disturbances on their caregivers. Geriatr Nurs. 2017;39(1):60–5.
10. Langa KM, Levine DA. The diagnosis and management of mild cognitive impairment: a clinical review. J Am Med Assoc. 2014;312(23):2551–61.
11. Alzheimer's research UK. Dementia symptoms. https://www.alzheimersresearchuk.org/about-dementia/helpful-information/symptoms/ Access 26/04/2020.
12. European Medicines Agency. Guideline on medicinal products for the treatment of Alzheimer's disease and other dementias. Pre-Authorisation Evaluation of Medicines for Human Use. London, 24 July 2008.Doc. Ref. CPMP/EWP/553/95 Rev. 1.
13. Peng WN, Zhou J, Xu M, et al. The effect of electro-acupuncture combined with donepezil on cognitive function in Alzheimer's disease patients: study protocol for a randomized controlled trial. Trials. 2017;18:301, 6 pages. https://doi.org/10.1186/s13063-017-2052-y.
14. Perng CH, Chang Y, Tzang RF. The treatment of cognitive dysfunction in dementia: a multiple treatments meta-analysis. Psychopharmacology. 2018;235:1571–80.
15. Tsoi K, Hirai H, Chan J, et al. Time to treatment initiation in people with Alzheimer disease: a meta-analysis of randomized controlled. J Am Med Dir Assoc. 2016;17(1):24–30.
16. Chen LP, Wang FW, Zuo F, et al. Clinical research on comprehensive treatment of senile vascular dementia. J Tradit Chin Med. 31:187–181 trials. J Am Med Dir Assoc. 2011;17:24–30.
17. Shan Y, Wang JJ, Wang ZQ, et al. Neuronal specificity of acupuncture in Alzheimer's disease and mild cognitive impairment patients: a functional MRI study. Evid Based Complement Alternat Med, 2018. Article ID 7619197, 10 pages.
18. Zhou J, Peng WN, Xu M, et al. The effectiveness and safety of acupuncture for patients with Alzheimer disease. Medicine. 2015;94(22):e933. 9 pages.
19. Qin WL, Su WL, Hu H, et al. The effect of medicated thread moxibustion combined with electro-acupuncture treatment on Montreal cognitive assessment (MoCA) of patients with vascular cognitive impairment of none dementia. Biomed Res. 2017;28(4):1871–7.
20. Unschuld PU. Huang Di Nei Jing Ling Shu: The ancient classic on needle therapy. University of California Press, 2016. eBook.
21. Wang B, Wu LS, Wu Q (Trans). Yellow Emperors cannon of internal medicine. Beijing: China Science & Technology Press, 1997.
22. Wang QR. Yi Lin Gai Cuo-correcting the errors in the forest of medicine. Blue Poppy Press; Bilingual edition. Boulder, 2007.
23. Asakawa Y, Ludwiczuk A, Nagashima F. Phytochemical and biological studies of bryophytes. Phytochemistry. 2013;91:52–80.
24. Peng J, Luo L, Xu L, et al. Therapeutic efficacy observation on electroacupuncture for Alzheimer's disease. J Acupunct Tuina Sci. 2015;13:171–4.
25. Liu ZB, Niu WM, Yang XH, et al. The clinical research of impact on cognitive function of patients with Alzheimer's disease by using 'Xiu Sanzhen'. Shan Xi J Tradit Chin Med. 2008;29:11–20.
26. Jia BH, Liu S, Min BQ, et al. The effects of acupuncture at real or sham acupoints on the intrinsic brain activity in mild cognitive impairment patients. Evid Based Complement Alternat Med. 2015. Article ID 529675, 9 pages. https://doi.org/10.1155/2015/529675.
27. Zhou YL, Jia JP. Effect of acupuncture given at the HT 7, ST 36, ST 40 and KI 3 acupoints on various parts of the brains of Alzheimer's disease patients. Acupunct Electrother Res. 2008;33(1–2):9–17.
28. Feng YY, Bai LJ, Ren YS, et al. FMRI connectivity analysis of acupuncture effects on the whole brain network in mild cognitive impairment patients. Magn Reson Imaging. 2012;30(5):672–82.

Chapter 10
Multiple Sclerosis

10.1 General Introduction

Multiple sclerosis (MS) is a progressive disease of the central nervous system in which communication between the Brain and other parts of the body is disrupted. Its effects can range from relatively benign in most cases, to somewhat disabling, and can become quite devastating for some people. During a MS attack, inflammation occurs in areas of the white matter of the central nervous system in random patches; these are called plaques. This is followed by the destruction of myelin. Myelin allows for the smooth, high-speed transmission of electrochemical messages between the Brain, the spinal cord, and the rest of the body. When myelin is damaged, neurological transmission of messages may be slowed or blocked completely, resulting in some body functions being diminished or lost [1, p. 25–26].

10.1.1 Basic Background of Multiple Sclerosis

Multiple sclerosis is the most common immune-mediated disorder affecting the central nervous system. Approximately 520,000 people in the Americas, 630,000 in Europe, 66,000 in the Eastern Mediterranean, 56,000 in the Western Pacific, 31,500 in south-East Asia, 11,000 in Africa, and 2.3 million people worldwide are diagnosed with MS [2, p. 14]. It primarily affects adults, with age of onset typically between 20 and 40 years, and is twice as common in women compared to men [3, p. 242].

10.1.2 The Aetiology and Pathogenesis of Multiple Sclerosis

Many risk factors for multiple sclerosis have been identified, but no definitive cause has been found. It likely occurs as a result of some combination of environmental and genetic factors such as infectious agents. The three main characteristics of MS

T. Wang, *Acupuncture for Brain*, https://doi.org/10.1007/978-3-030-54666-3_10

are the formation of plaques in the central nervous system, inflammation, and the destruction of myelin sheaths of neurons. These features interact in a complex and not yet fully understood manner to produce the breakdown of nerve tissue and in turn the signs and symptoms of the disease. Currently multiple sclerosis does not have a cure in terms of conventional treatments.

10.1.3   Typical Clinical Symptoms

Symptoms and signs of multiple sclerosis vary widely depending on the location of affected myelin sheaths. The most common symptoms of MS are weakness, spasticity in one or more limbs in one or more limb, seen in 50% of MS patient, followed by numbness, tingling, and fatigue, partial or complete loss of vision, double or blurred vision, incontinence of urine and dysfunction of bowel, pain, cognitive or behavioural problems, and sexual dysfunction. In the worst cases, persons with MS may be unable to write, speak, or walk. Multiple sclerosis is unpredictable and varies in severity. In some patients it is a mild disease, but it can lead to permanent disability in others. Multiple sclerosis may occur either in discrete attacks or slowly over time. Although systems may resolve completely between the episodes, permanent neurological problems usually persist, especially as the disease progresses.

10.1.4   Examination and Diagnosis of Multiple Sclerosis

Multiple sclerosis is typically diagnosed based on the presenting signs and symptoms, in combination with supporting medical imaging and laboratory testing. The McDonald criteria, which focus on clinical, laboratory, and radiologic evidence of lesions at different times and in different areas, is the most commonly used method of diagnosis with the Schumacher and Poser criteria being of mostly historical significance. In most people with relapsing-remitting MS, the diagnosis is fairly straightforward and based on a pattern of symptoms consistent with the disease and confirmed by Brain imaging scans, such as MRI. Currently, the United States National Multiple Sclerosis Society and the Multiple Sclerosis International Federation, describes four types of MS. Those are clinically isolated syndrome, relapsing-remitting MS, primary progressive MS, and secondary progressive MS.

10.1.5   The Treatment of Multiple Sclerosis
with Modern Medicine

Although there is no known cure for multiple sclerosis, several therapies have proven helpful. The primary aims of therapy focuses on returning function after an attack, preventing new attacks, slowing the progression of the disease, preventing disability, and managing MS symptoms. During symptomatic attacks, administration of high doses of intravenous corticosteroids, such as methylprednisolone, is the usual therapy. As of 2019, twelve disease-modifying medications are approved by regulatory agencies for relapsing-remitting multiple sclerosis. They are Interferon beta-1a, Interferon beta-1b, Glatirameracetate, Mitoxantrone, Natalizumab, Fingolimod, Teriflunomide, Imethylfumarate, Alemtuzumab, Ocrelizumab, Siponimod, and Cladribine. There is no cure for multiple sclerosis. Treatment typically focuses on speeding up the recovery from attacks, slowing the progression of the disease and managing MS symptoms.

A number of alternative or complementary therapies have been used globally to treat the disease symptomatically and convert MS into remission. The five most prevalent alternative or complementary approaches are diet and nutrition, acupuncture, herbal medicine, massage, and homeopathy.

10.2   TCM Understanding of Multiple Sclerosis

In Chinese medicine the main categorization of multiple sclerosis is Wei syndrome. It may be caused by external invasion of damp-heat, blood stagnation, Qi and blood deficiency, Liver and Kidney Yin deficiency, or Kidney Yang deficiency.

Invasion of external damp-heat is an important cause of disease in the acute stages. Damp-heat obstructs the meridians and causes heaviness sensation in legs, weakness, numbness and tingling. Stagnation of blood may cause weakness of the limbs, dizziness and vertigo. In remission stages of MS there is a progressive deficiency of Qi and Blood, deficiency of Liver and Kidney Yin, deficiency of Kidney Yang. The muscles, tendons, and bones failing to receive adequate moistening and nourishing result in weakness of limbs, blurring of vision, dizziness, fatigue, incontinence of bowel and urine, and loss of balance.

10.3   General Acupuncture Treatment for Multiple Sclerosis

Acupuncture has been used on the treatment of MS differently at the acute attack stage and the remission stage of MS. At the acute stage, acupuncture treatment mainly focuses on cleating Damp-Heat, dispersing Wind, and promoting Blood circulation. While at the remission stage acupuncture gives more attention to reinforcing Qi and blood, notifying Spleen, resolving Dampness, nourishing Liver and Kidney Yin, and warming Kidney Yang. The treatments based on the differentiation of patterns is as following [4, p. 325–336].

Acute attack stage of MS

10.3.1   Invasion of Damp-Heat in Meridians

Main manifestations: Flaccid paralytic limbs, swollen legs and ankles, general heaviness, constipation, dark urine, red tongue with yellow coating, rolling rapid pulse.

Treatment principle: Eliminate Damp, clear Heat, and move meridian Qi

Points selection: LI-4 Hegu, SJ-5 Waiguan, LI-11 Quchi, LI-15 Jianyu, BL-60 Kunlun, SP-6 Sanyinjiao, ST-36 Zusanli, ST-34 Liangqiu, SP-9 Yinlingquan, BL-20 Pishu.

10.3.2   Stagnation of Blood in Meridians

Main manifestations: rigid paralytic limbs, incontinence of bowel and urine, purplish tongue with thin white coating, wiry rolling or hesitant pulse.

Treatment principle: Promote Qi and Blood circulation and remove Blood stasis.

Points selection: LI-4 Hegu, SJ-5 Waiguan, LI-11 Quchi, LI-15 Jianyu, BL-60 Kunlun, SP-6 Sanyinjiao, ST-36 Zusanli, ST-34 Liangqiu, SP-10 Xuehai, BL-17 Geshu.

Chronic remission stage of MS

10.3.3   Deficiency of Qi and Blood

Main manifestations: flaccid paralytic limbs, poor appetite, abdominal distention after meals, loose stools, fatigue, dizziness, and weakness in the muscles. The tongue is usually swollen, with teeth-marks and a greasy coating and the pulse is slippery.

Treatment principle: Reinforce Qi, nourish Blood, and move meridian Qi.

Points selection: LI-4 Hegu, SJ-5 Waiguan, LI-11 Quchi, LI-15 Jianyu, BL-60 Kunlun, SP-6 Sanyinjiao, ST-36 Zusanli, ST-34 Liangqiu, ST- 40 Fenglong, BL-20 Pishu, REN-12 Zhongwan.

10.3.4   Liver and Kidney Yin Deficiency

Main manifestations: flaccid paralytic limbs, numbness and weakness, dizziness, and soreness in the lower back and knees, blurring of vision, insomnia, dry mouth, hot flush, red tongue with a little coated, thin wiry rapid pulse.

Treatment principle: Nourish Liver and Kidney Yin and move meridian Qi.

Points selection: LI-4 Hegu, SJ-5 Waiguan, LI-11 Quchi, LI-15 Jianyu, BL-60 Kunlun, SP-6 Sanyinjiao, ST-36 Zusanli, ST-34 Liangqiu, LV-8 Ququan, LV-3 Taichong, KI-6 Zhaohai.

10.3.5 Kidney Yang Deficiency

Main manifestations: flaccid paralytic limbs, cold hand and feet, lower back pain and knee weakness, diarrhea, frequent urine, pale tongue with thin white coated, weak pulse.

Treatment principle: Warm Kidney Yang and move meridian Qi.

Points selection: LI-4 Hegu, SJ-5 Waiguan, LI-11 Quchi, LI-15 Jianyu, BL-60 Kunlun, SP-6 Sanyinjiao, ST-36 Zusanli, ST-34 Liangqiu, REN-4 Guanyuan, KI-7 Fuliu, KI-3 Taixi. Moxibustion can enhance the therapeutic results of scalp acupuncture, especially for older or weak patients. Recommended points are ST-36 Zusanli, SP-6 Sanyinjiao, REN-4 Guanyuan, KI-1 Yongquan and BL-23 Shenshu.

In our practice with Western patients, the most commonly seen pattern of MS is Qi and Yin deficiency, meaning Spleen Qi deficiency and Liver and Kidney Yin deficiency. However, those patterns are often complicated by a combination of the above patterns. Some of these patients often have three or more concomitant patterns so that the practitioners should treat them accordingly.

10.4 Scalp Acupuncture Techniques for Multiple Sclerosis

Chinese scalp acupuncture is a contemporary acupuncture technique integrating traditional Chinese needling methods with Western medical knowledge of the cerebral cortex. Scalp acupuncture has been showed to be the most effective technique for treating central nervous system disorders ranging from multiple sclerosis, strokes [5, p. 159–165], Parkinson's disease, traumatic Brain injury, post-traumatic stress disorder to phantom pain and complex regional pain [6, p. 8]. The scalp somatotopic system appears to manifest the convergence of the central nervous system and the endocrine system. The scalp somatotopic system seems to operate as a miniature transmitter-receiver in direct contact with the central nervous system and endocrine system. By stimulating those reflex areas, acupuncture can have a direct effect on the cerebral cortex, cerebellum, thalamo-cortical circuits, thalamus, hypothalamus, and pineal body [7, p. 173–174]. Its unique neurologic and endocrinal composition makes the scalp an ideal external stimulating field for internal activities of the Brain. Using a small number of needles, scalp acupuncture can often produce remarkable results almost immediately, sometimes taking only several minutes to complete [8, p.5–7].

Scalp acupuncture treatment principle: Restore the Brain function and rewire neuron's connection.

Area selection: Motor Area, Sensory Area, Foot Motor and Sensory Area, Balance Area, Tremor, and Dizziness Area [9, p. 96–102]. Detail of scalp acupuncture, location and needling, please see Chap. 5 of this book.

Manipulation:

Motor Area, Sensory Area, and Foot Motor and Sensory Area should be inserted with needles and stimulated unilaterally or bilaterally, according to the patient's symptoms. Rotate the needles at least 200 times per minute with thumb and index finger for one to three minutes. The doctor should twirl the needles as vigorously as the patient can tolerate and repeat the stimulation every ten minutes. During treatment, some patients may have all or some of the following sensations: increase tingling or numbness, hot, cold, heaviness, distending, or the sensation of water or electricity moving along their spine, legs or arms. Those patients with some or all of these sensations usually respond and improve quickly. However, those who do not have such sensations could still have immediate positive results. Select the Balance Area or Dizziness Area according to the patient's symptoms, whether balance or dizziness and vertigo. The Tremor Area should be chosen if patient has tremor or limb spasm. Keep the needles in for 25–30 min; the treatment is given two to three times per week, and a therapeutic course consists of 10 treatments.

Recent studies have shown that scalp acupuncture can be a very effective modality in controlling MS. Scalp acupuncture often produces remarkable results after just a few needles are inserted. It usually relieves symptoms immediately, and sometimes only takes several minutes to achieve remarkable results. Scalp acupuncture areas may be chosen according to the patient's particular symptoms. The primary acupuncture areas for patients with motor problems such as paralysis, weakness of limbs or abnormal sensations in limbs, including tingling, numbness or pain, are the motor area and the sensory and foot-motor areas. Those areas should be inserted with needles and stimulated unilaterally or bilaterally, according to the patient's manifestations. Select the Balance Area or Dizziness Area of the scalp, respectively, depending on which symptom the patient manifests. The Tremor Area of the head should be chosen if patients have limb spasm. Many patients have a quick positive response in controlling urine and bowel functions when the Foot-Motor and Sensory Area is stimulated.

Scalp acupuncture has proven to have the most success in treating MS and other central nerve damage, as compared to other acupuncture modalities including acupuncture on the ear, body, and hand. It not only can improve the symptoms, and the patient's quality of life, yet has also slowly and reversed the progression of physical disability, while reducing the number of relapses. The patient should get acupuncture treatment as soon as possible; the earlier the patient receives treatment, the better the prognosis is. Scalp acupuncture treatment for MS has had much success in reducing numbness and pain, decreasing spasms, improving weakness and paralysis of limbs and improving balance. Many patients also have reported that their bladder and bowel control, fatigue and overall sense of wellbeing significantly improved after treatment.

There are many different acupuncture techniques to treat MS. Although scalp acupuncture has the fastest track record for improving symptoms, other techniques are also necessary for further improvement. Regular body acupuncture, electric acupuncture and moxibustion, as well as physical therapy and massage, can combine with scalp acupuncture to speed up the time of recovery. In addition to scalp acupuncture, it is important to use points on the Du meridian and Huatuojiaji point since the myelin sheath lesions are located in the Brain and around spine. Other regular acupuncture treatment has been found to have a positive therapeutic effect on the recovery of movement and reducing abnormal sensations of the hands, fingers, feet and toes. Commonly used points are GB-20 Fengchi, BL-9 Yuzhen, GB-19 Naokong. GB-30 Huantiao, GB-34 Yanglingquan, LV-3 Taichong, and KI-3 Taixi are used for lower limb, and LI-11 Quchi, LI-4 Hegu, and SJ-5 Waiguan are used for upper-limb (29). Electrical stimulation is very helpful if the practitioner has difficulty performing the needle rotation more than 200 times per minute. It is suggested that no more than two of the scalp needles be stimulated at any session so the Brain does not become too confused to respond. Moxibustion can enhance the therapeutic results of scalp acupuncture, especially for older or weak patients. Recommended points are ST-36 Zusanli, SP-6 Sanyinjiao, REN-4 Guanyuan, KI-1Yongquan and BL-23 Shenshu. When treating chronic progressive diseases like Multiple Sclerosis, Parkinsonism, and ALS, the effects are more often temporary sometimes. They may last for hours, days, weeks, or months, but follow-up treatments will be necessary on an ongoing basis.

Fatigue is one of the most common symptoms in multiple sclerosis and a complicated disorder affecting the central nervous system, immune system and other organs. It is characterized by extreme fatigue that does not abate with rest and worsens with physical or mental activities. While some patients are able to lead a relatively normal life, others are totally bed-bound and unable to care for themselves. Recently, stress and genetics have been found to be factors in the development of fatigue. Some research suggests that fatigue has been linked to an impaired stress response and emotional instability; and it may affect subtle dysfunctions of the hypothalamus-pituitary-adrenal axis. The majority of patients with fatigue begin experiencing it after a period of extreme stress in the year preceding the illness. It starts suddenly, and often is triggered by a flu-like viral or similar illness. For some patients the disease starts gradually and slowly, without a clear history of illness and sometimes it spans years. There is no specific treatment for fatigue in Western medicine. In general, treatments are aimed at relieving symptoms. Some dietary supplements and herbal remedies have been recognized as having potential benefits for patients with fatigue.

Scalp acupuncture has a fairly good track record for treating fatigue. Common scalp areas are Foot Motor and Sensory Area, Head Area, Sensory Area, Chest Area, Liver Area, Stomach Area, and Reproduction Area. The Foot Motor and Sensory Area should be inserted with needles bilaterally and the Head Area unilaterally. The selections of scalp acupuncture areas are usually based upon symptoms and diagnosis in western medicine. The internal organ areas on forehead are sometimes based on differentiation of patterns in Chinese medicine. It is a good technique to put one needle on Shenmen point on the ear to help the patient relax, and then reduce the sensitivity of the needle insertion and stimulation of the scalp. Use as few needles as possible in the scalp and rotate the needles at least 200 times per minute with the thumb and index finger for two minutes. The doctor should twirl the needles as gently as possible in the beginning so the patient can tolerate the intense sensations, and repeat the stimulation every ten minutes. During treatment, some patients may have some or all of the following sensations: hot, cold, tingling, numbness, heaviness, distending, or the sensation of water or electricity moving along their spine, legs or arms. Tell patients before the needles are inserted that these sensations are normal, and patients who experience them usually respond and improve quickly. This encourages patients to come back for additional treatments. However, it is important to also convey that patients who do not have such sensations could still have immediate positive results. Retain the needles in place for 10 to 20 minutes. The treatment is given two to three times per week, and a therapeutic course consists of 10 treatments.

The treatment of fatigue usually requires longer periods of treatment, and most patients need to receive 10 to 20 visits. It is very helpful if other acupuncture methods are utilized along with scalp acupuncture, such as body acupuncture and moxibustion. The selection of body points should be individualized based on the differentiation of patterns in Chinese medicine. For instance, ST-36 Zusangli, SP-6 Sanyinjiao, and REN-12 Zhongwan are used for deficiency of Spleen and Stomach, and KI-1 Yongquan, KI-3 Taixi, KI-6 Zhaohai and KI-7 Fuliu for deficiency of the Kidneys. Reports show that chronic fatigue syndrome may worsen with increased stress whether from physical, emotional, or psychological sources. Therefore, the scalp areas that have the function of relieving anxiety, irritability or depression should be combined with the foot motor and sensory area for best results. Other therapies that can promote relaxation and a sense of wellbeing may be helpful in relieving chronic fatigue syndrome, such as meditation, hypnosis, yoga, and herbs.

10.5   Research

There are a few ongoing researches looking for more effective, convenient, and tolerable acupuncture and moxibustion treatments for multiple sclerosis in China. Some sample studies of acupuncture for multiple sclerosis are listed below:

Dr. Wang's group [10] recruited 78 MS patients from four hospitals in Gansu, China. Scalp acupuncture Motor area and Sensory area and regular body points ST-40 Fenglong, SP-10 Xuehai, GV-20 Baihui, DU-26 Shuigou, LV-3 Taichong, LI-4 Hegu, HT-7 Shenmen, PC-6 Neiguan were stimulated, five sessions a week for 60 days, compared with Amitriptyline. The research showed both acupuncture group (38 people) and medication group (40 people) had improvements that helped with depression, anxiety, and their quality of life (QoL). They found no significant difference between the acupuncture group and Amitriptyline group on HAMD and HAMA outcome measure.

Dr. Li's team in Tiantan Hospital in Beijing, China [11] treated 21 MS patients with fatigue. Twenty-one patients were randomly divided into a treatment group (11 cases) and a control group (10 cases). Patients in treatment group were treated with acupuncture at ST-36 Zusanli, SP -6 Sanyinjiao, and GV-20 Baihui. Patients in the control group were treated with shallow acupuncture at the region nearby the above-mentioned points. All patients were treated once a day for continuous ten days. Before and after the treatment, all patients were evaluated with the rating scales of EDSS (expanded disability status *scale*) and FSS (fatigue severity scale). The concentration of IL-1α and IL-6 in serum was measured with ELISA (enzyme-linked immunosorbent assay). Results: EDSS score had no significant difference between two groups before or after acupuncture. The FSS after the treatment decreased significantly in the treatment group and the control group ($P < 0.01$, $P < 0.05$). There were no significant differences of FSS between two groups after the treatment. The concentration of serum IL-1α had no significant difference between two groups. The concentration of serum IL-6 after acupuncture decreased significantly in the treatment group and the control group ($P < 0.01$). There were no significant differences of serum IL-6 between two groups after the treatment. It showed that the treatment of acupuncture could effectively relieve the fatigue symptom of MS patients, and improve their life quality by decreasing serum IL-6, and the acupuncture is safe and reliable.

Donnellan and Sharley [12] compared the effects of two types of acupuncture on QoL measures in fourteen persons with secondary progressive MS. Using a single-blind randomized control design, subjects received either Chinese acupuncture or minimal acupuncture. Chinese medical acupuncture was defined as the insertion of needles to a specified depth into particular acupuncture points that were chosen based on identification of traditional Chinese medical patterns corresponding with MS. Minimal acupuncture, the control intervention, was defined as the superficial insertion of needles into points located away from real acupuncture points and away from points important in the treatment of MS. Outcomes included the Multiple Sclerosis Impact Scale 29 (MSIS-29) and the Fatigue Severity Scale (FSS). After ten treatments over five weeks the minimal acupuncture group reported significantly greater improvement in the MSIS-29 psychological subscale compared with those receiving Chinese medical acupuncture in an intention-to-treat analysis ($P < 0.04$), with mean change in Chinese acupuncture group of 6.0 and in minimal acupuncture group of 23.0. No change was noted in the FSS.

A few articles evaluated the use of acupuncture on animal models of MS using rats with experimental autoimmune encephalitis (EAE). EAE is an experimentally induced disease that results in demyelination of the central nervous system and is widely used as an animal model to study MS in humans. Liu et al. [13] found that rats with EAE treated with electroacupuncture had decreased disease severity, inhibited T-cell proliferation, and improved CD4+ T-cell balance as well as higher in vivo ACTH concentrations compared to the control group with rats. Huang et al. [14] found that demyelinated rats treated with electroacupuncture had increased production of oligodendrocyte precursor cells resulting in increased myelin formation. Spinal cord evoked potentials also improved in the experimental group. Liu et al. [15] did electroacupuncture on ST-36 (Zusanli) in every female Lewis rats, one for 21 days. It examined the mechanism by which electroacupuncture effectively treated EAE, finding that the anti-inflammatory effects of electroacupuncture on EAE were related to β-endorphin production that balances the Thl/Th2 and Th17/ Treg responses. These results suggest that β-endorphin could be an important component in the development of EA-based therapies used for the treatment of EAE.

A scalp acupuncture clinical case study [16] concludes that acupuncture benefits patients with multiple sclerosis. The study finds that acupuncture relieves the symptoms of multiple sclerosis, increases the patient's quality of life, slows the progression of physical disability and reduces the frequency of relapses. Scalp acupuncture was applied to several standard scalp zones: motor, sensory, foot motor and sensory, balance, hearing, dizziness, tremor. Acupuncture was applied once a week for the first ten weeks followed by once a month for the next six treatments. The patient in the study had multiple sclerosis (MS) for 20 years. After the application of 16 acupuncture treatments, standing and walking improved significantly. There was also a marked reduction in numbness and tingling in the limbs. Overall, the patient showed increased energy levels and reported less dizziness. The patient's condition went into remission after the acupuncture treatments. At the time the research was published, the patient had been in remission for 26 months.

10.6   Conclusion

Multiple sclerosis (MS) is a progressive disease of the central nervous system which has affected 520,000 people in the Americas and 2.3 million people worldwide. Currently, conventional treatments do not have a cure for MS. However, acupuncture is one of the major complementary or alternative therapies for MS. Our study shows that scalp acupuncture seems to be a more effective modality in bringing about quicker and often effective improvements to patients with MS compared to other acupuncture modalities such as acupuncture on the ear, body, and hand. Chinese scalp acupuncture is also more easily accessible, less expensive, entails less risk, can yield quicker responses, and often causes fewer side effects than some other forms of treatments.

In the West, most healthcare practitioners are familiar with acupuncture for pain management. However, scalp acupuncture, as a useful tool for the treatment of MS, is a relatively new concept. Even now, it is not surprising for a Western physician to claim that it is a natural remission or coincidence if a patient recover from MS after acupuncture. Scalp acupuncture can provide solutions in situations where Western medicine treatments are limited. It holds the potential to expand treatment options for MS in both conventional and complementary or integrative therapies. It not only can improve the symptoms, the patient's quality of life, and slow and reverse the progression of physical disabilities, but also can reduce the number of relapses and help patients stay in remission.

Although over the past 40 years there have been numerous hypotheses and research reports on scalp acupuncture for the central nervous system disorders and pain management in Western medical literature, there is still a long way to go in uncovering the mystery of the mechanisms of scalp acupuncture. Further study is needed to investigate the mechanisms underlying acupuncture's effect on the central nervous dysfunctions of patients with MS. If its scope were expanded, scalp acupuncture could have a significant impact on recovery on central nervous system disorders for thousands of patients. There is, therefore, a pressing need for Chinese scalp acupuncture to be studied and perfected using modern research methods, so that its potential can be fully explored and applied.

Although MS still is an incurable disease of the central nervous system, scalp acupuncture provides an important complementary/alternative in treatment approach for improving many of the MS symptoms and the patient's quality of life by slowing or reversing the progression of physical disability and reducing the number of relapses. By directly stimulating affected areas of the central nervous system, scalp acupuncture has shown to have more effective results compared to other acupuncture techniques. Our studies showed that 87 percent of the patients had immediate improvements after only one scalp acupuncture treatment. Scalp acupuncture treatment for MS is accessible, less expensive, safer, more effective, and causes fewer side effects than other treatments. Scalp acupuncture not only benefits patients with MS, but also significantly helps us to better understand the mechanisms that cause the condition. It may guide us to the discovery of new effective treatments and hopefully to a cure for this disease in the future.

References

1. Arslan OE. Neuroanatomical basis of clinical neurology. New York: The Parthenon Publishing Group; 2001.
2. World Health Organization, Atlas multiple sclerosis resources in the world, WHO Library Cataloguing in Publication Data, Geneva, Switzerland, 2008.
3. Blumenfeld H. Neuroanatomy through clinical cases. Sunderland, MA: Sinauer Associates; 2002.
4. Wang YY, Zhang BL. Brain diseases in Chinese medicine (Chinese). Beijing: People's Health Press; 2007.
5. Wang FC. Scalp acupuncture therapy (Chinese). In: People's Medical Publishing House. Beijing; 2007.
6. McMillan BB. Easing the pain, acupuncture program looks to help relieve discomfort of troops. Strip, February 17, 2006.
7. Lennard TA, Walkowski SA, Singla AK, et al. Pain procedures in clinical practice. Philadelphia, PA: Elsevier Saunders; 2011.
8. Jiao SF. Scalp acupuncture and clinical cases. Beijing: Foreign Languages Press; 1997.
9. Hao JJ, Hao LL. Chinese scalp acupuncture. Boulder, CO: Blue Poppy Press; 2011.
10. Wang JW, Huang SH, Fan SY, et al. Study on the treatment of multiple sclerosis with acupuncture. J New Chin Med. 2016;48(5):129–31.
11. Li KN, Fan YP, Wang WM, et al. Therapeutic effect and mechanism of acupuncture on the fatigue symptom of the patients with relapsing-remitting multiple sclerosis. China J Tradition Chin Med Pharm. 2016;31(11):4511–4.
12. Donnellan CP, Sharley J. Comparison of the effect of two types of acupuncture on quality of life in secondary progressive multiple sclerosis: a preliminary single-blind randomized controlled trial. Clin Rehabil. 2008;22(3):195–205.

13. Liu YM, Liu XJ, Bai SS, et al. The effect of electroacupuncture on T cell responses in rats with experimental autoimmune encephalitis. J Neuroimmunol. 2010;220(1-2):25–33.
14. Huang SF, Ding Y, Ruan JW, et al. An experimental electro-acupuncture study in treatment of the rat demyelinated spinal cord injury induced by ethidium bromide. Neurosci Res. 2011;70(3):294–304.
15. Liu YM, Wang HW, Wang XY, et al. The mechanism of effective electroacupuncture on T cell response in rats with experimental autoimmune encephalomyelitis. PLoS One. 2013;8(1):e51573. 10 pages. https://doi.org/10.1371/journal.pone.0051573
16. Hao JJ, Cheng W, Liu M, et al. Treatment of multiple sclerosis with Chinese scalp acupuncture. Global Adv Health Med. 2013;2(1):8–13.

Chapter 11
Traumatic Brain Injury

11.1 General Information

11.1.1 Basic Background of TBI

Traumatic brain injury (TBI) is a condition caused by blunt or sharp external forces on the head and Brain, which may lead to temporary or permanent Brain dysfunction [1]. TBI is a significant public health problem globally and one of the major causes of death and disability [2]. According to a survey from 195 countries by the World Health Organization in 2016, TBI will surpass many other factors as a main cause of death and disability by the year 2020 [3]. Traffic accidents and falls as the main causes [4]. Studies have indicated that the prevalence of TBI in the population is skewed towards younger people, in whom it has become a leading cause of death and disability [5].

Despite the continuous advances in neurosurgery and related medical management, numerous survivors suffer from TBI-related disabilities. It is estimated that 5.2 million people in the USA and 7.3 million people in the European Union have disabilities due to TBI [6, 7]. Among all the TBI patients, more than 75% of TBI are defined as mild (mTBI), which is a complex pathophysiologic process that can occur after trauma to the head. Some children with mTBI develop a cluster of cognitive, physical, and emotional problems commonly referred to as post-concussion syndrome (PCS) [8].

11.1.2 The Aetiology and Pathogenesis

TBI may lead a very complex physiopathology processes that results from initial and secondary injuries. The injuries may lead to temporary or permanent neurological deficits. The initial stage after TBI results from direct tissue damage and impaired

© Springer Nature Switzerland AG 2021
T. Wang, *Acupuncture for Brain*, https://doi.org/10.1007/978-3-030-54666-3_11

autoregulation of cerebral blood flow (CBF) along with disordered metabolism. This state, similar to ischemia, may lead to the accumulation of lactic acid, increased cell membrane permeability and subsequent oedema. Since anaerobic metabolism cannot sustain the demands of the Brain, Adenosine triphosphate (ATP) stores are depleted, which ultimately results in failure of the ATP-dependent membrane ionic pumps, which are essential for maintaining adequate homeostasis. The second stage of this cascade is characterized by sustained membrane depolarization, along with excitotoxicity (i.e., the excessive release of excitatory neurotransmitters such as glutamate and aspartate) and the activation of voltage-dependent Ca^{++} and Na^+ channels. The subsequent calcium and sodium influx results in the activation of lipid peroxidases, proteases and phospholipases, which trigger the apoptotic cascade and ultimately lead to membrane degradation and cell death [9, 10].

In addition, After TBI, the Brain injury produces a severe inflammatory response, leading to microglial activation, macrophage infiltration and astrocyte reactive hyperplasia. Microglia and astrocytes are not only the main immune cells of the central nervous system, but are also closely related to the formation of scar tissue after nerve injury [11]. The scar formation has two effects on Brain injury: (1) the formation of scar tissue around the lesions separates the inflammatory necrotic tissue from normal tissue in the early injury stage, preventing the inflammation from spreading; and (2) sustained scarring interferes with the growth of neuron axons in the later stage, which curbs the neuronal repair [12].

11.1.3   Typical Clinical Symptoms

The commonly seen symptoms related to TBI are disorders of consciousness (DOC) post-traumatic headache (PTH), insomnia, and various sequelae of TBI (e.g. aphasia, pain, facial palsy, post-concussive syndrome).

After TBI, regarding severe Brain damage, patients experienced varying degrees of DOC such as coma, a vegetative state, or a minimally conscious state, which is a prolonged cognitive impairment including the loss of awareness of oneself and environment. DOC seriously affects an individual's ability to perform the activities of daily living (ADL) and reduces the quality of life. The early recovery of consciousness is closely associated with recovery in other functional domains, and the duration of DOC is an important prognostic factor in patients who experience TBI [13].

Post-traumatic headache (PTH), also known as post-concussive headache, is one of the most common complaints after mild traumatic brain injury (mTBI). It occurs acutely in up to 90% of all individuals who sustain a concussion or mTBI. There are three patterns of PTHs: migraine-like, tension-like, and mixed symptomatology [14].

Insomnia is a frequent problem in the TBI population. Sleep disturbances can appear as soon as 24 h following injury and can continue for several years which impact 30% to 81% of TBI survivors. There are also some various sequelae of TBI, such aphasia, pain, facial palsy, post concussive syndrome [15].

11.1.4   Examination and Diagnosis

In the early stage of the assessment for the severe DOC after TBI, the Glasgow coma scale (GCS) is the most widely used method of recording the lever of consciousness in patients at presentation and at subsequent assessments, although it was original published in 1974 [9].

With the development of diagnostic tools such as functional magnetic resonance and electroencephalography, patients with severe TBI could be detected in early stage and commence early intervention [16].

More than 75% of the children TBI are defined as mild (mTBI). Mild TBI is a complex pathophysiologic process that can occur after trauma to the head. Some children with mTBI develop a cluster of cognitive, physical, and emotional problems commonly referred to as post-concussion syndrome (PCS) [8].

11.1.5   The Treatment of TBI with Modern Medicine

Brain Trauma Foundation (BTF) updated it guidelines in 2017 [17], which are protocol-based management strategies aimed at providing high quality care and improvements in outcomes for patients hospitalized with TBI. The cornerstone of the management of TBI is the intensive care treatment of these patients with careful attention paid to the airway, oxygenation and adequate hemodynamic support to avoid the secondary injuries that are associated with events such as hypoxia and hypotension.

Care of a TBI patient should begin at the site of the injury, with an aim to secure the patients' airway and maintain adequate ventilation and circulation. Patients with moderate or severe TBI should be transferred to a tertiary care centre with neurosurgical facilities as soon as possible. Outcomes in TBI patients have been found to be influenced by transport methods, the duration of transit and whether the responding team is led by a physician or a paramedic. The primary management goals are the prevention of hypoxia and hypotension, because even a single episode of hypotension has been found to be associated with a doubling of mortality and an elevated risk of morbidity [9].

The general management for TBI include airway control and ventilation, blood pressure and cerebral perfusion pressure (CPP), fluid management, sedation and analgesia, intracranial pressure (ICP) monitoring and management, osmotherapy, multimodal neuromonitoring, anticonvulsant therapy, temperature management, glycemic control, decompressive craniectomy, nutrition, antibiotic therapy, et al. [9].

The early management phase aims to achieve haemodynamic stability, limit secondary insults (e.g. hypotension, hypoxia), obtain accurate neurological assessment and appropriately select patients for further investigation [18]. Current therapeutic strategies for DOC include behavioral, pharmacological, and neurostimulatory approaches [16].

However, patients who experience TBI are still inadequately treated because of the lack of effective treatments. TBI survivors often experience severe neurological deficits. TBI has been suggested to trigger a series of secondary Brain injuries, such as regional ischaemia, blood flow decrease, DNA changes and eventually apoptotic cell death [19]. There is still lack of effective treatment for TBI recovery today [10].

11.2 TCM Understanding of TBI

Traditional Chinese medicine (TCM) understanding of TBI has a long history, similar to headache, coma, unconsciousness, and others. Its treatment principles are based on the different stages, such as coma period, wake-up period and recovery period. The commonly used treatment plan are Xing Nao Kai Qiao (Awake the Brain and Open Orifices) [20], particularly in the period of coma and wake-up. Other treatment principles include activate Blood circulation and clear stasis, clear Phlegm, nourish Heart and Spleen, and so forth. Chinese herb medicine and acupuncture are the two main therapies for TBI.

11.3 General Acupuncture Treatment for TBI

Acupuncture has been used in the treatment of stroke and its consequences for over 2000 years in China [21]. It has been used to promote the recovery of consciousness after coma or other DOCs (disorders of consciousness) for centuries [13]. A review suggest that acupuncture may have a beneficial effect on the recovery of consciousness after TBI. According to these findings, acupuncture may improve consciousness levels evaluated using GCS or GOS (Glasgow Outcome Score) scores, clinical efficacy, and lower mortality after TBI. Acupuncture may also help in rehabilitation [13]. In addition, acupuncture has a bidirectional modulatory effect on TBI [1]. Because of its safety, cost-effectiveness, and long-lasting benefits, adjunctive acupuncture should be offered to patients with chronic PTHs and may be a valuable primary treatment alternative for those with contraindications to pharmacotherapy [14].

According to the foundation of TCM theory, the principle of general acupuncture treatment would follow the pattern identification. As usual, below TCM patterns, symptoms and signs, and the points selection, are just sample suggestions. Clinic practice should follow the real individual patient.

11.3.1   Acute Stage

Due to the acute stage of a Brain injury being a critical period, it is suggested the combined management with modern western medical methods with acupuncture, if acupuncture involved in treatment during this acute stage [22, p. 179].

11.3.1.1   Blockage of Zangfu

Symptoms and Signs (SS): Coma after Brain injury, unconsciousness, unrespon-siveness, or severe confusion, agitation, restlessness, shortness of breath, may fever with flushed face, red or skewed tongue with yellow or black coat, rapid pulse.

Points selection: DU-20 Baihui, DU-26 Renzhong, Ex-Shixuan with bleeding, KI-1 Yongquan, LV-3 Taichong, PC-8 Laogong.

11.3.1.2   Exhaustion of Qi

SS: Deep coma after Brain injury, severe unconsciousness ad no response for call and pain at all, mouth opening, heavy breath, cold hands and feet, cool sweating, loss of bladder and bowel movement control; pale tongue, very weak and deep thin pulse.

Points selection: DU-26 Renzhong. REN-12 Zhongwan, REN-6 Qihai, REN-4 Guanyuan, with needle plus moxa, REN-8 Shenque with moxa only.

11.3.2   Wake-Up and Recovery Stage

11.3.2.1   Stagnation of Qi and Blood

SS: Headache after Brain injury, cognitive deficiency, hemiplegia, easy tired, purple tongue or purple spots with thin coat, wiry and thin pulse.

Points selection: DU-20 Baihui, LI-4 Hegu, LV-3 Taichong, SP-10 Xuehai, BL-17 Geshu, GB-20 Fengchi, plus local area points.

11.3.2.2   Deficiency of Heart and Spleen

SS: Dull headache worse with fatigue, vertigo and dizziness, palpitation, shortness of breath, insomnia with bad dreams, lassitude, wither face, pale tongue with thin white coat, thin and weak pulse.

Points selection: BL-15 Xinshu, BL-20 Pishu, HT-7 Shenmen, ST-36 Zusanli, SP-9 Yinlingquan.

11.3.2.3 Deficiency of Liver and Kidney

SS: Constant dull headache with empty felling, dizziness, poor memory, lack concentration, tinnitus, dry mouth and eyes, low back pain with weak knees, empty heat
sensation in palms, soles and chest, night sweating. Light red tongue less coat, thin
and fast pulse.

Points selection: BL-18 Ganshu, BL-23 Shenshu, DU-20 Baihui, LV-3 Taichong,
KI-3 Taixi, KI-6 Zhaohai.

Above pattern identifications may be separate used with general needling, better
combined with below unique Brain acupuncture techniques.

11.4   Unique Acupuncture Treatments for TBI

In TCM, the similar symptoms or pattern of trauma Brain injury (TBI) was separated in different Zangfu organs, such as Heart, Liver, Spleen, Kidney, and others.
With the development of TCM Brain theory, more TCM scholars believe the main
location of the disease in TBI is the Brain with other Zangfu organs involved. More
relevant acupuncture points selection and techniques are developed.

More clinical studies select Du Mai points as the major point to treat TBI [1],
particularly in the acute the stage, DU-26 Renzhong is widely used in patients with
stroke to prompt restoration of consciousness [16].

Influenced with neuroanatomy, neurophysiology, and bio-holographic principle
of modern medicine [23], scalp acupuncture is widely used for the neurological
diseases include TBI. Scalp acupuncture has been reported to (1) improve cerebral
blood circulation, promoting regional energy metabolism; (2) upregulate expression
of glial cell-line derived neurotrophic factor (GDNF), possibly promoting proliferation and differentiation of neural stem cells in the focal cerebral cortex and hippocampus; (3) reduce contents of excitatory amino acid and increase level of GABA,
thus lowering neurogenic toxicity; (4) ease cerebral vascular immunoinflammatory
reactions; (5) regulate blood lipid metabolism to resist cerebral free radical damage;
and (6) inhibit cerebral cortical apoptosis [21].

11.4.1   Scalp Acupuncture for Treating TBI (Detail of Scalp
Acupuncture, Location and Needling Please See
Chap. 5)

Some symptom treatments of scalp acupuncture are listed below:

- Hemiplegia: Opposite upper 1/5 and middle 2/5 Motor Area and Foot-Motor
  Sensory Area. During the needling, patients should move or helped to move their
  suffered limbs.

- Hemi- sensory disorder: Opposite upper 1/5 and middle 2/5 Sensory Area and Foot-Motor Sensory Area
- Hemianopia: Visual Area
- Motor aphasia: first Speech Area
- Anomic aphasia: second Speech Area
- Sensory aphasia: third Speech Area
- Dizziness: Vertigo and Auditory Area
- Ataxia: Balance Area
- Constipation: Intestine Area
- Frequently urination: Foot-Motor Sensory Area

11.4.2   Du Mai Dao-Qi Technique (Detail of Dao-Qi Technique on Du Mai, Points Location and Needling, Please See Chap. 6)

- DU-26 Renhong, DU-20 Baihui, DU-16 Fengfu, DU-15 Yamen, DU-14 Dazhui, DU-9 Zhiyang, DU-4 Mingmen, DU-3 Yaoyangguan
- DU-26 Renzhong Dao-qi needling: For coma or severe cases, oblique insertion upward 0.5 to 1 cun to the root of the nasal septum. Strong sensation may occur directly to the nose, or spread to the forehead, eyes and face. This restores consciousness should result in the tears out of the eyes or watery of eyes.

11.4.3   Ren Mai Dao-Qi Technique (Detail of Dao-Qi Technique on Ren Mai, Points Location and Needling, Please See Chap. 6)

- REN-12 Zhongwan plus 2–4 needles around it with 0.5–1 cm distance, REN-10 Xiawan, REN-6 Qihai, REN-4 Guanyuan, REN-17 Danzhong (Shanzhong).

Above unique Brain acupuncture techniques can be combined with syndrome differentiation treatment.

11.4.4   Brain Pattern Differentiation

The commonly clinical Brain patterns of TBI and its possible symptoms could be summarised as stated below, yet they are still in the development stage and have not been perfected at the moment.

- Acute Stage:

11.4.4.1   Blockage of Brain Shen

SS: Coma after Brain injury, unconsciousness, unresponsiveness, or severe confusion, agitation, restlessness, shortness of breath, may fever with flushed face, maybe mouth opening, heavy breath, cold hands and feet, cool sweating, loss of bladder and bowel movement control, red or skewed tongue with yellow or black coat, or pale tongue with less coat rapid pulse.

Scalp acupuncture areas selection as above Sect. 11.4.1.

Brain acupuncture points selection: DU-26 Renzhong Dao-qi needling, DU-20 Baihui, DU-16 Fengfu Dao-qi needling, DU-15 Yamen, REN-12 Zhongwan, plus Ex-Shixuan bleeding, KI-1 Yongquan, and so forth. May plus electric acupuncture.

Note: If acupuncture is involved in this critical stage, it should be combined with modern medicine management.

• Chronic Stage:

11.4.4.2   Stagnation of Brain Collaterals

SS: Hemiplegia, hemianopia, aphasia, Dizziness, headache, cognitive deficiency, easily fatigued, purple tongue or purple spots with thin coat, wiry and thin pulse.

Scalp acupuncture areas selection as above Sect. 11.4.1 plus Vasomotor Area.

Brain acupuncture points selection: DU-20 Baihui, DU-16 Fengfu, DU-15 Yamen, DU-14 Dazhui, REN-12 Zhongwan plus 2–4 needles, REN-6 Qihai, may plus LI-4 Hegu, LV-3 Taichong, and local area points.

11.4.4.3   Disorder of Brain Shen

SS: Depression, stress, anxiety, insomnia with bad dreams, poor memory, dull headache; light tongue with thin coating, wiry or slow pulse.

Scalp acupuncture: Spirit-Emotion Area.

Brain acupuncture points selection: DU-24 Shenting, DU-20 Baihui, DU-16 Fengfu, DU-10 Lingtai, DU-11 Shendao, REN-12 Zhongwan may plus 2–4 needles around.

11.4.4.4   Deficiency of Brain Marrow

SS: Chronic dull headache with empty felling, vertigo, dizziness, poor memory, lack of concentration, easily fatigued, lethargy, tinnitus, dry eyes or poor version. Light red tongue less coat, thin and slow pulse.

Scalp acupuncture areas selection as above Sect. 11.4.1 plus Vasomotor Area.

Brain acupuncture Points selection: DU-20 Baihui, DU-14 Dazhui, Ex-Bailaoxue, DU-4 Mingmen, REN-12 Zhongwan may plus 2–4 needles around, REN-4 Guanyuan, may plus KI-3 Taixi, GB-39 Xuanzhong, and local area points. Techniques could choose electric-acupuncture, Dao-qi technique, etc.

11.4.4.5   Deficiency of Brain Yang Qi

SS: Dull headache worse with fatigue, Fatigue, shortness of breath, vertigo and dizziness, sweating, palpitation, loose stool, swollen hands and feet, generally cold with particularly on suffered side or area, pale face. Light colour tongue with white coat with teeth marks on sides, deep and thin pulse.

Scalp acupuncture on related areas as above Sect. 11.4.1 plus Central Area.

Brain acupuncture points selection: DU-20 Baihui, DU-16 Fengfu, DU-14 Dazhui, DU-9 Zhiyang, DU-4 Mingmen, DU-3 Yaoyangguan, REN-12 Zhongwan, REN-10 Xiawan, REN-6 Qihai, REN-4 Guanyuan, plus local suffered area points. Moxa could be applied, with Dao-qi technique on 1–2 key points.

Notes
- *In acute stage, acupuncture should be combined with modern medicine emergency management.
- *For treatment of TBI, after life factors settled, the early involved the better are the results.
- *The treatment frequency: in the early stage, the more often the better. In acute stage, better with every day or every other day. Chronic stage, twice per week, then with time, move slow down to once per week followed by once in 2–4 weeks for maintenance.
- *Acupuncture can be combined with routine therapy such as physiotherapy, speech therapy, cognitive behaviour therapy (CBT), etc.
- *Above Brain related patterns for TBI can be identified separately for severe TBI, and combined with classic TCM pattern identifications.

11.5   Research

In China, acupuncture has been used for centuries to promote the recovery of consciousness after coma or other DOCs. It has been shown to be an effective method when applied to trauma brain injury (TBI) [13]. Systematic review suggested that acupuncture is efficacious in acute TBI [24].

Acupuncture contributes to recovery of mind, speech and motor function for the patient of acute severe craniocerebral injury [25]. Both auricular acupuncture [AA] and traditional Chinese acupuncture [TCA] improved headache-related QoL more than usual care (UC) did in Service members with TBI [26]. Acupuncture has a beneficial effect on perception of sleep or sleep quality and on cognition in our small sample of patients with TBI [15].

A review suggested that the main arms for acupuncture's effects in Brain injuries: (1) limit Brain secondary injury, by acting on systemic and local inflammation, oxidative stress, intracellular calcium overload, neuron regeneration, and growth factors release; (2) manage consequences, such as neuroendocrine and autonomic dysfunction, muscle spasticity, and pain [21].

There are some studies the possible mechanisms are increasing the excitability of nerve cells and the supply of oxygen and blood flow in the traumatized area of the Brain, which may be a potential mechanism for its rousing effects. Many animal experiments have investigated that acupuncture in promotes arousal in TBI patients, lowering the level of plasma D-dimer, which may be one of the therapeutic mechanisms of electroacupuncture in recovering consciousness [13].

Acupuncture has a bidirectional modulatory effect on TLR2/4-NF-κB signalling pathway-related genes TLR2, TLR4 and NF-κB in the injured cortex of rats with TBI, promoting their expression in the early stage and promoting glial scar repair; acupuncture also has had an inhibitory effect in the later stage, reducing glial scar hyperplasia, which is conducive to the regeneration of neurons. This may be one of the mechanisms by which acupuncture regulates scar repair in TBI [1].

Acupuncture significantly increases the expression of EGF and bFGF, and improves the repair of injured Brain tissues. This might be one of the mechanisms by which acupuncture can treat traumatic Brain injury and improve the nervous function [27]. Electric-acupuncture treatment on the points GV20 (DU-20 Baihui) and GV26 (DU-26 Renzhong) with 1 and 0.2 Hz, 1 mA EA for 60 min after TBI could increase the regional blood flow and attenuate the levels of TGIF in the injured cortex, might lead to a decrease in neuronal apoptosis and cell infarction volume, as well as represent one mechanism by which functional recovery may occur [19].

Mechanism studies using animal models have shown that electro-acupuncture may alleviate cerebral injuries via upregulation of transforming growth factor beta 1. Activation of large-conductance Ca^+-activated K+ channels is also likely involved in the protective effects of DU-26 [16].

In summary, lots of clinical trials have proved acupuncture benefit for TBI and its related symptoms. Increasing animal experiments have investigated the multi targets of the mechanism.

11.6   Conclusion

Traumatic brain injury (TBI) may lead to temporary or permanent Brain dysfunction. The commonly seen symptoms related to TBI are disorders of consciousness (DOC), post-traumatic headache (PTH), insomnia, and various sequelae of TBI, such as aphasia, pain, facial palsy, post-concussive syndrome, et al. Patients who experience TBI are still inadequately treated because of the lack of effective treatments. TBI survivors often experience severe neurological deficits.

Acupuncture may play an important role on the recovery of TBI, with centuries of history and experience. With the developing of acupuncture Brain theory, more practice and research will focus on the Brain and its affiliated channel which is Du Mai (Governor vessel). Du Mai points are the more commonly used acupuncture points. Scalp acupuncture and Dao-qi technique are the commonly used acupuncture techniques.

References

1. Lin SJ, Cao LX, Cheng SB, et al. Effect of acupuncture on the TLR2/4-NF-κB signalling pathway in a rat model of traumatic brain injury. Acupunct Med. 2018;36:247–53.
2. Feigin VL, Theadom A, Barker-Collo S, et al. Incidence of traumatic brain injury in New Zealand: a population-based study. Lancet Neurol. 2013;12(1):53–64.
3. GBD. Disease, injury incidence, and prevalence collaborators, global, regional, and national incidence, prevalence, and years lived with disability for 328 diseases and injuries for 195 countries, 1990-2016: a systematic analysis for the Global Burden of Disease Study 2016. Lancet (London, England). 2017;390:1211–59.
4. Taylor CA, Bell JM, Breiding MJ, et al. Traumatic brain injury-related emergency department visits, hospitalizations, and deaths - United States, 2007 and 2013. MMWR Surveill Summ. 2017;66(9):1–16.
5. Cuthbert JP, Harrison-Felix C, Corrigan JD, et al. Epidemiology of adults receiving acute inpatient rehabilitation for a primary diagnosis of traumatic brain injury in the United States. J Head Trauma Rehabil. 2015;30:122–35.
6. Langlois JA, Sattin RW. Traumatic brain injury in the United States: research and programs of the centres for disease control and prevention (CDC). J Head Trauma Rehabil. 2005;20:187 8.
7. Tagliaferri F, Compagnone C, Korsic M, et al. A systematic review of brain injury epidemiology in Europe. Acta Neurochir. 2006;148:255–68.
8. Babcock L, Terri Byczkowski T, Wade SL, et al. Predicting post-concussion syndrome after mild traumatic brain injury in children and adolescents who present to the emergency department. JAMA Pediatr. 2013;167(2):156–61.
9. Dash HH, Chavali S. Management of traumatic brain injury patients. Korean J Anesthesiol. 2018;71(1):12–21.
10. Galgano M, Toshkezi G, Qiu XC, et al. Traumatic brain injury: current treatment strategies and future endeavors. Cell Transplant. 2017;26(7):1118–30.
11. Kawano H, Kimura-Kuroda J, Komuta Y, et al. Role of the lesion scar in the response to damage and repair of the central nervous system. Cell Tissue Res. 2012;349:169–80.
12. Sheng XH, Song SL, Liang JF, et al. Protective effect of glial scar on central nervous system injury. Chem Life. 2011;2:272–6.
13. Tan L, Zeng LL, Wang N, et al. Acupuncture to promote recovery of disorder of consciousness after traumatic brain injury: a systematic review and meta-analysis. Evid Based Complement Alternat Med. 2019; https://doi.org/10.1155/2019/5190515.
14. Khusid MA. Clinical indications for acupuncture in chronic post-traumatic headache. Mil Med. 2015;180(2):132–6.
15. Zollman FS, Eric B, Larson BL, et al. Acupuncture for treatment of insomnia in patients with traumatic brain injury: a pilot intervention study. J Head Trauma Rehabil. 2012;27(2):135–42.
16. Liu J, Xue XS, Wu Y, et al. Efficacy and safety of electro-acupuncture treatment in improving the consciousness of patients with traumatic brain injury: study protocol for a randomized controlled trial. Trials. 2018;19:296. https://doi.org/10.1186/s13063-018-2687-3.
17. Carney N, Totten AM, O'Reilly C, et al. Guidelines for the management of severe traumatic brain injury, fourth edition. Neurosurgery. 2017;80:6–15.
18. Kolias AG, Guilfoyle MR, Helmy A, et al. Traumatic brain injury in adults. Pract Neurol. 2013;13:228–35.
19. Chuang CH, Hsu YC, Wang CC, et al. Cerebral blood flow and apoptosis-associated factor with electroacupuncture in a traumatic brain injury rat model. Acupunct Med. 2013;31:395–403.
20. Bai XY, Jiang GL. Comparative analysis of therapeutic effects of apoplexy treated by Xing Nao Kai Qiao acupuncture method and Western medicine. World J Acupunct Moxibustion. 1996;6(1):25–8.
21. Loredana Cavalli L, Briscese L, Cavalli T, et al. Role of acupuncture in the management of severe acquired brain injuries (sABIs). Evid Based Complement Alternat Med. 2018; https://doi.org/10.1155/2018/8107508.

22. Wingate DS. Healing brain injury with Chinese medical approaches: integrative approaches for practitioners. London and Philadelphia: Singing Dragon; 2018.
23. Liu Z, Guan L, Wang Y, et al. History and mechanism for treatment of intracerebral haemorrhage with scalp acupuncture. Evid Based Complement Alternat Med. 2012; https://doi.org/10.1155/2012/895032.
24. Wong V, Cheuk DKL, Lee S, et al. Acupuncture for acute management and rehabilitation of traumatic brain injury. Cochrane Database Syst Rev. 2013;3 https://doi.org/10.1002/14651858.
25. Ding J, Dong GF, Song YX, et al. Control observation on therapeutic effects of acupuncture treatment on acute severe craniocerebral injury. Chin Acupunct Moxibustion. 2002;22(7):445–7.
26. Jonas WB, Dawn M, Bellanti DM, et al. A randomized exploratory study to evaluate two acupuncture methods for the treatment of headaches associated with traumatic brain injury. Med Acupunct. 2016;28(3):113–30.
27. Zhang YM, Tang CZ, Cheng SB, et al. Effect of acupuncture on expression of EGF and bFGF in brain tissues of rats with traumatic brain injury. Chin Acupunct Moxibustion. 2012;28(6):1132–34,39.

Chapter 12
Autism

12.1 General Introduction

12.1.1 Basic Knowledge on Autism

Autism spectrum disorder (ASD) refers to a group of complex neurodevelopment disorders characterized by repetitive and characteristic patterns of behaviour impacting a person's perceptions, actions, and socialization cause problems in daily behaviour and difficulties with communication and interaction.

Autism was first described by Leo Kanner, a psychiatrist at John Hopkins Medical Centre in 1943 as a disease of the Brain. He studied 11 of his young patients who had remarkably similar behaviours of preoccupation with objects, monotonous repetitions, insistence on consistency, and deficiencies of language, among other behaviours and concluded that the characteristics of autistic behaviours started from birth and not from a gradual change in over time [1]. His finding led researchers to treat early infantile autism as a disorder resulting from abnormal development of the autistic child's Brain. However, not until the 1980s, was ASD accepted as an individual developmental disorder with a biological origin.

In the early 1980s, studies demonstrated the high heritability of ASD and its association with other genetic syndromes [2, 3], providing compelling evidence for a genetic ethology of ASD and fuelling the conceptualization of autism as a distinct neurodevelopmental disorder. From the definition of "childhood or early-onset schizophrenia" put forward by Kanner, autism was renamed "infantile autism" in 1980, "autism disorder" in 1987 and, more recently, "autism" or the umbrella term "ASD."

Some children and adults with ASD are fully able to perform all activities of daily living while others require substantial support to perform basic activities. The Diagnostic and Statistical Manual of Mental Disorders (DSM-5, published in 2013) includes Asperger syndrome, childhood disintegrative disorder, and pervasive developmental disorders not otherwise specified (PDD-NOS) as part of ASD rather

© Springer Nature Switzerland AG 2021
T. Wang, *Acupuncture for Brain*, https://doi.org/10.1007/978-3-030-54666-3_12

than as separate disorders. A diagnosis of ASD includes an assessment of intellectual disability and language impairment. Children with ASD is likely to have a unique pattern of behaviour and level of severity—from low functioning to high functioning. Some children with ASD have difficulty learning, and some have signs of lower than normal intelligence. Other children may have normal to high intelligence yet have trouble communicating and applying what they know in everyday life and adjusting to social situations. Because of the unique mixture of symptoms in each child, severity can sometimes be difficult to determine. It is generally based on the level of impairments and how they impact the ability to function.

ASD occurs in every racial and ethnic group, and across all socioeconomic levels. However, boys are significantly more likely to develop ASD than girls and most children with autistic syndrome usually have shown developmental abnormalities by 2 years of age. The latest analysis from the Centres for Disease Control and Prevention estimates that 1 in 68 children has ASD.

The American Academy of Paediatrics recommends that all children be screened for autism. Intensive and early treatments and services can improve a person's symptoms and ability to function, improving the lives of many children.

12.1.2   Aetiology and Pathogenesis

Autism spectrum disorders (ASDs) are complex, lifelong neurodevelopmental conditions, in which the causes are largely unknown. They are much more common than previously believed, second only to mental retardation in prevalence among the serious developmental disorders.

There is no known single cause for ASD, but it is generally accepted that it is caused by abnormalities in the central nervous system—the Brain function and the spinal cord. The developmental abnormalities could occur during fetal development, during birth, or even after birth. Conditions such as viral infections, metabolic imbalances, alcohol and drugs exposure, environmental chemicals, oxygen deprivation, and genetic/chromosomal factors can have an effect.

The Central Nervous System CNS functions as the computer for the body. Messages from the CNS control all aspects of learning, thinking, and movement that allows us to learn about the function in the world.

1. Exposure to alcohol and drugs-addicted babies
2. Genetic/chromosomal factors such as in Down syndrome
3. Exposure to environmental chemicals such as lead
4. Viral infections
5. Metabolic imbalance
6. Lack of oxygen

Scientists believe that both genetics and environment likely play a role in ASD, with occasionally non- genetic causes as well [4]. ASD can be associated with intellectual disability of various degree, dysmorphic features, malformations and epilepsy [5]. Imaging studies of people with ASD have found differences in the development of several regions of the Brain. Studies suggest that ASD could be a result of disruptions in normal Brain growth early-on in development. These disruptions may be the result of defects in genes that control Brain development and regulate how Brain cells communicate with each other.

Environmental factors may also play a role in gene function and development, but no specific environmental cause has yet been identified. The theory that parental practices are responsible for ASD has long been disproved. Multiple studies have shown that vaccination to prevent childhood infectious diseases does not increase the risk of autism in the population. There have been questions regarding where multiple vaccines received in one setting may increase the risk for autism.

12.1.3 Typical Clinical Symptoms

Some children show signs of ASD in early infancy, other children may develop normally for the first few months or years of life, but then suddenly become withdrawn or aggressive or lose language skills that they had already acquired. Signs usually are seen by the age of 2 years old.

For many children, symptoms may improve with behavioural treatment. During adolescence, some children with ASD may become depressed or experience behavioural problems, and their treatment may need some modification as they transition to adulthood. People with ASD usually continue to need services and supports as they get older, but depending on the severity of the disorder, people with ASD may be able to work successfully and live solely independent or within a supportive environment.

Numerous studies indicate gastrointestinal (GI) problems are unusually common among people with autism. In a 2014 study based on almost 300,000 children in the United States, children with autism are 67 percent more likely than typical children to have a diagnosis of Inflammatory Bowel Disease IBD [6].

Because of the unique mixture of symptoms in each child, severity can sometimes be difficult to determine. It is generally based on the level of impairments and how IBD may impact their ability to function.

Common symptoms of autism spectrum disorder include:

1. Challenges in social communication and interaction

   - Gestures
   - Spoken language
   - Expressing emotions
   - Eye contact
   - Recognizing emotions and intentions in others
   - Recognizing one's own emotions
   - Recognizing sensory stimuli
   - Feeling overwhelmed in social situations

- Taking turns in conversation
- Gauging personal space

2. Restricted and repetitive behaviours

- Repetitive body movements
- Repetitive motions with objects
- Staring at lights or spinning objects
- Ritualistic behaviours
- Narrow or extreme interests in specific topics
- Need for unvarying routine/resistance to change

3. Gastro-intestinal symptoms

- Crohn's disease
- Ulcerative colitis
- Constipation
- Diarrheal

12.1.4 Diagnosis

Currently, ASD is included in the diagnostic category of a neurodevelopmental disorders in the Diagnostic and Statistical Manual of Mental Disorders V [7]. The two defining symptoms: social-communication and interaction, and restricted and repetitive interests/behaviours are historically seen as integrally related [8]. Many individuals with ASD have co-occurring gastrointestinal (GI) symptoms. These GI symptoms often coincide with problem behaviours and internalizing symptoms, which reduces the quality of life for these individuals [9].

Autism is also associated with various comorbidities, including sensory and motor abnormalities, sleep disturbance, epilepsy, attention deficit/hyperactivity disorder (ADHD)-like hyperactivity, intellectual disability, and mood disorders such as anxiety and aggression [10–12].

The most significant scientific challenge to the concept of autism as one "disease" or even "diseases" is the heterogeneity of the genetic findings [13] because many different genetic patterns associated with autism are also associated with numerous other psychological and psychiatric disorders [14]. Hope for understanding autism has pointed to genetic and neurobiological approaches but the lack of an "autistic gene" makes it hard to specify the genetic aetiologies for all individuals with autism. Predictions of the ability account for 30–40 percent [15] of cases of autism through identifiable genetic variation. From this point of view, behavioural diagnosis is considered valuable primarily as providing quantifiable measures that can be linked to potential biomarkers that provide objective, and biologically meaningful associations to underlying pathophysiological factors or other strong risk factors [16].

ASD is diagnosed by clinicians based on symptoms, signs, and testing according to the Diagnostic and Statistical Manual of Mental Disorders-V, a guide created by the American Psychiatric Association used to diagnose mental disorders. Children should be screened for developmental delays during periodic check-ups and specifically for autism at 18- and 24-month well-child visits.

These are the early behavioural indicators that require evaluation by an expert [17]:

- Have no babbling or pointing by age 1
- Have no single words by age 16 months or two-word phrases by age 2
- Have no response to name
- Loss of language or social skills previously acquired
- No eye contact or poor eye contact
- Excessive lining up of toys or objects
- Have no smiling or social responsiveness

Later indicators include:

- Impaired ability to make friends with peers
- Impaired ability to initiate or sustain a conversation with others
- Absence or impairment of imaginative and social play
- Repetitive or unusual use of language
- Abnormally intense or focused interest
- Preoccupation with certain objects or subjects
- Inflexible adherence to specific routines or rituals

High-Functioning Autism Spectrum
High-Functioning Autism spectrum are individuals that are abler, near normal, mildly autistic. However, research has shown that "high-functioning" is misleading, giving the illusion that the problems are mild and little support will be needed. They have similar problems as their lower-functioning peers. Sometimes confused with learning disabilities and emotional disturbances.

12.1.5 Modern Medicine Treatment, Possible Disadvantages

There are many different types of treatment for ASD, including medication management, education, rehabilitation training, sensory integration, and dietary approaches [18]. Since the early 1970s, Chinese medicine, in the form of scalp acupuncture made great stride in combining a modern understanding of neuroanatomy and neurophysiology with traditional techniques of Chinese acupuncture to develop a radical new tool for treating the functions of the central nervous system [19, p. 5].

Although there are no treatments for the core features of ASD, certain behavioral and medication therapies have been identified in Western medical practices for the management of hyperactivity, depression, inattention, obsessive-compulsive disorder (OCD), sleep disturbances, or seizures [20, 21]. Most health care professionals agree that the earlier the intervention the better.

The treatments a child can benefit from most depends on his situation and needs, but the goal is the same: to reduce his symptoms and improve his learning and development.

Intervention applicable to children with autism includes:

- Behaviour and Communication Therapy is used to develop social skills, combined with speech language and occupational therapy. This treatment uses highly structured and intensive skill-oriented training sessions to help children develop social and language skills, such as applied behavioural analysis, which encourages positive behaviours and discourages negative ones. In addition, family counselling for the parents and siblings of children with ASD often helps families cope with the particular challenges of living with a child with ASD [22].
- Dietary Approaches: Some dietary treatments have been developed by reliable therapists. But many of these treatments do not have the scientific support needed for widespread recommendation.
- Many biomedical interventions call for changes in diet. Such changes include removing certain types of foods from a child's diet and using vitamin or mineral supplements. Dietary treatments are based on the idea that food allergies or lack of vitamins and minerals cause symptoms of ASD. Some parents feel that dietary changes make a difference in how their child acts or feels [22].
- Cognitive Behavioural Therapy (CBT) aims to define the triggers of a particular behaviours, so that a child starts to recognize those moments himself. CBT helps with concerns common to autism, such as being overly fearful or anxious [23].
- Medical and pharmacologic intervention: While no medications can cure the core symptoms of ASD, some drugs approved by FDA are prescribed by doctors to address seizures, depression, obsessive-compulsive disorder, and disturbed sleep. Antipsychotic medications are used to treat severe behavioral problems [24]. Seizures can be treated with one or more anticonvulsant drugs. Medication used to treat people with attention deficit disorder can be used effectively to help decrease impulsivity and hyperactivity in people with ASD [25]. Drug treatments have largely been ineffective or less effective in subjects with ASDs than in those with the prototypical disorders. In addition, the tolerability of these drugs has been reduced in the subjects with ASDs. These results suggest that fundamental biological mechanisms may be quite different between disorders despite similarities in aspects of clinical presentation. Differences in response to drugs have also been identified across development in subjects with ASDs; the same has been observed with regarding to drug tolerability [26]. Parents, caregivers, and people with autism should use caution before adopting any unproven treatments.

The development of effective treatment methodology requires ongoing evaluation of the child's current strengths and needs and other factors relating to health.

12.2 TCM Understanding of Autism

Traditional Chinese medicine (TCM) interventions—There are creative and effective methods for helping children with ASD to develop appropriate social behaviours administered by traditional and alternative medical practitioners. In the area of TCM, the practice of neuro-acupuncture is a specialty that combines western study of neurology and Chinese scalp acupuncture. It has had great influence over the treatment and research of neurological disorders worldwide. The volume of research into herbal medicines, a form of Complementary and Alternative Medicine (CAM), shows fewer adverse effects, which has increased this treatment for children with ASD. Chinese herbal medicine have pharmacological effects, which mainly resulted in immune system improvement, memory enhancement, gastrointestinal tract improvement, and calming of the nerves [27, 28].

In Chinese medicine, reason and awareness, which are strongly affected by autism, are primarily ruled by three organ systems: Kidney, Heart, and Liver.

The Heart holds the Mind or Shen and rules the mental functions, including the emotional state of the individual and short-term memory. The heart is most important in governing the blood and housing the mind.

The Liver ensures the smooth flow of Qi. Its influence extends all over the body and to many different Ying and Yang organs. Liver helps the spleen to transform and transport food essences and the stomach to rot and ripen food. The Liver-Qi also helps Spleen-Qi to ascend and the Stomach-Qi to descend. Problems in the emotional life are by far the most important cause of Liver-Qi stagnation.

The Kidneys are the essence of energy that plays an extremely important role in human physiology, controlling the growth of bones in children, and normal Brain development. Kidney essence is the organic substance that forms the basis for growth, reproduction, and development. Kidney-Qi rules over long-term memory. A disturbance in these areas can lead to displays of any autism characteristic.

TCM identifies ASD to have the following basic clinical symptoms:

1. Social communication disorder
2. Developmental disorder in language and speech
3. Special behaviours
4. Different degrees of intelligence function

Theory in Chinese Medicine of Autism
In Chinese medicine, autism belongs to the category of "Brain disorder", relentlessness, implacability, inflexibility, rigidity, obstinacy.

In essence, Qi deficiency, Kidney deficiency, weak uterus.

Deficiency of Heart Qi and Blood, blockage of Heart orifice, not nourishing the Brain.

Liver Qi stagnation.

Slower to develop language, have no language at all, or have significant problems with understanding or using spoken language.

According to the ancient book, Yellow Emperor's Classic: "The Brain is the sea of essence. Acupoints reside as high as on top of the skull, and goes as low as on Feng Fu." Therefore, acupuncture points for Brain disorders are located on the scalp.

The Chinese Medicine's Concept of Brain Function
Brain controls the essence and the intelligence of human being
The Brain controls memory, thought process, and cognition.
The Brain controls mobility and the senses.
The Brain self regulates and controls all body functions, balances the physical and psychological wellbeing.
The Brain commands the wholeness of the spirit of a human being.

12.3 General Acupuncture Treatment

Body acupuncture has been used in the treatment and prevention of disorders for over 2000 years. Acupuncture has been used in the treatment and prevention of disorders for over 2000 years. In order to make a treatment plan based on acupuncture, a doctor will need to make a diagnosis based on four components: inspection, auscultation, inquiry, and palpation.

Acupuncture has been used for the treatment of ASD. The basic theory of acupuncture starts with the meridian system and flow of energy, or Qi. There are 12 regular and eight supplemental meridians that run either longitudinally along the body surface or from the interior to the exterior of the body to the surface of the body. Meridians connect the Zangfu organs to each other and to the surface of the body [29].

Acupuncture Treatment for autism symptom disorders can be grouped into the following modalities.

12.3.1 Body Acupuncture Principle

A. Aim and Treatment Principles

- Dredging the channel
- Circulating Qi and Blood
- Adjusting Yin and Yan

B. Indications

- Language disorders
- Social communication disorders.
- Emotional disorders.

C. Principles of Compatibility of Points

- Deficiency of Kidney be treated with acupuncture mainly by tonifying method.
- Liver Qi stagnation be treated with acupuncture by method of relieving Liver and soothing Qi.

- Heat in the Heart and Liver be treated with clearing the Fire of Heart and Liver.
- Insufficiency of Heart and Spleen be treated with tonifying Spleen, tranquilizing mind, and nourishing Heart.

12.3.2   Body Acupuncture Points

Chinese medicine believes that the head is the meeting area of all Yang meridians. Hence, scalp acupuncture is specifically effective for Brain diseases.

Treatment Principle and Point Selection for adults:

- In case of adults, the initial treatment is done with scalp acupuncture, followed by ear and body acupuncture, depending on the major symptom, usually within the same session.

Scalp acupuncture area selection on adult patient is similar to points selections on children. However, the body acupuncture points selection on adult patient is as shown as below:

- Deficiency of Kidney Essence and Liver Yin deficiency: KI-3 Taixi, KI-7 Fuliu, ST-36 Zusanli, Ex-Yintang.
- Liver Qi stagnation: LV-3 Taichong, SP-6 Sanyinjiao.
- Heat in the Heart and Liver: PC-6 Neiguan, LI-11 Quchi.
- Insufficiency of Heart and Spleen Qi: PC-6 Neiguan, SJ-5 Waiguan.
- Damp-heat pattern: SI-3 Houxi, BL-62 Shenmai, LI-4 Hegu, GB-41 Zulinqi.

12.3.3   Auricle Acupuncture

Commonly use ear acupuncture point Shenmen for calming.

12.4   Unique Brain Acupuncture Techniques

Chinese medical theory can be traced back to 100 BCE, the classical medical text, Huang Di Nei Jing: The Yellow Emperor's Classic of Internal Medicine, which described the relationship between the Brain and the body in physiology, pathology, and treatment as it was understood at that time, and citation of acupuncture on the head can be found throughout classical Chinese literature [30, p. 72, 77, 428].

Scalp acupuncture is a well-documented in natural science and incorporates extensive knowledge of both the past and present, years of clinical experience has contributed to its recent discoveries and developments. Scalp acupuncture has 50 years of history, it often produces remarkable results with just a few needles and usually brings about immediate improvement, sometimes taking only several seconds to a minute. The central nervous system (CNS) functions as the computer for the body. Messages from the CNS control all aspects of learning, thinking, and movement that allows us to learn about the function in the world.

Autism is a syndrome, or condition, with many possible causes, anything that makes the CNS develop abnormally can cause autism. The result of scalp acupuncture has rendered great improvement in clinical and research settings.

Several pioneers in scalp acupuncture history, including Drs. Fang-S, Tang-S, and Zhu-S created special therapeutic bands on the scalps. These scalp locations are formulated by penetrating several regular head points.

Internationally recognized as the modern founder of scalp-acupuncture, Dr. Shun-Fa Jiao, systematically undertook the scientific exploration and charting of scalp acupuncture modality and efficacy. He later combined the understanding of neuroanatomy and neurophysiology with traditional techniques of Chinese acupuncture to develop a radical new tool for affecting the functions of the central nervous system.

This technique differs from the conventional one needle to one single point placement; instead, scalp acupuncture needles are subcutaneously inserted into whole section of various zones, through which the functions of the central nervous system, endocrine system, and channels are transported to and from the surface of the scalp. From a Western perspective, these zones correspond to the cortical areas of the cerebrum and cerebellum responsible for central nervous system functions such as motor activity, sensory input, vision, hearing, and balance.

Scalp acupuncture areas are frequently used in the rehabilitation of paralysis due to stroke, multiple sclerosis, automobile accident, and Parkinson's disease. These areas may also be effectively employed for pain management, especially those caused by the central nervous system such as phantom pain, complex regional pain, and residual limb pain.

Dr. Linda Hao started treating children with neurological and Brain disorders by using scalp acupuncture over 25 years ago in the United States. She developed the theory 5-Rs of treatment for neurological disorders in children with difficult and complex neurological issues. The method is a result of many years of teaching and practice. From her experience, the mechanisms can be refined into the following: Repair, Remap, Rewire, Reprogram, and Reset. Starting with Repair, the orders of the 5-Rs steps do not need to be in the exact order, it depends on the patient's Brain functions and progress [31].

12.4.1   Scalp Acupuncture Principle and Treatment

Chinese scalp acupuncture is a contemporary acupuncture technique integrating traditional Chinese needling methods with Western medical knowledge of representative area of the cerebral cortex. It has been proven to be the most effective technique for treating acute and chronic centre nervous system disorders. Scalp acupuncture, also called Neuro-acupuncture, is a modern innovation and development. The nervous system is the most complex system in the body. The scalp is the softer tissue envelope of the cranial vault. It extends from the superior nuchal line on the posterior area of the supraorbital margins [32].

Commonly Used Scalp Acupuncture Areas

- Motor Area
- Sensory Area
- Speech I Area
- Speech III Area
- Balance Area
- Chorea and Tremor Area
- Head Area
- Vertigo and Hearing Area
- Foot Motor & Sensory Area
- Auricular Acupuncture
- Body Acupuncture

Due to its proven efficacy, scalp acupuncture is the highly recommended needling method for children. The established pattern, by Dr. Linda Hao, are enumerated as followed.

12.4.2 Clinical Procedures of Scalp Acupuncture

Use disposable and sterilized stainless needles of 0.18–0.30 mm diameter. The size of Chinese needles is number 32 (0.25 mm) to number 36 (0.20 mm). For children, generally, needle # 34 (0.22 mm) is inserted alone. Insert needles at a 15- to 25-degree angle and 1 to 2 inches in depth. Each treatment uses 4 to 5 needles for most common symptoms. Needles inserted do not need stimulation.

Ideal position for scalp acupuncture treating is sitting.

12.4.3 Treatment Principle and Selection Areas with Children

- 4.3.1 If child has aphasia who is diagnosed with genetic disorders, often combined with no eye contact: Head Area, Foot Motor & Sensory Area, Speech I Area, 5 points in total.

- 4.3.2 If child has limited speech ability, speaking only words without completing a sentence: Motor Area, Speech I Area, 4 points in total.
- 4.3.3 If child has problems in acquiring knowledge and understanding, attention, memory, and reasoning: Modifying 4.3.1, add DU-20 Baihui.
- 4.3.4. If child has problems with communication and social interaction problems: Modifying 4.3.1, add Ex-Sishenchong.
- 4.3.5 If child has motor issue, walking, running, balance issues: Modifying 4.3.2, add Balance Area.
- 4.3.6 If child has sleep and digestive issues: Modifying 4.3.3, add Ex-Yintang and Stomach Area.
- 4.3.7 If child has emotional problems: Apply 4.3.3 and 4.3.4, plus or minus.

12.4.4   Unique Features of Scalp-Acupuncture for Children

Compared to the regular acupuncture techniques, scalp-acupuncture for children has its unique features such as: short needles, thin needles, less needles, quick insertion, light stimulation, no stimulation, short retention, mobility during needling, et al.

12.4.5   Keys to Working with Children Successfully

Compared to adult patients, children patients often have special needs. To be successful when communicating, we need to be able to build relationships, taking into consideration their age, psychological and emotional conditions to attend to their needs. Based on many years of clinical experience, the following key points are followed to work with children successfully:

- knowledgeable, skilful, compassionate, loving, fervent, patient, thorough, empathetic, attentive, appreciative, concentrated, credible and honest.

12.5   Research

There have been a wide variety of techniques and treatment protocols used in the treatment of ASD. Our research focuses on integrating Chinese medical concepts and diagnostic parameters for their usefulness and relevancy in treating neurological diseases.

We followed the success of Dr. Linda Hao who developed and established the specialty in treating neurological disorders utilizing scalp acupuncture. Her teaching, research, and practice in the field of scalp-acupuncture contributed much to the world of acupuncture that impacts people worldwide.

Considerable clinical evidence showed scalp acupuncture to be most commonly used to treat Brain and neurological disorders including Autism syndromes, cerebral palsy, paralysis, stroke, Parkinson's, multiple sclerosis, traumatic Brain injury, post-traumatic stress disorder, chorea, attention deficit hyperactivity disorder, Down syndrome, coma, and Alzheimer's disease. Scalp acupuncture is used for post-stroke and Brain surgery therapy. The speed and amount of recovery vary with the individual and the severity of damage, but progress is usually readily seen with treatment. Long-term conditions and expectations need to be realistic, although some patients will occasionally surprise practitioners. Scalp acupuncture has the best and fastest response [32].

12.6 Conclusion

Acupuncture is frequently used to treat a variety of disorders including those with neurological dysfunction. Chinese scalp acupuncture has greatly enhanced the practice of acupuncture in the last 45 years. Worldwide, there is increased recognition of acupuncture as a treatment modality. Evidence with recent discovery that patients can recover from Brain damage even decades after the trauma, in contrast to the common assumption that only immediate treatment would be effective.

There is a great need, and a great challenge to find the most effective treatment for children with neurological disorders. Evidences for the efficacy and safety of scalp acupuncture in children with ASD has been proven in clinical experiences and studies.

Scalp acupuncture is an extremely effective methodology for treatment, which often produces remarkable even surprising results with just a few needles and usually brings about immediate improvement. There is a pressing need for Chinese scalp acupuncture to be studied and perfected using modern research methods, to further enhance the practice and development so that its potential can be fully explored and applied.

References

1. Kanner L. Autistic disturbances of affective contact. J Psychopathol Psychother Mental Hyg Guid Child. 1943;2:217–50.
2. Gilbert C, Wahlström J. Chromosome abnormalities in infantile autism and other childhood psychoses. A population study of 66 cases. Dev Med Child Neurol. 1985;27:293–304.
3. Wahlström J, Gilbert C, Gustavsson KG, et al. Infantile autism and the Fragile-X-syndrome. A Swedish population multicenter study. Am J Med Genet. 1986;23:403–8.
4. Muhle R, Trentacoste SV, Rapin I. The genetics of autism. Pediatrics. 2004;113:e472–86.
5. Robert C, Pasquier L, Cohen D, et al. Role of genetics in the aetiology of autistic spectrum disorder: towards a hierarchical diagnostic strategy. Int J Mol Sci. 2017;18:618. https://doi.org/10.3390/ijms18030618.

6. Nylund CM, Eide M, Gorman GH. Association of *clostridium difficile* infections with acid suppression medications in children. J Pediatr. 2014;165(5):979–84.
7. Grzadzinski R, Huerta M, Lord C. DSM-5 and autism spectrum disorders (ASDs): an opportunity for identifying ASD subtypes. Mol Autism. 2013;4:12. https://doi.org/10.1186/2040-2392-4-12.
8. Fein D, Helt M. Facilitating autism research. J Int Neuropsychol Soc. 2017;23:903–15.
9. Ferguson BJ, Dovgan K, Takahashi N, et al. The relationship among gastrointestinal symptoms, problem behaviors, and internalizing symptoms in children and adolescents with autism spectrum disorder. Front Psych. 2019;10:194. https://doi.org/10.3389/fpsyt.2019.00194.
10. Goldstein S, Schwebach AJ. The comorbidity of pervasive developmental disorder and attention deficit hyperactivity disorder: results of a retrospective chart review. J Autism Dev Disord. 2004;34:329–39.
11. Simonoff E, Pickles A, Charman T, et al. Psychiatric disorders in children with autism spectrum disorders: prevalence, comorbidity, and associated factors in a population-derived sample. J Am Acad Child Adolesc Psychiatry. 2008;47:921–9.
12. Geschwind DH. Advances in autism. Annu Rev Med. 2009;60:367–80.
13. Veenstra-Vanderweele J, Christian SL, Cook EH. Autism as a paradigmatic complex genetic disorder. Annu Rev Genomics Hum Genet. 2004;5:379–405.
14. Guilmatre A, Dubourg C, Mosca AL, et al. Recurrent rearrangements in synaptic and neurodevelopmental genes and shared biologic pathways in schizophrenia, autism, and mental retardation. Arch Gen Psychiatry. 2009;66(9):947–56.
15. Geschwind DHG. Autism genetics and genomics: brief overview and synthesis. In: Amaral DG, et al., editors. Autism spectrum disorders. Oxford: Oxford University Press; 2011. p. 812–24.
16. Lee H, Marvin AR, Watson T, et al. Accuracy of phenotyping of autistic children based on internet implemented parent report. Am J Med Genet B Neuropsychiatric Genet. 2010;153(6):1119–26.
17. National Institute of Neurological Disorders and Stroke. Autism spectrum disorders fact sheet. National Institutes of Health. 2019. https://www.ninds.nih.gov/disorders/patient-caregiver-education/fact-sheets/autism-spectrum-disorder-fact-sheet. Accessed 26 Apr 2020
18. Bang MR, Lee SH, Cho SH, et al. Herbal medicine treatment for children with autism spectrum disorder: a systematic review. Evid Based Complement Alternat Med. 2017; https://doi.org/10.1155/2017/8614680.
19. Hao JJ, Hao LL. Chinese scalp acupuncture. Boulder, CO: Blue Poppy Press; 2011.
20. Wink LK, Erickson CA, McDougle CJ. Pharmacologic treatment of behavioural symptoms associated with autism and other pervasive developmental disorders. Curr Treat Options Neurol. 2010;12:529–38.
21. Accordino RE, Kidd C, Politte LC, et al. Psychopharmacological interventions in autism spectrum disorder. Expert Opin Pharmacother. 2016;17(7):937–52.
22. Centre for Disease Control and Prevention. Treatment for autism spectrum disorders. 2019. https://www.cdc.gov/ncbddd/autism/treatment.html. Accessed 26 Apr 2020.
23. O'Rourke-Lang C, Mark B. Which behaviour therapy works best for children with autism? Attitude's ADHD Med Rev. January 20, 2020. https://www.additudemag.com/which-behavior-therapy-works-best/. Accessed 26 Apr 2020.
24. Nazeer A. Psychopharmacology of autistic spectrum disorders in children and adolescents. Pediatr Clin N Am. 2011;58(1):85–97.
25. LeClerc S, Easley D. Pharmacological therapies for autism spectrum disorder: a review. P T. 2015;40(6):389–97.
26. Doyle CA, McDougle CJ. Pharmacologic treatments for the behavioural symptoms associated with autism spectrum disorders across the lifespan. Dialogues Clin Neurosci. 2012;14(3):263–79.
27. Cai JL, Lu JQ, Lu G, et al. Autism spectrum disorder related TCM symptoms and TCM herbs prescriptions: a systematic review and meta-analysis. N Am J Med Sci. 2015;8(1):20–30.

28. Lee MS, Choi TY, Shin BC, et al. Acupuncture for children with autism spectrum disorders: a systematic review of randomized clinical trials. J Autism Dev Disord. 2012;42(8):1671–83.
29. Ming X, Chen X, Wang XT, et al. Acupuncture for treatment of autism spectrum disorders. Evid Based Complement Alternat Med. 2012; https://doi.org/10.1155/2012/679845.
30. Maciocia G. The foundations of Chinese medicine: a comprehensive text for acupuncturists and herbalists. 2nd ed. London and New York: Churchill Livingstone; 1989.
31. Bennett M. The point of hope: Journal North Reporter. Albuquerque J. 3 February 2019. www.abqjournal.com/1276344/the-point-of-hope-ex-neuroacupuncture-is-giving-patients-new-freedoms.html. Accessed 26 April 2020.
32. Hao JJ, Hao LL. Review of clinical applications of scalp acupuncture for paralysis: an excerpt from Chinese scalp acupuncture. Glob Adv Health Med. 2012;1(1):102–21.

Chapter 13
Cerebral Palsy

13.1 General Information of Cerebral Palsy

13.1.1 Basic Background

Cerebral palsy (CP) is a group of disorders that affect a person's ability to move and maintain balance and posture. CP is the most common motor disability in childhood [1]. The condition of CP was first described by William Little in 1861 [2]. The term 'cerebral palsics' was first coined by William Osler [3, p. 103]. In the 2007 consensus definition, the term 'cerebral palsy' was defined as "a group of permanent disorders of the development of movement and posture, causing activity limitation, that are attributed to non-progressive disturbances that occurred in the developing fetal or infant Brain" [4]. The proposition of "cerebral palsy spectrum disorder" now suggested as a more accurate and beneficial term [5].

Epidemiological studies have found that the global prevalence of CP is 1.5–4 per 1000 live births, and the prevalence is higher in poor areas. As an incurable illness, CP not only brings significant economic burdens to families, but the disease if also associated with additional psychological problems. Compared to healthy individuals, CP is associated with a higher frequency of autism spectrum disorders, sclerotic deformity, and the incidence of fractures [6].

Cerebral palsy is a lifelong condition attributed to a non-progressive disturbance that occurs in the developing fetal or infant Brain [7]. The disorder can occur at any time during pregnancy, delivery, or the first 3–5 years of age [8]. Cerebral palsy results from Brain malformation that arises early in life and subsequently interferes with normal motor development [9]. Cerebral palsy may be accompanied by disturbances in sensation, cognition, communication, perception, and behaviour, as well as seizure disorder [10]. Due to the motor dysfunction present, children with CP show restricted activities of daily living (ADL) and social participation, which greatly influence the quality of life (QoL) and their ability to adapt to society [11].

© Springer Nature Switzerland AG 2021 179
T. Wang, *Acupuncture for Brain*, https://doi.org/10.1007/978-3-030-54666-3_13

Based on the CDC data in 2008, CP was more common among boys than among girls [1]. Most (77.4%) of the children identified with CP had spastic CP. Many of the children with CP also had at least one co-occurring condition—41% had co-occurring epilepsy and 6.9% had co-occurring ASD [1].

The prevalence of CP has a modest increase in the last two decades of the twentieth century owing largely to the greatly increased survival of very premature infants as a result of the success of the new technology [12]. Cerebral palsy is not a disease entity in the traditional sense but a clinical description of children who share features of a non-progressive Brain injury or lesion acquired during the antenatal, perinatal or early postnatal period [13].

13.1.2   The Aetiology and Pathogenesis

CP is caused by abnormal development of the Brain or damage to the developing Brain that affects a child's ability to control his or her muscles. There are several possible causes of the abnormal development or damage. People used to think that CP was mainly caused by lack of oxygen during the birth process. Now, scientists think that this causes only a small number of CP cases [1].

The Brain damage that leads to CP can happen before birth, during birth, within a month after birth, or during the first years of a child's life, or even the first 3–5 years of age [8] while the Brain is still developing. CP related to Brain damage that occurred before or during birth is called congenital CP. The majority of CP (85%–90%) is congenital. In many cases, the specific cause is not known. A small percentage of CP is caused by Brain damage that occurs more than 28 days after birth. This is called acquired CP, and usually is associated with an infection (such as meningitis) or head injury. There are several risk factors, such as low birthweight and premature birth, disruption of blood and oxygen supply to the developing Brain, and infection among mothers [1]. But the exact cause is still unclear [12], they overlap and interact with each other in ways that are not easy to dissect [14].

13.1.3   Typical Clinical Symptoms

Cerebral palsy mainly affects how the Brain controls muscles and movement. Sometimes it can also affect other ways the Brain works, such as how we see, hear, communicate, feel, understand and think. The Brain can't send messages to different parts of the body properly, and this causes problems with things like balance, movement and coordination, talking, chewing and swallowing. Everyone with cerebral palsy is affected differently – symptoms vary widely and the effects can range from minor problems to severe disability. Around 1 in 3 children with cerebral palsy have epilepsy [15].

All people with CP have problems with movement and posture. Many also have related conditions such as intellectual disability, seizures; problems with vision, hearing, or speech; changes in the spine (such as scoliosis); or joint problems (such as contractures) [1].

Types of Cerebral Palsy [1]

CP could be classified according to the main type of movement disorder involved. Depending on which areas of the Brain are affected, one or more of the following movement disorders can occur, stiff muscles (spasticity), uncontrollable movements (dyskinesia) or poor balance and coordination (ataxia).

There are four main types of CP: Spastic Cerebral Palsy, Dyskinetic Cerebral Palsy, Ataxic Cerebral Palsy, Mixed Cerebral Palsy.

13.1.3.1   Spastic Cerebral Palsy

The most common type of CP is spastic CP. Spastic CP affects about 80% of people with CP.

People with spastic CP have increased muscle tone. This means their muscles are stiff and, as a result, their movements can be awkward. Spastic CP usually is described by what parts of the body are affected.

13.1.3.2   Dyskinetic Cerebral Palsy

Also includes athetoid, choreoathetoid, and dystonic cerebral palsies.

People with dyskinetic CP have problems controlling the movement of their hands, arms, feet, and legs, making it difficult to sit and walk. The movements are uncontrollable and can be slow and writhing or rapid and jerky. Sometimes the face and tongue are affected and the person has a hard time sucking, swallowing, and talking. A person with dyskinetic CP has muscle tone that can change (varying from too tight to too loose) not only from day to day, but even during a single day.

13.1.3.3   Ataxic Cerebral Palsy

People with ataxic CP have problems with balance and coordination. They might be unsteady when they walk. They might have a hard time with quick movements or movements that need a lot of control, like writing. They might have a hard time controlling their hands or arms when they reach for something.

13.1.3.4   Mixed Cerebral Palsy

Some people have symptoms of more than one type of CP. The most common type of mixed CP is spastic-dyskinetic CP.

There are some early signs may be noticed by parents and in their child as they develop. Below are some examples [15].

- Unusual movements as a baby
- Lmbs seem either too floppy or too stiff

- Difficulties with feeding
- Late in sitting (after 8 months) or walking (after 18 months)
- Use 1 hand more than the other before they are 12 months' old
- Often walk on tip-toes.

Patients, children and adult, with CP may also suffer learning disabilities, behavioural problems, and attention deficit hyperactivity disorder, etc. [16].

13.1.4   Examination and Diagnosis

CP may be formally diagnosed and classified following a complete history and neurological examination. Severity is variable depending on the affected limbs, the degree of movement impairment, speech problems, balance and other symptoms [7].

There are several groups of CP. Spastic cerebral palsy is characterized by a combination of tight, stiff, and weak muscles, making control of movement difficult. It is the most common type of cerebral palsy, accounting for 70% of affected children. It can be further subcategorized into diplegia, characterized primarily by involvement of the lower limbs; quadriplegia, in which all four limbs are affected; and hemiplegia, in which the limbs on one side of the body are affected [17].

Diagnosing CP at an early age is important to the well-being of children and their families. Diagnosing CP can take several steps [1].

Developmental Monitoring
Developmental monitoring (also called surveillance) means tracking a child's growth and development over time. If any concerns about the child's development are raised during monitoring, then a developmental screening test should be given as soon as possible.

Developmental Screening
During developmental screening a short test is given to see if the child has specific developmental delays, such as motor or movement delays. If the results of the screening test are cause for concern, then the doctor will make referrals for developmental and medical evaluations.

Developmental and Medical Evaluations
The goal of a developmental evaluation is to diagnose the specific type of disorder that affects a child.

For the clinical observation and study, the Gross Motor Function Measure-66 (GMFM-66) and Fine Motor Function Measure (FMFM) are commonly used to measure change over time or following interventions [18].

Unfortunately, there are several barriers for recognize CP, which include: (a) a lack of definitive biomarkers; (b) uneasiness about false positives; (c) the difficult conversation of giving the diagnosis and the resultant grief and perceived stigma; (d) the desire to rule out the differential diagnosis of every treatable condition first; (e) the lack of curative treatments and evidence for early interventions; and (f) making a diagnosis when faced with a lack of definitive signs on traditional clinical examination [19].

13.1.5   The Treatment of CP with Modern Medicine

Although there is no cure for CP, treatment and support can be given to help children and young people cope with their symptoms and become as independent as possible [15]. Children with CP and their families seek multiple forms of therapy, particularly those that have the potential to improve the way in which the children function or feel [20]. Various therapies have been found to improve activities of daily living (ADL). These include physical therapy and occupational therapy, as well as speech and language therapy. Surgical approaches for treatment of spastic cerebral palsy also exist, these include orthopedic surgery and selective posterior rhizotomy (cutting of a spinal nerve root) [7].

No single treatment is the best one for all children with CP. Before deciding on a treatment plan, it is important to talk with the child's doctor to understand all the risks and benefits [1].

Safer and more effective interventions have been invented for children with cerebral palsy in the last decade, as a consequence of an exponential growth in high-quality cerebral palsy research, including prevention research and the discovery of activity-based rehabilitation interventions that induce neuroplasticity [21].

13.2   TCM Understanding of CP

According to the signs and symptoms, in traditional Chinese medicine (TCM), CP is equivalent to "Wu Chi (Five delayed developments)", "Wu Ruan (Five Softs)", "Wu Ying (Five stiffness)" and "Wei Zheng (Paralysis)", et al. Mostly due to insufficient innate endowment, or acquired less or Brain injury, et al.

The commonly used TCM therapies for CP are acupuncture, Chinese herbal medicine and Tuina massage.

13.3   General Acupuncture Treatment for CP

In China, acupuncture has been widely used as a treatment for children with CP in combination with the standard conventional treatment, showing promising effectiveness in improving clinical symptoms, such as drooling, sleep, bowel function, spasm, motor function and daily life activities [11]. In western countries, acupuncture has increasing being integrated into paediatric health care, including CP. Although the actual mechanisms of acupuncture are still unknown, TCM acupuncture theory believes that health is achieved by maintaining an uninterrupted flow of Qi. Qi flows through a network of 14 channels, called "meridians", which run along the surface of the human body. There are nearly 400 acupuncture points (acupoints) on the body surface, which linked through the 14 meridians to various organs or viscera. By stimulating various meridian points, acupuncture is thought to correct the imbalance of energy in the body and restore natural internal homeostasis [22].

According to the TCM theory about CP classifications, the principle of general acupuncture treatment would be followed the pattern identification. As usual below patterns, symptoms and signs, and the points selection, are just sample suggestions. Clinic practice should follow the real individual patient.

13.3.1   Insufficient of Kidney and Marrow

Signs and symptoms (SS): Low intelligent, reflected sluggishness, limb paralysis with thin and unused, stunted development, delayed fontanel closure, unclear speech, delayed movement development, difficulty raising head and sitting. Light red tongue, thin and weak pulse.

Points selection: BL-23 Shenshu, KI-1 Yongquan, GB-39 Xuanzhong (Juegu), ST-36 Zusanli, plus local area points.

13.3.2   Yin Deficiency and Wind Movement

SS: Paralysis of the limbs, forced or stiff neck, slow movements of hands and feet, foot spasms, unstable foot movements, eye and face restraints, unfavourable speech, and seizures. Red tongue, thin and fast pulse.

Points selection: BL-18 Ganshu, BL-23 Shenshu, GB-20 Fengchi, LI-4 Hegu, ST-36 Zusanli, plus local area points.

13.3.3   Spleen Qi Deficiency

SS: Fatigue, paralysis of the limbs, lazy speech, weak chewing, drooling, tongue often extension, poor appetite, abdominal distension, loose stool. Light tongue, thin and weak pulse.

Points selection: BL-20 Pishu, BL-21 Weishu, DU-20 Baihui, ST-36 Zusanli, SP-6 Sanyinjiao, SP-9 Yinlingquan, plus local area points.

13.3.4   Stagnation of Internal Blood

SS: Paralysis of the limbs, mental retardation, thinning hair, exposed blue vessel, cold limbs. Purple tongue, thin pulse.

Points selection: BL-17 Geshu, BL-18 Ganshu, DU-20 Baihui, DU-14 Dazhui, LI-4 Hegu, ST-36 Zusanli, plus local area points.

Above pattern identifications may be separate used with general needling, or combined with below unique Brain acupuncture techniques.

13.4   Unique Brain Acupuncture Techniques for CP

Above traditionally general acupuncture treatment for CP has been widely practiced and still often practice in most acupuncture clinics. In the last a few decades, with the development of TCM Brain theory, it is believed that TCM Brain has played a unique role of CP, on its ethology, pathology, and treatment strategy. It is believed that the internal and external pathological factors, cause Brain channels stagnation, Brain Yin and Yang imbalance, may lead to damage of Brain marrow and result of CP. The major organ location of CP is no doubt in the Brain, and involved other Zangfu organs such as Kidney, Liver, Spleen, et al.

In terms of the unique acupuncture treatment, due to the Brain is the main location of disease, the treatment principle will be more focus on the rebalance the Brain and regulating Du Mai. Thus scalp acupuncture and Du Mai Dao-qi technique are mostly used in acupuncture practice for CP. Tongue acupuncture is another unique treatment for cerebral palsy [23].

Chinese scalp acupuncture is a microsystem technique in which the acupuncture needle is inserted into various areas of the scalp. Specific manipulations of the needle are conducted to regulate and strengthen various functional activities of the Brain and body.

Within the scalp acupuncture stimulation areas, the Motor Area of Jiao's scalp acupuncture is mostly choice in scalp acupuncture for the treatment of motor dysfunction in CP. Jiao's scalp acupuncture combines a modern understanding of neuroanatomy and neurophysiology with traditional techniques of Chinese acupuncture to develop a radical new tool for affecting the functions of the central nervous system and accepts a central theory that incorporates Brain functions into Chinese medicine principles [24]. The Motor Area of Jiao's scalp acupuncture specifically used for the treatment of motor dysfunction in CP is the equivalent of the precentral gyrus of the cerebral cortex used for scalp projection [7]. In addition, Scalp acupuncture therapy does not increase the risk of onset or epileptiform discharges in the children with cerebral palsy combined with epilepsy or epileptiform discharges. Scalp acupuncture combined with rehabilitation is better than simple rehabilitation for those with cerebral palsy and epilepsy onset [25].

13.4.1   Scalp acupuncture for Treating CP (Detail of Scalp Acupuncture, Location and Needling, Please See Chap. 5)

- Hemiplegia: Opposite upper 1/5 and middle 2/5 of Motor Area and Foot-Motor Sensory Area.
- Motor aphasia: first Speech Area
- Ataxia: Balance Area

13.4.2   Du Mai Dao-Qi Techniques (Detail of Dao-Qi Technique on Du Mai, Points Location and Needling, Please See Chap. 6)

- DU-20 Baihui, DU-16 Fengfu, DU-15 Yamen, DU-14 Dazhui, DU-9 Zhiyang, DU-4 Mingmen, DU-3 Yaoyangguan

13.4.3   Ren Mai Dao-Qi Technique (Detail of Dao-Qi Technique on Ren Mai, Points Location and Needling, Please See Chap. 6)

- REN-12 Zhongwan plus 2–4 needles around it with 0.5–1 cm distance, REN-10 Xiawan, REN-6 Qihai, REN-4 Guanyuan, REN-17 Dangzhong and REN-23 Lianquan.

Above unique Brain acupuncture techniques can be combined with syndrome differentiation treatment.

13.4.4   Brain Pattern Differentiation

The commonly clinical Brain patterns of CP and its possible symptoms could be summary as below and they are on the way for developing and not perfect at the moment.

13.4.4.1   Deficiency of Brain Marrow

SS: Mental retardation, reflected sluggishness, limb paralysis with thin and unused, slow development, delayed fontanel closure, slurred speech, delayed movement development, difficulty raising head and sitting. Light red tongue, thin and weak pulse.

Scalp acupuncture areas: Motor Area, Foot Motor-Sensory Area, Balance Area, etc.

Brain acupuncture points selection: DU-20 Baihui, DU-14 Dazhui, DU-24 Shenting, DU-4 Mingmen, KI-3 Taixi, GB-39 Xuanzhong, and local area points. Techniques could choose electric-acupuncture, Dao-qi technique, etc.

13.4.4.2   Deficiency of Brain Yang Qi

SS: Paralysis of the limbs with cold, low intelligent, easy tired, lazy speech, weak chewing with drooling, tongue often extension, poor appetite, loose stool. Light tongue, thin and weak pulse.

Scalp acupuncture areas: Motor Area, Foot Motor-Sensory Area, Central Area, etc.

Brain acupuncture points selection: DU-20 Baihui, DU-16 Fengfu, DU-14 Dazhui, DU-9 Zhiyang, DU-4 Mingmen, DU-3 Yaoyangguan, REN-12 Zhongwan, REN-10 Xiawan, REN-6 Qihai, REN-4 Guanyuan, plus local suffered area points. Moxa could be applied. Dao-qi technique on 1–2 key points may be added.

13.4.4.3 Stagnation of Brain Collaterals

SS: Paralysis of the limbs, mental retardation, thinning hair, exposed blue vein on face and head, neck stiffness. Purple tongue, thin pulse.

Scalp acupuncture areas: Motor Area, Foot Motor-Sensory Area, Vasomotor Area, etc.

Brain acupuncture points selection: DU-20 Baihui, DU-16 Fengfu, DU-14 Dazhui, DU-9 Zhiyang, DU-3 Yaoyangguan, REN-12 Zhongwan, REN-10 Xiawan, REN-6 Qihai, plus local suffered area points. Moxa could be applied. Dao-qi technique on 1–2 key points may be added.

Notes

*For treatment CP, the early involved the better results. Even before formally diagnosed of CP acupuncture may start earlier for some CP related symptoms.

*The treatment frequency: in the early stage, the often the better. In western countries, suggest start with twice per week, then with time, move slow down to once per week followed by once in 2–4 weeks for maintenance. If in some areas and some occasions, possible start with every day.

*Acupuncture can be combined with routine therapy such as physiotherapy, speech therapy, etc.

*Above Brain related patterns for CP can be identified separately, and combined with classic TCM pattern identifications.

*Scalp acupuncture, compared with other body acupuncture, is more convenience for children, including CP. It can be remaining 20–30 min without any attention for children, as they can watch interesting movies, play in ground, etc.

13.5 Research

Acupuncture-cantered rehabilitation as part of a unified treatment plan including conventional therapies has been proposed as an appropriate strategy for overcoming disability associated with cerebral palsy. This remains the main method practiced in both top-grade hospitals and national research institutes in China. Acupuncture has been found to improve motor activity, sensation, speech, and other neurological functions in children with cerebral palsy [7]. Several systematic reviews have shown acupuncture to be clinically effective in children with cerebral palsy [22].

A recently meta-analysis [3], included 21 studies and 1718 children with CP, found that the pooled effect size showed positive results for improvements in GMF FMF, MAS, ADL, and total effective rate. No serious adverse events related to acupuncture were confirmed. The present meta-analysis supports acupuncture for children with cerebral palsy as a potentially beneficial alternative and complementary therapy in the domain of modern western medicine. Thus, acupuncture may have benefits in both practical and research settings as an alternative and complementary therapy. In addition, most of the studies were conducted by Chinese researchers. Only one study [26], use laser acupuncture as an adjunctive therapy for spastic cerebral palsy in children, was conducted by non-Chinese researchers [7].

Scalp acupuncture is an important means of rehabilitation of cerebral palsy in traditional Chinese medicine. It is a contemporary acupuncture technique integrating traditional Chinese needling methods with Western medical knowledge of representative areas of the cerebral cortex [12, 25, 27].

Motor dysfunction is the most significant clinical symptom in children with CP. The upper 1/5 and middle 2/5 regions of the motor area on the scalp were selected as the primary areas for scalp acupuncture stimulation while taking into account the motor dysfunction typically seen in CP [11].

Scalp acupuncture combined with exercise therapy and conventional rehabilitation training can significantly improve gross motor function and the ability to perform ADLs (activities of daily living) in children with spastic cerebral palsy compared to conventional rehabilitation training alone. Systematic reviews show that acupuncture is a safe intervention for pediatric patients, and no severe side effects, including CP [6].

For investigate the risk of epilepsy onset by scalp acupuncture, a recently study has found scalp acupuncture therapy does not increase the risk of onset or epileptiform discharges in the children with cerebral palsy combined with epilepsy or epileptiform discharges. Scalp acupuncture combined with rehabilitation is better than simple rehabilitation for those with cerebral palsy and epilepsy onset [25].

In addition to the clinic studies, there are some researches try to find the mechanism of acupuncture for CP.

Preliminary reports have suggested that acupuncture can increase the supply of blood and oxygen to blood vessels, and that acupuncture may repair, activate, and regenerate injured neurons in the Brain. Modern neuroimaging methods (magnetic resonance imaging MRI) confirmed the activation of subcortical and cortical centres after acupuncture and confirmed the ability of acupuncture to increase cerebral blood flow and cerebral oxygen supply in children with cerebral palsy [7]. Based on fMRI studies, scalp acupuncture has also been shown to have effects on movement regulation. Moreover, the curative effect of scalp acupuncture has been shown to be correlated with the cerebral activating reaction in motor dysfunction in stroke patients [28, 29].

One study reported that the physiological effect of tongue acupuncture might result from the modification of neural signaling in the motor/ somatosensory cortex, resulting in improved motor function [23].

Studies have demonstrated that scalp acupuncture therapy may have the potential to treat epilepsy by increasing the blood flow speed of microchannel architecture, and upregulate anticardiolipin levels [30]. Decreased expression levels of cystathionine beta-synthase, and increased expression levels heme-oxygenase-1 and hypoxia-inducible factor-1α, have been observed in perinatal rat cortex cells after electrical acupuncture treatment, implicating a novel protective mechanism for CP [31].

13.6 Conclusion

Cerebral palsy (CP) is a permanent non-progressive cerebral disorder, which is one of the most severe Brain diseases that a child can have. CP has a high disability rate, which can cause physical and mentally burden and a possible decrease in the quality of life for children. The goal of cerebral palsy treatment is to help children work on their own, improving their quality of life.

Acupuncture, as one the major therapies of TCM, has been partly of the rehabilitations for CP widely used, particularly in China. Increasing evidence have support acupuncture can improve motor activity, sensation, speech, and other neurological functions in children with CP. Scalp acupuncture is one the unique acupuncture techniques which focus on the stimulations areas on the scalp. It can play as a monotherapy or as integrate treatment with general acupuncture and other rehabilitation therapies might benefits for CP.

There are some preliminary studies have indicated that acupuncture may increase cerebral blood flow and cerebral oxygen supply in CP children, may repair, activate, and regenerate injured neurons in the Brain, and other novel protective mechanism for CP.

References

1. CDC. What is Cerebral palsy. https://www.cdc.gov/ncbddd/cp/facts.html. Accessed 26 Apr 2020.
2. Pakula AT, Van Naarden Braun K, Yeargin-Allsopp M. Cerebral palsy: classification and epidemiology. Phys Med Rehabil Clin N Am. 2009;20:425–52.
3. Osler W. The cerebral palsies of children: a clinical study from the infirmary for nervous diseases. London: H.K. Lewis; 1889.
4. Rosenbaum P, Paneth N, Leviton A, et al. A report: the definition and classification of cerebral palsy. Dev Med Child Neurol Suppl. 2007;109:8–14.
5. Shevell M. Cerebral palsy to cerebral palsy spectrum disorder: time for a name change? Neurology. 2019;92:233–5.
6. Guo TP, Zhu BW, Zhang Q, et al. Acupuncture for children with cerebral palsy: a systematic review protocol. JMIR Res Protoc. 2017;6(1):e2. https://doi.org/10.1002/14651858. CD007127.
7. Li LX, Zhang MM, Zhang Y, et al. Acupuncture for cerebral palsy: a meta-analysis of randomized controlled trials. Neural Regen Res. 2018;13(6):1107–17.
8. Morris S. Ashworth and Tardieu scales: their clinical relevance for measuring spasticity in adult and paediatric neurological populations. Phys Ther Rev. 2002;7:53–62.
9. Verma H, Srivastava V, Semwal BC. A review of cerebral palsy and its management. J Sci. 2012;2:54–62.
10. Bax M, Goldstein M, Rosenbaum P, et al. Executive committee for the definition of cerebral palsy, proposed definition and classification of cerebral palsy. Dev Med Child Neurol. 2005;47:571–6.
11. Wang J, Shi W, Khiati D, et al. Scalp acupuncture treatment for motor dysfunction in children with cerebral palsy: study protocol for a multi-centre randomized controlled trial. Trials. 2020;21:29. https://doi.org/10.21203/rs.2.12483/v1.
12. Lee GE, Lee PT, Ran N, et al. Scalp acupuncture for children with cerebral palsy: a protocol for a systematic review. Medicine. 2019;98(48):e18062. https://doi.org/10.1097/MD.0000000000018062.

13. Graham HK, Rosenbaum P, Paneth N, et al. Cerebral palsy. Nat Rev Dis Primers. 2016;2 https://doi.org/10.1038/nrdp.2015.82.
14. Korzeniewski SJ, Slaughter J, Lenskiet M, et al. The complex aetiology of cerebral palsy. Nat Rev Neurol. 2018;14(9):528–43.
15. NICE. Cerebral palsy in under 25s: assessment and management. National Institute for Health and Care Excellence. 25 Jan 2017. https://www.nice.org.uk/guidance/ng62. Accessed 27 Apr 2020.
16. Dove D, Reimschisel T, McPheeters M, et al. Developmental disabilities issues exploration forum: cerebral palsy. Research white paper (Prepared by the Vanderbilt evidence-based practice Centre under contract no. 290-2007-10065-I). AHRQ Publication No. 11(12)-EHC078-EF. Rockville, MD: Agency for Healthcare Research and Quality, October 2011. https://effectivehealthcare.ahrq.gov/sites/default/files/pdf/cerebral-palsy-issues_white-paper.pdf. Accessed 27 Apr 2020.
17. Pountney D. Identifying and managing cerebral palsy. Br J Neurosci Nurs. 2013;6:20–3.
18. Harvey AR. The gross motor function measure (GMFM). J Physiother. 2017;63(3):187.
19. Velde AT, Morgan C, Novak I, et al. Early diagnosis and classification of cerebral palsy: an historical perspective and barriers to an early diagnosis. J Clin Med. 2019;8:1599. https://doi.org/10.3390/jcm8101599.
20. Liptak GS. Complementary and alternative therapies for cerebral palsy. Ment Retard Dev Disabil Res Rev. 2005;11:156–63.
21. Novak I. Evidence-based diagnosis, health care, and rehabilitation for children with cerebral palsy. J Child Neurol. 2014;29(8):1141–56.
22. Yang CS, Hao ZL, Zhang LL, et al. Efficacy and safety of acupuncture in children: an overview of systematic reviews. Syst Rev. 2015;78(2):112–9.
23. Sun JG, Ko HC, Wong V, et al. Randomised control trial of tongue acupuncture versus sham acupuncture in improving functional outcome in cerebral palsy. J Neurol Neurosurg Psychiatry. 2004;75:1054–7.
24. Duncan B, Shen K, Zou LP, et al. Evaluating intense rehabilitative therapies with and without acupuncture for children with cerebral palsy: a randomized controlled trial. Arch Phys Med Rehabil. 2012;93(5):808–15.
25. Li SY, Liu ZH, Zhao WJ, et al. Scalp acupuncture for epileptiform discharges of children with cerebral palsy. Zhongguo Zhen Jiu. 2017;37(3):265–8.
26. Dabbous OA, Mostafa YM, Noamany E, et al. Laser acupuncture as an adjunctive therapy for spastic cerebral palsy in children. Lasers Med Sci. 2016;31:1061–7.
27. Hao JJ, Hao LL. Review of clinical applications of scalp acupuncture for paralysis: an excerpt from Chinese scalp acupuncture. Glob Adv Health Med. 2012;1:102–21.
28. Romeo Z, Marta M, Barbara T. Modulation of hand motor-related area during motor imagery and motor execution before and after middle 2/5 of the MS6 line scalp acupuncture stimulation: an fMRI study. Brain Cogn. 2016;103:1–11.
29. Cui FY, Zou YH, Tan ZJ, et al. Rehabilitation of motor function and curative effect of scalp acupuncture in patients with hemiplegia after stroke: studies on fMRI and DTI. J Beijing Univ Trad Chinese Med (Clin Med). 2013;20(4):34–8.
30. Xiang L, Wang H, Li Z. TCD observation on cerebral blood flow dynamics inference of cerebral palsy with scalp therapy. Zhen Ci Yan Jiu. 1996;21(4):7–9.
31. Liu YC, Li ZH, Shi XY, et al. Neuroprotection of up-regulated carbon monoxide by electrical acupuncture on perinatal hypoxic-ischemic brain damage in rats. Neurochem Res. 2014;39(9):1724–32.

Chapter 14
Epilepsy, Headache and Pain Associated with Neurological Disorders

The previous chapters in this book have introduced several of the most commonly seen neurological diseases in practice, namely stroke, Parkinson's disease, Alzheimer's disease and other dementias, multiple sclerosis, traumatic Brain injury, autism and cerebral palsy. Some other commonly seen neurological diseases will be briefly introduced in this chapter, i.e. epilepsy, headache and pain associated with neurological disorders.

Unlike the previous chapters on the most commonly seen neurological diseases, which explain in detail the basic background, aetiology and pathogenesis, typical clinical symptoms, examination and diagnosis, treatment with modern medicine, TCM understanding of the disease, general acupuncture treatment, unique acupuncture treatment and relevant research, among other things, this chapter will only focus on general information and unique acupuncture treatment for some sample neurological diseases.

In order to simplify the treatment principle and make it easy to follow for clinical practice, the Brain acupuncture treatment section of this chapter will start with general basic treatment and move on to several additional treatments.

14.1 Epilepsy

14.1.1 General Background of epilepsy

Epilepsy is a neurological disorder consisting of recurrent seizures resulting from excessive, uncontrolled electrical activity in the Brain [1]. The WHO has defined epilepsy as "a disorder of the Brain characterized by an enduring predisposition to generate epileptic seizures, and by the neurobiological, cognitive, psychological

© Springer Nature Switzerland AG 2021
T. Wang, *Acupuncture for Brain*, https://doi.org/10.1007/978-3-030-54666-3_14

and social consequences of this condition. The definition of epilepsy requires the occurrence of at least one epileptic seizure" [2, p. 56].

In 2017, the International League Against Epilepsy (ILAE) published in two articles an updated classification of seizures and different types of epilepsy, together with an instructional manual on how to apply the classification of a seizure. These were the first new official papers on classification from the ILAE since 1989. There are three types of seizure, namely focal, generalized and unknown, and four epilepsy types, i.e. focal, generalized, combined generalized and focal, and unknown [3].

Because there are many types of seizure and epilepsy, there is no single cause. The most common causes of epilepsy are structural causes, genetic causes, infectious causes, metabolic causes, immune causes and unknown causes [2, p. 57].

The primary focus of care for patients with epilepsy is the prevention of further seizures, which may, in fact, lead to additional morbidity or even mortality. The goal of treatment should be the maintenance of a normal lifestyle, preferably free of seizures and with minimal side effects from the medication used [2, p. 62].

Most epilepsies can be well controlled by conventional anti-epileptic drugs (AEDs), however the medications available have adverse effects and long-term impacts. In addition, about one-third of epilepsy patients are resistant to AEDs [4].

Due to the growing efforts to invoke electrical stimulation to treat refractory epilepsy, neuromodulation is becoming one of the most vigorous fields in neurosurgery. In general, aberrant Brain activities can be restored via electrical stimulation at either the peripheral nerve(s) or the very Brain itself. Neurostimulation therapies, including vagus nerve stimulation (VNS), deep brain stimulation (DBS), trigeminal nerve stimulation (TNS) and others, are reported to provide some palliation for refractory epilepsies, but, with different risk profiles, relatively low clinical efficiency (~30%), and less likeliness of seizure freedom [4]. Moreover, and unfortunately, many patients remain totally unresponsive to such interventions [5, 6].

14.1.2   General Acupuncture for Epilepsy

Acupuncture has been used for the suppression of epileptic seizure for more than 2000 years in Chinese medicine. Significant progress towards elucidating the biological basis of acupuncture suppression has been made in the past several decades, including biochemical, molecular, electrophysiological and immunological techniques, as well as electroencephalogram and power spectra. Accumulating data have shown that acupuncture suppresses epileptic seizure through the regulation of several neurotransmitters/modulators and their receptors, including excitatory and inhibitory amino acids, and neuropeptides such as cholecystokinin, somatostatin, enkephalin, dynorphin and nitric oxide. However, the cellular and molecular basis of acupuncture therapy for epilepsy is far from being well understood [7, p. 326–364].

The commonly used acupoints are those along the Du Mai (Governor Vessel) and the Ren Mai (Conception Vessel) meridians. Most reports have shown that acupuncture is remarkable effective, although there was negative evidence in some studies. Optimizing acupuncture conditions, including methods of delivery, acupoints and stimulation parameters, may further improve the efficacy of acupuncture therapy for epilepsy. Since TCM considers that the purpose of the Du Mai (Governor Vessel GV), which is located in the posterior midline rising from the perineum to the head, is to govern the whole Yang of the body, the most frequently used anti-epileptic acupoints are selected from this meridian [8, p. 227].

One clinical study demonstrated that a therapy combining scalp acupuncture with body acupuncture and medication is superior to medication only [9]. A recent trial indicated that acupuncture treatment was associated with a decreased risk of epilepsy in stroke patients [10].

14.1.3 Brain Acupuncture for Epilepsy

14.1.3.1 Basic Treatment

Scalp acupuncture (SA) Spirit-Emotion Area, Foot Motor Sensory Area, Manic Control Area, Central Area, plus DU-20 Baihui, DU-24 Shenting, DU-16 Fengfu (Dao-qi), REN-12 Zhongwan (Dao-qi or plus two to four needles), electric acupuncture may add on DU-24, DU-20 and DU-16.

14.1.3.2 Additional Treatment

Deficiency of Brain Marrow

Signs and Symptoms (SS): Chronic epilepsy accompanied by dizziness and vertigo, stopping activities abruptly, temporary confusion, dropping objects suddenly, staring upward, can't recall incident after consciousness returns, insomnia, poor memory and concentration, irritability, weak body or limbs, tinnitus, dry eyes and mouth, thirst, especially at night, light-colored or light red tongue, thin and deep pulse.

Additional treatment: SA Reproduction Area, Ex-Bailaoxue, DU-4 Mingmen (Dao-qi), REN-4 Guanyuan, KI-3 Taixi, LV-3 Taichong, GB-39 Xuanzhong, BL-23 Shenshu, etc.

Deficiency of Brain Yang Qi

SS: Chronic epilepsy, fatigue and tiredness, temporary confusion, dizziness and vertigo, poor appetite, lustreless complexion, heavy head and limbs, cold hands and feet, light-coloured tongue with white and thick coat with teeth marks on sides, deep and thin pulse.

Additional treatment: SA Stomach Area, DU-14 Dazhui, DU-9 Zhiyang, DU-3 Yaoyangguan, REN-10 Xiawan, REN-6 Qihai, REN-4 Guanyuan, ST-36 Zusanli, SP-9 Yinlingquan, etc. Moxa could be applied. Dao-qi technique May be added on one or two key Du Mai or Ren Mai points, such as DU-16, DU-14, REN-12 and REN-6.

Stagnation of Brain Collaterals

SS: Sudden onset, falling down or fainting, contraction of limbs, habitual fixed headache, worse at night or stopping activities abruptly, dropping objects suddenly, forward bending of the neck, staring upward after consciousness returns, patient does not recall incident, maybe purplish face, extremities, lips and fingers, can be triggered by anger or strong emotional stimulation, possible history of injury to the head, purple tongue with light or greasy coat, wiry or slippery pulse.

Additional treatments: SA Vasomotor Area, Head Area, DU-26 Renzhong, DU-15 Yamen, DU-14 Dazhui, REN-10 Xiawan, REN-6 Qihai, ST-36 Zusanli, SP-10 Xuehai, LV-3 Taichong, LI-4 Hegu, GB-20 Fengchi, etc. Moxa could be applied, may add Dao-qi technique on one or two key points, such as DU-16 and REN-12.

Brain Shen Disorder

SS: Sudden onset, falling down or fainting, contraction of limbs, temporary confusion, insomnia, nightmares, waking up in the early morning or sleeping lightly, frequently feeling anxious or stressed, dreaming, easily startled, poor concentration and memory, dizziness and vertigo, general headache, etc., light tongue with thin coating, wiry or slow pulse.

Additional treatment: SA Head Area, DU-26 Renzhong, Ex-Yintang, DU-14 Dazhui, HT-7 Shenmen, BL-15 Xinshu, etc. Electric acupuncture may be added, Dao-qi technique on one or two key points such as DU-16, DU-14 and REN-12.

Notes
- Acupuncture treatment for epileptic patients, mainly treating for seizures and secondarily generalized chronic seizures, and a possible decrease in status epilepticus severity.
- Electric acupuncture (EA): no EA-related adverse effect was reported from either experiments or clinical studies. In contrast, EA could reduce the seizure.

14.2   Headache

Headache is one of the most common disorders encountered in medicine. Interest in headache extends back almost as far as recorded history. The lifelong prevalence of headache is 96%, with a female predominance [11]. Despite the widespread and incapacitating nature of headache, it is underestimated in terms of scope and scale, and headache disorders remain under-recognized and under-treated everywhere, despite causing substantial disability in populations throughout the world [2, p. 71].

The International Classification of Headache Disorders (ICHD) was first published in 1988 and has now gone through two revisions, most recently in 2013. Based on the ICHD 2013, the most common primary headaches, which have no known underlying cause, include migraine, tension-type headache and cluster headache. The most common secondary headaches are headaches related to infection, vascular disease and trauma [12].

14.2.1   General Background of Headache

14.2.1.1   Migraine

According to the International Headache Society, chronic migraine is defined as "headache lasting more than four hours each day for more than 15 days per month and for at least 3 months, with at least eight days of headache meeting diagnostic criteria for episodic migraine" [12, p. 650]. Migraine is the third most prevalent disorder and the seventh-highest cause of disability worldwide [13]. Migraine almost certainly has a genetic basis, but environmental factors play a significant role in how the disorder affects those who suffer from it [12, p. 72]. The main subtypes are migraine with and without aura. An aura is a fully reversible set of nervous system symptoms, most often visual or sensory symptoms, that typically develops gradually, recedes and is then followed by headache accompanied by nausea, vomiting, photophobia and phonophobia [11, 14]. Chronic migraine is also associated with a significantly greater degree of health-care burden and psychiatric co-morbidity, such as depression and anxiety.

Most people with migraine require drugs for an acute attack. These may be symptomatic or specific [2, p. 78]. Topiramate, as an anti-epileptic medication (AED), is Food and Drug Administration approved and widely accepted as a treatment for chronic migraine prevention. Several placebo-controlled randomized clinical trials have shown that Topiramate significantly reduces the number of migraine headache days in patients with chronic migraine [14].

14.2.1.2   Tension-Type Headache

The mechanism of tension-type headache is poorly understood, though it has long been regarded as a headache with muscular origins. It may be stress related or associated with musculoskeletal problems in the neck [12, p. 73]. Tension-type headache has distinct subtypes. As experienced by very large numbers of people, episodic tension-type headache occurs, like migraine, in attack-like episodes.

Tension-type headache is a dull, bilateral, mild- to moderate-intensity pressure/pain without associated features that may be categorized as infrequent, frequent or chronic and is easily distinguished from migraine [11].

14.2.1.3 Cluster Headache

Cluster headache is one of a group of primary headache disorders (trigeminal autonomic cephalalgias) of uncertain mechanism that are characterized by frequently recurring, short-lasting but extremely severe headache [2, p. 73]. Cluster headache, often referred to as "suicide headache" because of the intensity of the pain, occurs more commonly in men and is usually episodic, characterized by "clusters" of from 2 weeks to 3 months. The pain is extremely severe, with one to eight episodes per day, often wakening the patient from sleep shortly after falling asleep [11].

There is good evidence that very large numbers of people troubled, even disabled, by headache do not receive effective health care. A lack of knowledge among health-care providers is the principal clinical barrier to effective headache management [2, p. 76].

Examination in headache is based on the general neurologic examination. Additional features include examination of the superficial scalp vessels, neck vessels, dentition and bite, the temporomandibular joints, and cervical and shoulder musculature. Pericranial muscle tenderness is thought to be an important physical finding in the diagnosis of tension-type headache [12, p. 766].

The treatment of migraine and other primary headaches is not uniform but is proportional to the severity of the symptoms and disability. Mild and infrequent symptoms may be initially treated with lifestyle modification, stress management techniques and over-the-counter abortive medications [11]. Even with the recent advancement in the diagnosis and treatment of different headache disorders, many patients with headaches are still suffering due to the lack of effective treatment [15].

14.2.2   General Acupuncture for Headache

As an alternative to traditional treatment, acupuncture is one of the more commonly researched and widely accepted complementary and alternative medicine (CAM) therapies in the treatment of migraines [16].

A review in 2000 showed that the use of acupuncture for the treatment of headache seems promising because the majority of the clinical trials (23 out of 27) reported positive conclusions regarding its effectiveness [17].

An RCT study concluded that acupuncture was more effective than Topiramate in reducing the number of monthly moderate/severe headache days [18]. There is moderate-quality evidence that whole-body acupuncture is effective for preventing migraine. Compared with usual care, acupuncture is at least 50% more effective at reducing headache frequency [13].

A very recent study systematically reviewed the evidence on the use of acupuncture for acute and preventive treatment of migraine with a view to gaining further awareness of the effect of acupuncture on migraine. It was concluded that using acupuncture for treating migraine has the advantage of reducing pain and improving safety [19].

In a recent study protocol the main points used for migraine were: GV20 (Baihui DU-20), GV24 (Shenting DU-24), bilateral GB13 (Benshen), bilateral GB8 (Shuaigu) and bilateral GB20 (Fengchi) [14].

The particular mechanism through which acupuncture affects migraine has not been fully revealed [14]. According to gate control theory, once fine acupuncture needles have been inserted into body points, delta fibres may be stimulated to close the pain gates in the central nervous system, therefore the sensation of pain will not be perceived due to its failure to reach the thalamus [20].

In addition, many researchers have held the view that acupuncture may influence calcium signalling and the opioid system. The acupuncture stimulations may produce and release endogenous opioids, which bind to opiate receptors in the Brain and mediate analgesia through the descending pain inhibitory system [21].

Acupuncture could be a tool for treating patients with episodic and chronic headache, especially if we bear in mind that these patients are usually subjected to chronic abuse of drugs at a considerable social and economic cost [22].

14.2.3 Brain Acupuncture for Headache

14.2.3.1 Basic Treatment

Scalp acupuncture (SA) Vasomotor Area, Foot-Motor Sensory Area, Spirit-Emotion Area, Central Area, plus DU-20 Baihui, DU-16 Fengfu (Dao-qi), REN-12 Zhongwan (Dao-qi or plus two to four needles).

14.2.3.2 Additional Treatment

Deficiency of Brain Marrow

SS: Mild to moderate chronic headache with a sensation of emptiness of the head, worse with exertion, dizziness and vertigo, weakness and aching of the neck, low back and knees, fatigue, tinnitus, insomnia, light-coloured or light red tongue, thin, weak and deep pulse.

Additional treatment: SA Reproduction Area, Ex-Bailaoxue, DU-4 Mingmen (Dao-qi), REN-4 Guanyuan, KI-3 Taixi, LV-3 Taichong, GB-39 Xuanzhong, BL-23 Shenshu, etc.

Deficiency of Brain Yang Qi

SS: Constant dull headache, heaviness, aggravated by overexertion or cold, weakness, fatigue, loss of appetite, general cold, particularly four limbs, light colour or pale tongue, thin white coating, maybe teeth marks on sides, weak, thin and deep pulse.

Additional treatment: SA Stomach Area, DU-14 Dazhui, DU-9 Zhiyang, DU-3 Yaoyangguan, REN-10 Xiawan, REN-6 Qihai, REN-4 Guanyuan, ST-36 Zusanli, SP-9 Yinlingquan, BL-20 Pishu, etc. Moxa could be applied, Dao-qi technique on one or two key Du Mài or Ren Mai points, such as DU-16, DU-14, REN-12 and REN-6.

Stagnation of Brain Collaterals

SS: Headache with repeated and long-lasting, fixed and stabbing pain, worse at night. Possible head trauma history, may be accompanied by numbness, pain in limbs, even paralysis on one side of the body. Purple tongue or light tongue with purple spots, light coat, wiry, choppy or slippery pulse.

Additional treatments: SA Head Area, Vasomotor Area, DU-14 Dazhui, REN-10 Xiawan, REN-6 Qihai, ST-36 Zusanli, SP-10 Xuehai, LV-3 Taichong, LI-4 Hegu, GB-20 Fengchi, BL-17 Geshu, BL-18 Ganshu, etc. Moxa could be applied, maybe with Dao-qi technique on one or two key points such as DU-16 and REN-12.

14.3 Pain Associated with Neurological Disorders

14.3.1 General Background

Pain is an unpleasant sensory and emotional experience associated with actual or potential tissue damage, or described in terms of such damage [23]. Pain can be a direct or indirect consequence of a neurological disorder. The former is seen in neurological conditions where there has been a lesion or disease of pathways that normally transmit information about painful stimuli either in the peripheral or in the central nervous system (CNS). These types of pain are known as "neuropathic pains" [2, p. 128].

It is useful to distinguish between acute and chronic pain. Pain frequently begins as an acute experience, but for physical and often psychological reasons, it becomes a long-term or chronic problem, which means any pain lasting for longer than 3 months [2, p. 128].

In contrast to nociceptive pain, which is the result of stimulation of primary sensory nerves, neuropathic pain results when a lesion or disruption of function occurs in the nervous system. Neuropathic pain is often associated with marked emotional changes, especially depression, and disability in activities of daily life. If the cause is located in the peripheral nervous system, it gives rise to peripheral neuropathic pain, and if it is located in the CNS (Brain or spinal cord), it gives rise to central neuropathic pain. Painful diabetic neuropathy and the neuralgia that develops after herpes zoster are the most frequently studied peripheral neuropathic pain conditions. Diabetic neuropathy has been estimated to afflict 45–75% of patients with diabetes mellitus. About 10% of these develop painful diabetic neuropathy, particularly when the function of small nerve fibres is impaired. Pain is a normal symptom of acute herpes zoster, but disappears in most cases with the healing of the rash. In 9–14% of patients, pain persists chronically beyond the healing process (post-herpetic neuralgia). Neuropathic pain may also develop after peripheral nerve trauma as in the condition of chemotherapy-induced neuropathy. Central post-stroke pain is the most frequently studied central neuropathic pain condition. It occurs in about 8% of patients who suffer an infarction of the Brain. The incidence is higher for infarctions of the Brain stem. Two-thirds of patients with multiple sclerosis have chronic pain, half of which is central neuropathic pain [2, p. 128].

The causes of neuralgia can vary greatly. Trauma, chemical irritation, inflammation, compression of nerves by nearby structures (for instance, vertebral subluxations) and infections may all lead to neuralgia [24, p. 307]. Chronic pain also occurs in neurological conditions of unknown aetiology, e.g. idiopathic neuropathies [25].

Clinically, pain assessment includes a full history of the development, nature, intensity, location and duration of pain. In addition to clinical examination, self-report measures of pain are often used. In clinical practice, however, there is widespread use of a 0–10 scale, a visual analogue scale, which is easy to understand and use and is not affected by differences in language. Pain drawings are another technique used in clinical assessment, and these allow the patient to mark the location of pain and its qualities using a code on a diagram of the body. A pain diary is used by patients to record levels of pain throughout the day, using a visual analogue scale [2, p. 130].

According to the International Association for the Study of Pain (IASP) [23], chronic peripheral neuropathic pain and chronic central neuropathic pain are the two major types of pain. The former includes trigeminal neuralgia, chronic neuropathic pain after peripheral nerve injury, painful polyneuropathy, post-herpetic neuralgia, painful radiculopathy, and other specified and unspecified chronic peripheral neuropathic pain. The latter includes chronic central neuropathic pain associated with spinal cord injury, chronic central neuropathic pain associated with Brain injury, chronic central post-stroke pain, chronic central neuropathic pain caused by multiple sclerosis, and other specified and unspecified chronic central neuropathic pain [23].

Trigeminal neuralgia is the most common form of neuralgia and is the result of inflammation or compression of the trigeminal nerve, which runs along the side of the face. A related but rather uncommon neuralgia affects the glossopharyngeal nerve, which provides sensation to the throat. Symptoms of this neuralgia are short, shock-like episodes of pain located in the throat. The occipital nerve can also be affected, causing occipital neuralgia in the back of the neck and scalp. In cases where partial or full paralysis occurs or there is a loss of sensation to a nerve area, pain can occur along a nerve trajectory [24, p. 307].

Neurogenic pain or discomfort may actually increase temporarily as feeling and/ or the range of motion increases with treatment. This is similar to a body part that has "fallen asleep", and discomfort can occur as it "wakes up" until full neural signalling is re-established [24, p. 307].

The mechanistic underpinnings of pain hypersensitivity and spontaneous pain in these conditions are complex, and their relationship with the underlying pathological disease process often remains unclear [25].

Therapeutic management is challenging. Medications recommended as first-line treatments provide less than satisfactory relief in many patients [25]. The range of treatments available for pain directly caused by diseases of the nervous system includes pharmacological, physical, interventional (nerve blocks, etc.) and psychological therapies. Treatments for pain are used in association with other forms of treatment for the primary condition, unless, of course, pain itself is the primary disorder [2, p. 134]. Similar to other chronic pain conditions, only a small proportion of trial participants experience a good response to treatment for neuropathic pain [26].

14.3.2 Acupuncture for Pain Associated with Neurological Disorders

Acupuncture has been increasingly used to treat chronic pain (including neuropathic pain) and is considered to be one of the most popular types of complementary alternative medicine available in Western health care [27]. The most commonly studied chronic neuropathic pain conditions treated with acupuncture include (but are not limited to): cancer-related neuropathy; central neuropathic pain; complex regional pain syndrome (CRPS) type II; HIV neuropathy; painful diabetic neuropathy (PDN); phantom limb pain; post-herpetic neuralgia (PHN); post-operative or traumatic neuropathic pain; spinal cord injury; and trigeminal neuralgia [28].

A recent randomized controlled clinical trial compared acupuncture plus usual medication (methylcobalamin) with medication only for chemotherapy-induced peripheral neuropathy (CIPN) in patients with multiple myeloma (MM). The results showed that acupuncture combined with methylcobalamin in the treatment of CIPN showed a better outcome than methylcobalamin administration alone, based on the visual analogue scale (VAS) pain score, daily activity and electromyographic (EMG) nerve conduction velocity (NCV) determination [29].

14.3.3 Brain Acupuncture for Neuropathic Pain

14.3.3.1 Basic Treatment

Scalp acupuncture (SA) Foot Motor Sensory Area, Sensory Area, Spirit-Emotion Area, DU-20 Baihui, DU-16 Fengfu (Dao-qi), REN-12 Zhongwan.

14.3.3.2   Additional Treatment

Deficiency of Brain Marrow

SS: Mild to moderate chronic pain in limbs or face, with a sensation of emptiness of the head and back, worse with exertion, dizziness and vertigo, weakness and aching of the neck, low back and knees, fatigue, tinnitus, insomnia, light-colored or light red tongue, thin, weak and deep pulse.

Additional treatment: SA Reproduction Area, Ex-Bailaoxue, DU-4 Mingmen (Dao-qi), REN-4 Guanyuan, KI-3 Taixi, LV-3 Taichong, GB-39 Xuanzhong, BL-23 Shenshu, etc.

Deficiency of Brain Yang Qi

SS: Constant dull headache, heaviness, aggravated by overexertion or cold, weakness, fatigue, loss of appetite, general cold, particularly four limbs, light-coloured or pale tongue, thin white coating, maybe teeth marks on sides, weak, thin and deep pulse.

Additional treatment: SA Stomach Area, DU-14 Dazhui, DU-9 Zhiyang, DU-3 Yaoyangguan, REN-10 Xiawan, REN-6 Qihai, REN-4 Guanyuan, ST-36 Zusanli, SP-9 Yinlingquan, BL-20 Pishu, etc. Moxa could be applied, May add Dao-qi technique on one or two key Du Mai or Ren Mai points, such as DU-16, DU-14, REN-12 and REN-6.

Stagnation of Brain Collaterals

SS: Headache with repeated and long-lasting, fixed and stabbing pain, worse at night. Possible head trauma history, may be accompanied by numbness, pain in limbs, even paralysis on one side of the body. Purple tongue or light tongue with purple spots, light coat, wiry, choppy or slippery pulse.

Additional treatments: SA Head Area, Vasomotor Area, DU-14 Dazhui, REN-10 Xiawan, REN-6 Qihai, ST-36 Zusanli, SP-10 Xuehai, LV-3 Taichong, LI-4 Hegu, GB-20 Fengchi, BL-17 Geshu, BL-18 Ganshu, etc. Moxa could be applied. May add Dao-qi technique on one or two key points, such as DU-16 and REN-12.

Spine Marrow Stagnation

SS: Stiffness and pain in neck and back, limited movement of spine and limbs, spinal curvature straightened, segmented skin and muscle pain, or chronic flaccidity and weakness of the limbs with muscular atrophy, numbness of the limbs, dark-coloured skin, purple or purple spots on tongue, wiry or unsmooth pulse.

Points selection: SA Vasomotor Area, DU-20 Baihui, DU-16 Fengfu, DU-14 Dazhui, DU-9 Zhiyang, DU-8 Jinsuo, DU-7 Zhongshu, DU-3 Yaoyangguan, Ex-Shiqizhuixia, REN-11 Jianli, REN-10 Xiawan, REN-6 Qihai, REN-4 Guanyuan, plus local affected area points. Scalp acupuncture may be added as well. Moxa could be applied, with Dao-qi technique on one or two key points.

Clinical Notes

- *There are many different types of pain associated with neurological disorders. Clinical practice should be based on individual disease and symptoms to select individual treatment plan.
- *Brain acupuncture technique includes scalp acupuncture, Du Mai and Ren Mai Dao-qi needling, which could be combined with other general techniques such as electric acupuncture, moxibustion, et al.

References

1. He W, Rong PJ, Li L, et al. Auricular acupuncture may suppress epileptic seizures via activating the parasympathetic nervous system: a hypothesis based on innovative methods. Evid Based Complement Alternat Med. 2012; https://doi.org/10.1155/2012/615476.
2. WHO. Neurological disorders: public health challenges. Geneva, Switzerland: World Health Organization; 2006.
3. Brodie MJ, Zuberi SM, Scheffer IE, et al. The 2017 ILAE classification of seizure types and the epilepsies: what do people with epilepsy and their caregivers need to know? Epileptic Disord. 2018;20(2):77–87.
4. Chen SP, Wang SB, Rong PJ, et al. Acupuncture for refractory epilepsy: role of thalamus. Evid Based Complement Alternat Med. 2014; https://doi.org/10.1155/2014/950631.
5. DeGiorgio CM, Soss J, Cook IA, et al. Randomized controlled trial of trigeminal nerve stimulation for drug-resistant epilepsy. Neurology. 2013;80(9):786–91.
6. Fisher RS. Therapeutic devices for epilepsy. Ann Neurol. 2012;71(2):157–68.
7. Yang R, Cheng JS. Effect of acupuncture on epilepsy. In: Xia Y, Cao XD, Wu GC, et al., editors. Acupuncture therapy for neurological diseases: a neurobiological view. Beijing, China: Springer-Tsinghua Press; 2010.
8. Cheng XN. Chinese acupuncture and moxibustion. 2nd ed. Beijing, China: Foreign Language Press; 2010.
9. Niu XX. Clinical observation on treating 30 cases of epilepsy by head and body acupuncture. Clin J Chin Med. 2014;6(4):65–7.
10. Weng SW, Liao CC, Yeh CC, et al. Risk of epilepsy in stroke patients receiving acupuncture treatment: a nationwide retrospective matched-cohort study. BMJ Open. 2016;6:e010539. https://doi.org/10.1136/bmjopen.
11. Rizzoli P, Mullally WJ. Headache. Am J Med. 2018;131:17–24.
12. HIS (Headache Classification Committee of the International Headache Society). The international classification of headache disorders, 3rd edition (beta version). Cephalalgia. 2013;33(9):629–808.
13. Arnold MJ, McIntyre JM. Acupuncture for migraine prevention. Cochrane Clin. 2017;96:23–4.
14. Liu L, Zhao L, Zhang CS, et al. Acupuncture as prophylaxis for chronic migraine: a protocol for a single-blinded, double-dummy randomised controlled trial. BMJ Open. 2018;8:e020653. https://doi.org/10.1136/bmjopen-2017-020653.
15. Chen L. The role of acupuncture in pain management. Acupunct Mod Med. 2013;2013:235–53. https://doi.org/10.5772/56259.

16. Plank S, Goodard J. The effectiveness of acupuncture for chronic daily headache: an outcomes study. Mil Med. 2009;174(12):1276–81.
17. Manias P, Tagaris G, Karageorgiou K. Acupuncture in headache: a critical review. Clin J Pain. 2000;16(4):334–9.
18. Yang CP, Chang MH, Liu PE, et al. Acupuncture versus topiramate in chronic migraine prophylaxis: a randomized clinical trial. Cephalalgia. 2011;31:1510–21.
19. Zhang XT, Li XY, Zhao C, et al. An overview of systematic reviews of randomized controlled trials on acupuncture treating migraine. Pain Res Manag. 2019; https://doi.org/10.1155/2019/5930627.
20. Zhao ZQ. Neural mechanism underlying acupuncture analgesia. Prog Neurobiol. 2008;85:355–75.
21. Vijayalakshmi I, Shankar N, Saxena A, et al. Comparison of effectiveness of acupuncture therapy and conventional drug therapy on psychological profile of migraine patients. Indian J Physiol Pharmacol. 2014;58:69–76.
22. Granato A, Grandi FC, Stokelj D, et al. Acupuncture in tension-type headache. Neuroepidemiology. 2010;35:160–2.
23. IASP (International Association for the Study of Pain). Pain terms. https://www.iasp-pain.org/terminology. Accessed 20 Feb 2020.
24. Wingate DS. Healing brain injury with Chinese medical approaches: integrative approaches for practitioners. London and Philadelphia: Singing Dragon; 2018.
25. Scholz J, Finnerup NB, Attal N, et al. The IASP classification of chronic pain for ICD-11: chronic neuropathic pain. Pain. 2019;160:53–9.
26. Moore RA, Derry S, Eccleston C, et al. Expect analgesic failure; pursue analgesic success. BMJ. 2013;346:f2690. https://doi.org/10.1136/bmj.f2690.
27. Barnes PM, Bloom B, Nahin RL. Complementary and alternative medicine use among adults and children: United States, 2007. Natl Health Stat Rep. 2008;12:1–23.
28. Ju ZY, Wang K, Cui HS, et al. Acupuncture for neuropathic pain in adults. Cochrane Database Syst Rev. 2017; https://doi.org/10.1002/14651858.CD012057.pub2.
29. Han XY, Wang LJ, Shi HF, et al. Acupuncture combined with methylcobalamin for the treatment of chemotherapy-induced peripheral neuropathy in patients with multiple myeloma. BMC Cancer. 2017;17:40. https://doi.org/10.1186/s12885-016-3037-z.

Chapter 15
Depression

15.1 General Introduction

Depression is a mood disorder or affective disorder caused by various factors, featured by depression as the main clinical manifestation. There are a group of symptoms characterized by persistent mood depression, decreased ability and various physical symptoms, such as decreased interest, psychomotor retardation, sleep disorders, appetite and weight loss, various physical discomforts, etc. As estimated 15% of patients with severe major depression eventually die from suicide [1] and major depressive episode is the most common current psychiatric diagnosis among suicide victims with attempters (56–87%) [2]. These figures have indicated that depression has a great impact on social stability and economic development.

Due to the economic and social development, the pressure of life and employment is increasing, and the depression is gradually increasing worldwide. The treatment of depression is long course, but slow effect. This disease has become one of the conditions that seriously damages human health.

15.1.1 Basic Background of Depression

Depression is considered as one of the major public health disorders that affects 8–20% of the worldwide population [3]. According to WHO reports, depression is predicted to become the second leading contributor to disease worldwide by 2020, the first disease of female death and disability, affecting at least 350 million people [4], and the leading cause of the global disease burden by 2030 [5]. Almost one million lives are lost yearly due to suicide, which translates to 3000 suicide deaths every day. For every person who completes a suicide, 20 or more may attempt to end his or her life [5].

© Springer Nature Switzerland AG 2021
T. Wang, *Acupuncture for Brain*, https://doi.org/10.1007/978-3-030-54666-3_15

World Health Organization estimated that depression would occupy a growing share in the global burden of disease, rising from third place in 2004 with 4.3% of the total to first place by 2030 with 6.2% of the total (followed by ischemic heart disease, road traffic accidents, cerebrovascular disease and chronic obstructive pulmonary disease). WHO found that depression was already the leading cause of lost years of healthy life for women in the 15–44 age groups. We should act to address the upward trend of this widespread illness. Depression has significant socioeconomic costs. European studies have shown that early retirement accounted for 47% of the cost of depression, and sick leave a further 32%, compared with just 3% for the cost of drugs to treat the illness [6].

It is also usually highly recurrent, with at least 50% of those who recover from a first episode of depression having one or more additional episodes in their lifetime, and approximately 80% of those with a history of two episodes having another recurrence [7].

15.1.2   The Aetiology and Pathogenesis of Depression

Studies to date suggest that the cause of depression is related to genetic factors, psychosocial factors, endocrine disorders, and Neuro-structural changes, et al. [6].

The pathogenesis of depression is not well understood, and there are various hypotheses, including catecholamine and receptor hypothesis, serotonin and receptor hypothesis, multiple amine metabolic disorder hypotheses, and cholinergic-adrenergic function balance. Disorder hypothesis, neuroendocrine hypothesis, HPA axis hypo-function theory, emotional disorder neural structure and functional changes, Brain function changes, and so on. At present, the most valued and clinically used is the theory of decreased of serotonin (5-HT) in depression. This hypothesis is that depression occurs in the central nervous system with a decrease in 5-HT release and a decrease in synaptic clearance. Selective serotonin reuptake inhibitors (SSRIs) studied and used according to this hypothesis are currently the most commonly used first-line antidepressants.

15.1.3   Typical Clinical Symptoms

The clinical manifestations of depression can be divided into three groups: core, psychological and physical symptoms. Core symptom group: low mood, lack of interest, lack of energy; psychological symptoms group: including psychological accompanying symptoms (anxiety, self-blame, guilt, Psychiatric symptoms, cognitive symptoms, suicidal ideation and behaviour, self-knowledge) and psychomotor symptoms (psychomotor excitability and psychomotor retardation); somatic symptoms: sleep disorders (difficulty falling asleep and early awakening), appetite disorders (decreased appetite and weight loss), sexual dysfunction, loss of energy, morning lightness, non-specific physical symptoms such as: chronic pain, general discomfort, gastrointestinal dysfunction, palpitation, shortness of breath, etc [4].

Typical symptoms of depression include persistent emotion depression or low, emotional discomfort, unable expression emotion, lack of energy, disorders of autonomic and somatic function, endocrine and physical dysfunction.

15.1.4 Examination and Diagnosis of Depression

The commonly used clinical diagnostic criteria include the 4th Edition American Diagnostic Manual for Mental Disorders (DSMIV), and the International Classification of Diseases, 10th Edition, Clinical Description and Diagnostic Points (ICD-10) [7].

Clinical symptoms for the diagnosis of depression: the main symptoms must be met with low mood, and include at least 4 items from the following list and at least lasted 2 weeks almost every day:

1. loss of interest, no feeling of happiness
2. energy loss or fatigue
3. mental retardation or agitation
4. self-evaluation too low, self-blame, or guilty
5. association difficulties or conscious thinking ability decline
6. repeated thoughts of wanting to die or suicidal, self-injury behaviour
7. sleep disorders, such as insomnia, early sleep or excessive sleep;
8. Loss of appetite or significant weight loss
9. loss of libido.

For the purpose of clinical observation and research, a variety of diagnostic scales have been widely used in clinical, especially clinical research. These are: Beck Depression Inventory (BDI), Self-rating Depression Scale (SDS) and Depression Status Questionnaire. (DSI), Depression Experience Questionnaire (DEQ), Carroll Depression Self-Assessment Scale (CRSD), Geriatric Depression Scale (GDS), Hamilton Depression Rating Scale (HAMD, HRSD), and a composite international diagnostic conversation check core (CIDI-C), Neuropsychiatric Clinical Assessment Form (SCAN), etc. The Hamilton Depression Scale (HAMD, HRSD) is the most standard depression scale on all depression scales. It can also reflect the psychopathological characteristics of patients with depression through factor analysis [7].

15.1.5 The Treatment of Depression with Modern Medicine

The standard treatment for depression of west medicine are psychotherapy and antidepressant. Current pharmacological and psychological interventions have limited acceptability and effectiveness. Up to 50%–60% of patients do not adequately respond to pharmacological antidepressant treatment [8].

Commonly used antidepressants include monoamine oxidase inhibitors, tricyclic antidepressants, and non-tricyclic antidepressants. Commonly used tricyclic antidepressants such as imipramine, amitriptyline, doxepin, protriptyline, clomipramine, trimethylamine and so on.

The most commonly used non-tricyclic antidepressants in the clinic are selective serotonin reuptake inhibitors (SSRIs), represented by fluoxetine. They are a new class of high-efficiency antidepressants. It selectively inhibits the reabsorption of 5-HT by the presynaptic membrane, increases the concentration of 5-HT in the synaptic gap, acts on the postsynaptic membrane receptor, enhances conduction, and acts as an antidepressant and anti-anxiety agent. Commonly used SSRI antidepressants in clinical practice include fluoxetine, paroxetine, sertraline, citalopram and levofloxacin. Compared with monoamine oxidase inhibitors and tricyclic antidepressants, SSRIs have the advantages of high efficacy, convenient use and low side effects. However, slow onset is a common deficiency of these drugs. The average effective time of fluoxetine, paroxetine and fluvoxamine is 3–4 weeks.

Moreover, because of the high incidence of adverse effects, the clinical use of these drugs is limited. An evaluation of the use of pharmacotherapy in depression showed that only 7% of patients kept taking antidepressants, while the majority did not continue the medication because of the occurrence of side-effects [9].

The antidepressants may cause a wide range of side effects within a few weeks, some can occasionally persist. Commonly seen side effects of selective serotonin reuptake inhibitors (SSRIs) can include [10]:

- feeling and being sick
- feeling agitated, shaky or anxious
- indigestion and stomach aches
- diarrhoea or constipation
- loss of appetite
- dizziness
- not sleeping well (insomnia), or feeling very sleepy
- headaches
- low sex drive
- difficulties achieving orgasm during sex or masturbation
- in men, difficulties obtaining or maintaining an erection (erectile dysfunction)

15.2   TCM Understanding of Depression

Depression in Chinese medicine has a long history which called Yu Zhen (depression). In the classic book "The Yellow Emperor's Internal Classic" 'Man has the five depots; they transform the five Qi, thereby generating joy, anger, sadness, anxiety, and fear' [11, p. 103].

If the intensity of internal and external stimuli is too strong, the duration is too long, or the stimulating nature is serious, exceeding the individual's ability to endure the threshold and adjust, it can make people's seven emotions (anger, joy, sadness, worry, pensiveness, fear, shock) excessive, and thus hurt the function of viscera and blood, and generate emotions disease. There are also internal and external stimuli that are not strong, the duration of action is not long-lasting, and the stimulating nature is not serious, but due to the patient's personal quality, the patient's experience and reaction to these stimuli are excessive. Emotions could become a cause of disease when they are either long lasting or very intense [12, p. 243].

In addition to strong stimulation of internal and external, if the five visceral Qi unbalances, deficiency and excess, which can increase the sensitivity of people to stimulations and lead to excessive seven emotions. As NJLS Chap 8-Ben Shen (To Consider the Spirit as the Foundation) point out: [11, p. 150–151].

> The Liver stores the blood. The blood hosts the hun soul.
> The Liver Qi:
> If depleted, then fear results.
> If replete, then rage results.

> The spleen stores the camp [Qi]. The camp [Qi] host the intentions.
> The spleen Qi:
> If depleted, then the four limbs are useless.
> The five long-term depots are not in peace.
> If replete, then the abdomen will be distended. Neither menses nor urine flow freely.

> The heart stores the vessels. The vessels host the spirit.
> The heart Qi:
> If depleted, then [the patient] will be grieved.
> If replete, then he will laugh without end.
> The lung stores the Qi. The Qi hosts the po soul.
> The lung Qi:
> If depleted, then the nose will be blocked. The [breath Qi] do not flow freely, with shortness of [breath] Qi.
> If replete, then [the patient] will cough with loud noises, a feeling of fullness in the chest, and breathing with the face directed upward.

> The Kidneys store the essence. The essence hosts the mind.
> The Kidneys Qi:
> If depleted, then this results in receding [Qi].
> If replete, then this results in distention.

"Huangdi Neijing-Lingshu Chapter 54-Tian Nian (Years Given by Heaven)" also stated: 'all five long-term depots are depleted. The spirit Qi have all left. Only the physical appearance and the skeleton remain, and that is the end.' [11, p. 491].

It is believed that the main reason of depression is over-thinking without achieving the goal, leading to Qi stagnation, particularly Liver Qi stagnation. Qi stagnation cause Spleen dysfunction that results in the production of Phlegm-Damp. Phlegm and Qi congeal to obstruct the Heart and Brain and cause stress and depression.

The process of syndrome differentiation is the process of understanding the nature of the disease. The status of syndrome differentiation of depression can reflect the current level of understanding of depression in Chinese medicine. There are many different syndrome differentiations of depression, two major samples in western English books are listed below:

- Wingate states nine patterns is his book "Healing Brain Injury with Chinese Medical Approaches: Integrative Approaches for Practitioners" [13, p. 528–34]: Stagnation of Liver Qi, Qi Stagnation turning into Fire, Obstruction of Static Qi and Phlegm, Phlegm Dampness Obstruction, Blood Stasis Obstructing Internally, Yin and Blood Deficiency (Restless Organ Disorder), Heart and Spleen Dual Deficiency (Qi and Blood), Spleen–Kidney Yang Deficiency, Heart and Kidney Disharmony,
- Maciocia explained 12 patterns in his book 'The Psyche in Chinese Medicine_ Treatment of Emotional and Mental Disharmonies with Acupuncture and Chinese Herbs' [14, p. 358–376], which are Liver-Qi stagnation, Heart and Lung-Qi stagnation, Stagnant Liver-Qi turning into Heat, Phlegm-Heat harassing the Mind, Blood stasis obstructing the Mind, Qi stagnation with Phlegm, Diaphragm Heat, Worry injuring the Mind, Heart and Spleen deficiency, Heart-Yang deficiency, Kidney- and Heart-Yin deficiency, Empty Heat blazing and Kidney-Yang deficiency.

15.3   General Acupuncture Treatment for Depression

Acupuncture treatment and research for the disease of depression has started from early 1980' in China (for details see below Sect. 15.5 Research in this chapter). It has been increased in many areas, the basic theory to understand depression, classic texts discussed about depression, the five-element theory on depression, Shen (Spirit) with depression, Ghost point with depression, internal organs with depression, etc. In particular, the development of TCM Brain theory has provided a brand-new view to understanding depression, the basic aetiology and pathology, the Brain and Shen, the channel of Brain, the points selection of treating depression, scalp acupuncture and the Dao-qi technique for treating depression, et al. These developing areas have been enriched TCM and traditional acupuncture theory and clinical practice and increased the treatment confidence for depression.

The below syndrome differentiation is based on the commonly seen clinical patterns. They might be separated or mixed together.

15.3.1   Liver Qi Stagnation

Signs and symptoms (SS): Depression, fullness at chest, rib area and stomach, helium and sigh, impatient and irritability, dry month and bitter, with headache, red eyes, tinnitus, constipation, or foreign body sensation at throat, irregular period, red tongue, light and yellow coat, wiry pulse.

Treatment principle: Sooth the Liver, remove Qi and reduce Fire.

Points selection: LV-3 Taichong, LI-4 Hegu, LV-13 Qimen, GB-34 Yanglingquan, SJ-6 Zhigou, DU-20 Baihui,

15.3.2   Spleen Qi Deficiency

SS: Depression, overthinking, suspicious, sign, poor appetite, easy fatigue, loose stool, cold body, light and white tongue coating, thin weak and slippery pulse.

Treatment principle: Nourish Spleen Qi.

Points selection: REN-12 Zhongwan, REN-10 Xiawan, REN-6 Qihai, SP-15 Daheng, SP-9 Yinlingquan, SP-6 Sanyinjiao, BL-20 Pishu.

15.3.3   Heart and Gallbladder Qi Deficiency

SS: Depression, Emotional restlessness, timed and fear, palpitation and easy tired, Inferiority and despair, Difficult to make decision, insomnia and dreaming, disturbed sleep, light tongue, thin and white coat, deep, thin and weak pulse.

Treatment principle: nourish Heart and Gallbladder Qi, soothe and quite the mind.

Points selection: HT-7 Shenmen, REN-6 Qihai, GB-34 Yanglingqun, GB-40 Qiuxu, BL-15 Xinshu, BL-19 Danshu.

15.3.4   Both Spleen and Heart Deficiency

SS: Depression, overthinking, easily worried, dizziness, tired, palpitation, insomnia, forgetful, poor appetite, fatigue, burnout, pale complexion, light tongue, thin white coat, thin and slow pulse.

Treatment principle: nourish Heart and Spleen, replenish Qi and Blood.

Points selection: DU-20 Baihui, HT-7 Shenmen, HT-3 Shaohai, SP-9 Yinlingquan, REN-6 Qihai, REN-12 Zhongwan, BL-15 Xinshu, BL-20 Pishu.

15.3.5   Both Kidney and Liver Deficiency

SS: Depression, Irritability, bored, poor concentration, forgetful, worry, back pain, know pian, low libido, light tongue, deep and weak pulse.

Points selection: KI-10 Yingu, KI-3 Taixi, SP-6 Sanyinjiao, LV-3 Taichong, REN-4 Guanyuan, BL-15 Xinshu, BL-18 Ganshu. Ex-Sishencong.

15.4   Unique Brain Acupuncture Techniques for Depression

Traditionally, TCM and acupuncture treatment for depression was mainly focused on the organs of Liver, Heart, Spleen, Kidney, etc. Above general acupuncture treatment has a long history to treating depression symptom, with plenty of experiences and good results for some depression patients.

Recently with the development of TCM Brain theory, it is believed that TCM Brain theory has played a unique role of the depression occurrence, developments and recovery. Due to the Brain Shen disorder, the ability of regulating other Zangfu organs has been decreased or lost. When one Zangfu organ disordered, it can be regulated or re-balanced. But when two or more Zangfu organs are disharmonised, then it will be very difficult to be rebalance. Brain, the highest regulator, is needed to coordinate the disorder of Zangfu organs.

Depression disorder, with such complex clinical manifestation, persistent emotion depression or low, emotional discomfort, unable to express emotion, lack of energy, disorders of autonomic and somatic function, endocrine and physical dysfunction, et al. There are definitely more than two organs involved, particularly in their moderate or later severe stage.

In terms of the acupuncture treatment, during the middle and later stage, the Brain will be the main location of the disease. The treatment principle will be more focused on regulating Du Mai and rebalance the Brain. Thus, Du Mai Dao-qi technique and scalp acupuncture are mostly used in acupuncture practice.

15.4.1   Scalp Acupuncture for Treating Depression (Detail of Scalp Acupuncture, Location and Needling, Please See Chap. 5)

Spirit-Emotion Area, Head Area, Central Area. With anxiety, plus Mania Control Area.

15.4.2   Du Mai Dao-Qi Techniques (Detail of Dao-Qi Technique on Du Mai, Points Location and Needling, Please See Chap. 6)

DU-16 Fengfu, DU-14 Dazhui, DU-9 Zhiyang, DU-4 Mingmen.

15.4.3   Ren Mai Dao-Qi Technique (Detail of Dao-Qi Technique on Ren Mai, Points Location and Needling, Please See Chap. 6)

REN-12 Zhongwan may plus 2–4 needle around it with 0.5–1 cm distance, REN-6 Qihai, REN-4 Guanyuan, REN-17 Danzhong (Shanzhong).

Above unique Brain acupuncture techniques can be combined with syndrome differentiation treatment.

15.4.4   Brain Acupuncture Patterns

Based on the review of TCM classify books and the new developments of the Brain, the commonly clinical patterns of depression and its possible symptoms could be summarized as below and are being developed and are not perfect at the moment [15].

15.4.4.1   Deficiency of Brain Marrow

SS: Depression, chronic vertigo, tinnitus, dizziness, stress, visual dim, insomnia or lethargy, infantile retardation of growth and closure of fontanel, Physical stunting, amnesia and dull facial expression, light-colored or light red tongue, thin and deep pulse.

Brain acupuncture points selection: DU-20 Baihui, DU-14 Dazhui, Ex-Bailaoxue, DU-4 Mingmen, KI-3 Taixi, GB-39 Xuanzhong, and local area points. Techniques could choose electric-acupuncture, scalp acupuncture, Dao-qi technique, etc.

15.4.4.2   Deficiency of Brain Yang Qi

SS: Chronic Stress, mental depression, insomnia or lethargy, amnesia and dull facial expression, general cold sensation, cold limbs and body, dispiritedness, fatigue, whitish or pail tongue, weak and deep pulse.

Brain acupuncture points selection: DU-20 Baihui, DU-16 Fengfu, DU-14 Dazhui, DU-9 Zhiyang, DU-3 Yaoyangguan, plus local area points. Moxa could be applied, or add scalp acupuncture, Dao-qi technique, etc.

15.4.4.3   Disorder of Brain Shen

SS: Mental depression, stress, anxiety, restlessness, insomnia or lethargy, delirium, murmuring, abnormal behavior, anorexia, polyphagia, dementia, drooling, schizophrenia, etc. light tongue with thin coating, wiry or slow pulse.

Brain acupuncture points selection: DU-24 Shenting, DU-20 Baihui, DU-16 Fengfu, DU-14 Dazhui, Ex-Yintang, HT-7 Shenmen plus local area points. Techniques could select electric acupuncture, scalp acupuncture, Dao-qi techniques, etc.

Above Brain related patterns for depression can be identified separately for severe depression, and combined with classic TCM pattern identifications.

15.5 Research

From early 1980s, Prof. Hechun Luo [16], from Mental Health Institute of Beijing Medical University, started to study electro-acupuncture on DU-20 Baihui and Extraordinary point Yintang, to treat major depression and compared with antidepressant. After that, there are increasing studies published, including Prof Lingling Wang and her team from Nanjing University of Chinese Medicine [17]. The researches have proved that, acupuncture, or combined with antidepressant, can effectively help depression patients, with the similar clinical results with antidepressant, but less side effects.

There are different styles of researches design for depression including acupuncture, particularly electro-acupuncture, compare with different kind of antidepressant, acupuncture combined with antidepressant compared with antidepressant, and acupuncture combined with other treatments, et al. Some sample studies of acupuncture for depression are listed below:

Luo et al. [18] recruited 241 depression patients (aged 32–64) from three psychiatric hospitals, who scored over 20 on the Hamilton Rating Scale. Two acupuncture points (DU-20 Baihui and Extraordinary point Yintang) were stimulated with electro acupuncture (EA), six sessions a week for 6 weeks, compared with Amitriptyline. They found no significant difference between EA and Amitriptyline on primary outcome measure. Biochemical markers were different for intervention and control. Hamilton Rating Scale for Depression, Clinical Global Impression Chart, Asberg Rating Scale for Side-effects. Grading System for assessment of therapeutic effects commonly used in China (cured, markedly improved, improved, failed/deteriorated).

Chen et al. [19] used Dredging Governor Meridian and Regulating Shen therapy (DGRS) combined with fluoxetine to treat depression and compared with fluoxetine only. The main points were DU-16, DU-20, DU-24 and Ex-Yintang. The results indicated that DGRS plus antidepressant were much better than antidepressant only. Wang et al. [20] compared acupuncture combined with an SSRI antidepressant for the patients with depression in hospital with antidepressant only. The 17-item Hamilton Depression Rating Scale (HDRS-17) was used to quantitatively assess patients after 1, 2, 4 and 6 weeks of treatment. The conclusion was acupuncture combined with an SSRI showed a statistically significant benefit for patients with depression in hospital over the 6-week period compared with SSRIs alone. The reduction in symptoms started in the first week and continued to the end of the study. These two studies from the same research group, used the similar treatment protocol and reported similar results as well.

Yang and colleagues [21] compared electro-acupuncture treatment (ET) and fake acupuncture control (FC) for depression patients on HAMD-24, SDS. In additional they monitored plasm ACTH, serum CORT and fMRI. They found there was a significant difference between the two groups, the ET group was greater than FC group. The plasm ACTH and serum CORT were lower than before. The Brain functional activities of two group patients were significant as well. They concluded that electro-acupuncture can effectively regulate the endocrine function of major depression patients, improve symptoms, and thus enhance the compensatory function and the quality of life.

Sun et al. [22] compared the therapeutic effects of electro-acupuncture (EA) and Fluoxetine, one of the SSRIs, for depression disorder (DD) patients and focusing on the serum level of Glial Cell Line-Derived Neurotrophic Factor (GDNF). After the treatments of 6 weeks and five times per week, they found EA and Fluoxetine had similar curative effects on DD patients. EA had a faster onset of action, better response rate and better improvement rate than fluoxetine. Both EA and fluoxetine restored the normal concentration of GDNF in the serum of DD patients. They concluded that EA treatment for depression is as effective as a recommended dose of fluoxetine.

Vazquez et al. [23] conducted a study aim to establish the effect of a low frequency electro-acupuncture point formula on the clinical improvement of depressed patients and tested the relation with changes on salivary cortisol. They found a major effect on the reduction of the depression symptoms and salivary cortisol levels of depression patients studied compared to the sham control group.

MacPherson et al. [24] recruited 755 patients who suffered with depression and had consulted their primary health care provider within the last 5 years and who had a score of more than 20 on the BDI-II (Beck Depression Inventory-II), a score that is defined as moderate-to-severe depression on this depression rating scale, at the start of the study. Patients were randomized to receive up to 12 weekly sessions of acupuncture plus usual care (302 patients), up to 12 weekly sessions of counselling plus usual care (302 patients), or usual care alone (151 patients). Both the acupuncture protocol and the counselling protocols allowed for some individualization of treatment. Usual care, including antidepressants, was available according to need and monitored in all three groups. Compared to usual care alone, there was a significant reduction (a reduction unlikely to have occurred by chance) in the average PHQ-9 (Patient Health Questionnaire) scores at both 3 and 6 months for both the acupuncture and counselling interventions. The difference between the mean PHQ-9 score for acupuncture and counselling was not significant. At 9 months and 12 months, because of improvements in the PHQ-9 scores in the usual care group, acupuncture and counselling were no longer significantly better than usual care.

The meta-analysis conducted by Zhang et al. [25] analysed eligible six RCTs and revealed that the combination of SSRIs and electro-acupuncture were associated with superior on HAMD, SDS, and SERS measures compared with SSRIs alone after 1–4 weeks of treatment. They concluded that the evidence suggests that the early treatment of primary depression using the combination of electro-acupuncture with SSRI is more effective that SSRIs alone and leads to a better and earlier benefits of depression symptoms.

15.6 Conclusion

Depression is one of the challenge diseases of clinical practice, wherever in conventional medicine or Chinese medicine. Acupuncture has a long history to treating depression symptom, according to the TCM pattern identification and following treatment principles. The common patterns of classic TCM are Liver Qi stagnation, Spleen Qi deficiency, Heart and Gallbladder Qi deficiency, both Spleen and Heart deficiency and both Kidney and Liver deficiency. The specific Brain patterns for depression are: Deficiency of Brain Marrow, Deficiency of Brain Yang-qi and Disorder of Brain Shen. These two pattern differentiations could be applied combination.

Except traditional acupuncture needling, there are some special Brain related techniques, scalp acupuncture and Dao-qi techniques as two unique samples.

There are increasing evidences to suggest acupuncture are benefit for depression, wherever separately use, or combined with antidepressant. Electric acupuncture is the mostly commonly selected technique. Du Mai points are mostly selected acupoints for major depression. Scalp acupuncture is increasingly used and studied for depression.

References

1. Ganda X, Fountoulakis KN, Kaprinis G, et al. Prediction and prevention of suicide in patients with unipolar depression and anxiety. Ann General Psychiatry. 2007;6:23. https://doi.org/10.1186/1744-859X-6-23.
2. Rihmer Z, Gonda X. Prevention of depression-related suicides in primary care. Psychiatry Hung. 2012;27(2):72–81.
3. Ferrari AJ, Somerville AJ, Baxter AJ, et al. Global variation in the prevalence and incidence of major depressive disorder: a systematic review of the epidemiological literature. Psychol Med. 2012;25:1–11.
4. World Health Organization (WHO). Depression, a global public health concern. 2012. http://www.who.int/mental_health/management/depression/who_paper_depression_wfmh_2012.pdf. Accessed 28 Apr 2020.
5. World Health Organization (WHO). Global burden of mental disorders and the need for a comprehensive, coordinated response from health and social sectors at the country level. 2011. http://apps.who.int/gb/ebwha/pdf_files/EB130/B130_9-en.pdf. Accessed 28 Apr 2020.
6. World Health Organization. Depression: a global crisis world mental health day, October 10 2012. https://www.who.int/mental_health/management/depression/wfmh_paper_depression_wmhd_2012.pdf. Accessed 28 Apr 2020.
7. American Psychiatric Association. Diagnostic and statistical manual of mental disorders. Text revision. 4th ed. Washington, DC: American Psychiatric Association; 2000.
8. Fava M. Diagnosis and definition of treatment resistant depression. Biol Psychiatry. 2003;53:649–59.
9. Pigott HE, Leventhal AM, Alter GS, Boren JJ. Efficacy and effectiveness of antidepressants: current status of research. Psychother Psychosom. 2010;79(5):267–79.
10. NHS. Antidepressant side effects. https://www.nhs.uk/conditions/antidepressants/side-effects/. Accessed 28 Apr 2020.
11. Unschuld PU, Tessenow H, Zheng JS. Huang Di Nei Jing Su Wen: an annotated translation of Huang Di's inner classic – basic questions: Volume II eBook. Berkeley, CA.: University of California Press; 2011.
12. Maciocia G. The foundations of Chinese medicine. 2nd ed. Edinburgh: Churchill Livingstone; 2005.
13. Wingate DS. Healing brain injury with Chinese medical approaches: integrative approaches for practitioners. London and Philadelphia: Singing Dragon; 2018.
14. Maciocia G. The psyche in Chinese medicine-treatment of emotional and mental disharmonies with acupuncture and Chinese herbs. Edinburgh: Churchill Livingstone; 2009.

15. Wang TJ. A new understanding of the brain and its clinical application. EJOM. 2015;8:28–31.
16. Luo HC, Jia YK, Zhan L. Electro-acupuncture versus amitridtyline in the treatment of depressive states (in Chinese). J Trad Chin Med. 1985;5:3–8.
17. Wang LL, Liu LY, Lv M. Clinical thinking of acupuncture treatment for depression (Chinese). J Acupunct Clin. 2003;19(7):7–9.
18. Luo HC, Meng FQ, Jia YK, et al. Clinical research on the therapeutic effect of the electro-acupuncture treatment in patients with depression. Psychiatry Clin Neurosci. 1998;52:S338–S40.
19. Chen L, Wang XJ, Wang LL. Clinical observation of dredging governor vessel and regulating Shen acupuncture method combined with fluoxetine treatment for 30 depression patients (in Chinese). Jiangsu J Chin Med. 2011;12:57–9.
20. Wang TJ, Wang LL, Tao W, et al. Acupuncture combined with an antidepressant for patients with depression in hospital: a pragmatic randomised controlled trial. Acupunct Med. 2014;32:308–12.
21. Yang MZ, Zhou YM, Wu YF, et al. Clinical observation of electro-acupuncture for depression and its brain response monitored by fMRI. Sichuan Mental Health. 2016;29(2):132–6.
22. Sun H, Zhao H, Ma C, et al. Effects of electro-acupuncture on depression and the production of glial cell line–derived neurotrophic factor compared with fluoxetine: a randomized controlled pilot study. J Altern Complement Med. 2011;19(9):733–9.
23. Vazquez RD, González-Macías L, Berlanga C, et al. Effect of acupuncture treatment on depression: correlation between psychological outcomes and salivary cortisol levels. Salud Mental. 2011;34:21–6.
24. MacPherson H, Richmond S, Bland M, et al. Acupuncture and counselling for depression in primary care: a randomised controlled trial. PLoS Med. 2013;10(9):e1001518. https://doi.org/10.1371/journal.pmed.1001518.
25. Zhang Y, Qu SS, Zhang JP, et al. Rapid onset of the effects of combined selective serotonin reuptake inhibitors and electro-acupuncture on primary depression: a meta-analysis. J Altern Complement Med. 2016;22(1):1–8.

Chapter 16
Anxiety

16.1 General Information

16.1.1 Basic Background of the Disease

The WHO's ICD-11 defines anxiety as "Anxiety and fear-related disorders are characterized by excessive fear and anxiety and related behavioural disturbances, with symptoms that are severe enough to result in significant distress or significant impairment in personal, family, social, educational, occupational or other important areas of functioning." [1].

Anxiety-associated disorders are very common and include panic disorder with or without agoraphobia, generalized anxiety disorder, social anxiety disorder, specific phobias and separation anxiety disorder, which are the major parts of the most prevalent mental disorders. According to a review of large population-based surveys worldwide, up to 33.7% of the population are affected by an anxiety disorder during their lifetime [2]. In the UK, women are twice as likely to be diagnosed with anxiety disorders as men [3].

Anxiety in the UK is on the rise. A 2007 survey covering Great Britain indicated that over a period of 14 years, there was a 12.8% increase in the number of cases, with 1.7% more of the population of England experiencing an anxiety-related mental health disorder in 2007 than in 1993, meaning 800,000 more UK adults would have qualified for a diagnosis of an anxiety disorder in 2007 than in 1993 [3]. In 2013, there were 8.2 million cases of anxiety in the UK [4]. As a result, anxiety-related mental health conditions are associated with immense health-care costs [5].

In a 2016 statistics report on mental health in England, it was stated that most mental disorders were more common in people living alone, in poor physical health and not employed. Claimants of Employment and Support Allowance (ESA), a benefit aimed at those unable to work due to poor health or disability, experienced particularly high rates among all the disorders assessed [6].

© Springer Nature Switzerland AG 2021
T. Wang, *Acupuncture for Brain*, https://doi.org/10.1007/978-3-030-54666-3_16

Several types of anxiety disorder exist:

1. **Agoraphobia** is a type of anxiety disorder in which people fear and often avoid places or situations that might induce panic and feelings of being trapped, helpless or embarrassed.
2. **Anxiety disorder due to a medical condition** includes symptoms of intense anxiety or panic that are directly caused by a physical health problem.
3. **Generalized anxiety disorder** includes persistent and excessive anxiety and worry about activities or events—even ordinary, routine issues. The worry is out of proportion to the actual circumstance, is difficult to control and affects how the person feels physically. It often occurs along with other anxiety disorders or depression.
4. **Panic disorder** involves repeated episodes of sudden feelings of intense anxiety and fear or terror that reach a peak within minutes (panic attacks). People may have feelings of impending doom, shortness of breath, chest pain, or a rapid, fluttering or pounding Heart (Heart palpitations). These panic attacks may lead to worrying about them happening again or avoiding situations in which they have occurred.
5. **Selective mutism** is a consistent failure of children to speak in certain situations, such as school, even when they can speak in other situations, such as at home with close family members. This can interfere with school, work and social functioning.
6. **Separation anxiety disorder** is a childhood disorder characterized by anxiety that is excessive for the child's developmental level and related to separation from parents or others who have parental roles.
7. **Social anxiety disorder (social phobia)** involves high levels of anxiety, fear and avoidance of social situations due to feelings of embarrassment, self-consciousness and concern about being judged or viewed negatively by others.
8. **Specific phobias** are characterized by major anxiety when you are exposed to a specific object or situation and a desire to avoid it. Phobias provoke panic attacks in some people.
9. **Substance-induced anxiety disorder** is characterized by symptoms of intense anxiety or panic that are a direct result of misusing drugs, taking medications, being exposed to a toxic substance or withdrawal from drugs.
10. **Other specified anxiety disorder and unspecified anxiety disorder** are terms for anxiety or phobias that don't meet the exact criteria for any other anxiety disorders but are significant enough to be distressing and disruptive.

Previously, anxiety disorders included obsessive compulsive disorder (OCD) and post-traumatic stress disorder (PTSD), as well as acute stress disorder. However, these mental health difficulties no longer come under the anxiety category.

16.1.2   The Aetiology and Pathogenesis

The exact cause of anxiety isn't fully understood, although it's likely that a combination of several factors plays a role. Possible causes include:

1. Environmental stress, such as difficulties at work, relationship problems or family issues
2. Genetics, as people who have family members with an anxiety disorder are more likely to experience one themselves
3. Medical factors, such as the symptoms of a different disease, the effects of a medication, or the stress of an intensive surgery or prolonged recovery
4. Brain chemistry, as psychologists define many anxiety disorders as misalignments of hormones and electrical signals in the Brain
5. Withdrawal from an illicit substance, the effects of which might intensify the impact of other possible causes

16.1.3   Typical Clinical Symptoms

Anxiety can have both psychological and physical symptoms. Psychological symptoms can include:

- Feeling worried or uneasy a lot of the time
- Having difficulty sleeping (insomnia), which may result in further tiredness
- Not being able to concentrate
- Being irritable
- Being extra alert
- Feeling on edge or not being able to relax
- Needing frequent reassurance from other people
- Feeling tearful

Physical symptoms can include:

- A pounding heartbeat
- Breathing faster
- Palpitations
- Feeling sick
- Chest pains
- Headaches
- Sweating
- Loss of appetite
- Feeling faint
- Needing the toilet more frequently
- "Butterflies" in the abdomen

16.1.4 Examination and Diagnosis

Anxiety, mostly seen as generalized anxiety disorder (GAD), can be difficult to diagnose. In some cases, it can also be difficult to distinguish from other mental health conditions, for example depression and addiction-related conditions like alcohol or drug misuse.

Therefore, the diagnosis of GAD/anxiety is not an examination-oriented conclusion but is based on the patient's symptoms, such as:

A. Significant worry, which affects daily life, including job and social life
B. Extreme worry, which is stressful and upsetting
C. Worrying negatively about all sorts of things and having a tendency to think the worst
D. Worrying about being overwhelmed and out of control
E. Suffering from worry nearly every day for at least six months

Physical examinations or Blood tests are used to rule out other conditions that may be causing the same symptoms, such as anaemia (a deficiency in iron or vitamin B12 and folate), or overactive thyroid gland (hyperthyroidism).

16.1.5 The Modern Medicine Treatment for Anxiety, and Possible Disadvantages

Other problems alongside anxiety, such as depression or alcohol misuse, may need to be treated before specifically treating anxiety.

Anxiety is a long-term condition, and the treatments for it in modern medicine include:

16.1.5.1 Medication

Selective Serotonin Reuptake Inhibitors (SSRIs)

This type of medication works by increasing the level of serotonin in the Brain. The most commonly prescribed SSRIs are: Sertraline; Citalopram or Celexa; Paroxetine; Fluoxetine or Prozac. SSRIs can be taken on a long-term basis but, as with all antidepressants, they can take several weeks to start working. Common side effects of SSRIs include: feeling agitated; feeling or being sick; indigestion; diarrhoea or constipation; loss of appetite and weight loss; dizziness; blurred vision; a dry mouth; excessive sweating; headaches; insomnia or drowsiness; low sex drive; difficulty achieving orgasm during sex or masturbation; erectile dysfunction.

Serotonin and Noradrenaline Reuptake Inhibitors (SNRIs)

This type of medicine increases the amount of serotonin and noradrenaline in the Brain. These medications include Venlafaxine and Duloxetine. Common side effects of SNRIs include: feeling sick; headaches; drowsiness; dizziness; a dry mouth; constipation; insomnia; sweating; raised Blood pressure.

Pregabalin (Anticonvulsant/Antiseizure)

Pregabalin is an anticonvulsant that is used to treat conditions such as epilepsy, but it has also been found to be beneficial in treating anxiety. Side effects of Pregabalin may include: drowsiness; dizziness; increased appetite and weight gain; blurred vision; headaches; a dry mouth; vertigo. Pregabalin is less likely to cause nausea or a low sex drive than SSRIs or SNRIs.

Benzodiazepines

Benzodiazepines are a type of sedative that may sometimes be used as a short-term treatment during a particularly severe period of anxiety. Among the most commonly prescribed is Diazepam. Benzodiazepines are fast working—believed to help ease symptoms within 30 to 90 min of taking the medication. Benzodiazepines can become addictive if used for longer than four weeks. They also start to lose their effectiveness after this time. To avoid potential addiction to the medicine, it is advised not to take it for any longer than four weeks at a time. Side effects of Benzodiazepines can include: drowsiness; difficulty concentrating; headaches; vertigo; tremor; low sex drive.

Other additional drugs include monoamine oxidase inhibitors (MAOIs), beta-blockers and Buspirone.

16.1.5.2 Psychological Therapies for Anxiety

Cognitive Behavioural Therapy (CBT)

Cognitive behavioural therapy (CBT) is a talking therapy that can help manage people's problems by changing the way a person thinks and behaves. CBT aims to help deal with overwhelming problems in a more positive way by breaking them down into smaller parts, and is believed to be one of the most effective treatments for GAD. Studies of different treatments for GAD have found that the benefits of CBT may last longer than those of medication, but no single treatment works for everyone. It usually involves meeting with a specially trained and accredited therapist for a one-hour session every week for three to four months.

Applied Relaxation

Applied relaxation focuses on relaxing muscles in a particular way during situations that usually cause anxiety. The technique also needs to be taught by a trained therapist. The Alexander Technique is one of the best-known applied relaxation techniques in the West.

The two therapies described above are non-invasive treatments for GAD, therefore there are no side effects. But a root treatment that looks into the radical cause of GAD is still not available.

16.2 TCM Understanding of Anxiety

Due to the chronicity, the high relapse rates and the need for a long-term maintenance treatment, there is an urgent need for an effective treatment for anxiety, with less undesirable side effects. In recent years, non-conventional therapies such as acupuncture have become more popular for treating this mental health problem. Several studies have proved that acupuncture is a safe therapy with rare adverse side effects [7, 8]. In the view of traditional Chinese medicine, anxiety is mainly the result of an impairment of the functions of internal organs, such as the Heart and Kidneys' Yin/Yang flow (and lack of communication between them) and a hyperactivity of Liver Yang (overly active and vitalizing force). Acupuncture, through the stimulation of specific trigger points (acupoints), can, therefore, improve and alleviate this condition [9].

Pathology in TCM [10, p. 103] [11, p. 463–7].

"Huangdi Neijing-Simple Question—Chapter 5" states 'Heaven has its four seasons and five agents, it is through (the former that heaven causes) generations, growth, gathering and storage, it is through (the latter it) generates cold, summer heat, dampness, dryness and wind; Man has the five depots, they transform the five Qi, therefore generate joy, anger, sadness, anxiety and fear'. Anxiety as a mental disorder condition has a very close relation with the internal five Yin organs and six Yang organs.

While there has been no particular diagnostic name for anxiety-related conditions in the history of TCM, anxiety-related symptoms were recorded in disease names like: Yu Zheng/depression, Bu Mei/insomnia, Bai He Bing, Zang Zao/restless organ disorder and Zheng Chong/palpitations, which can help provide clues to the differential patterns and relevant treatment. Our understanding on the pathology starts with the functions of related organs.

Heart: According to the theory of TCM, the Heart is in charge of the Shen, Heart-mind, which is connected to general mental activities. The symptoms of anxiety, restlessness, panic, insomnia and Heart-racing, etc. are believed to be mainly linked to the Heart's pathology. The most common Heart-associated patterns are: Heart Blood deficiency, Heart Yin deficiency and Heart Fire.

Heart Blood deficiency: anxiety with palpitations, dizziness, insomnia, dream-disturbed sleep, anxiety, easily startled, poor memory, poor concentration, dull pale complexion, lips are likely to be pale. Tongue diagnosis: pale, possibly thin and maybe dry. Pulse diagnosis: thin or choppy (often felt in the Heart position).

Heart Yin deficiency: similar to Blood deficiency but with more anxiety and restlessness, palpitations, insomnia, dream-disturbed sleep, easily startled, poor memory, fidgeting, malar flush, night sweats, five-palm heat, a dry mouth. Tongue diagnosis: red or peeled with or without coat. Pulse diagnosis: floating, empty or thin, fast.

Heart Fire: anxiety with palpitations, thirst, tongue/mouth ulcers, restlessness, red complexion, bitter taste in the mouth, esp. if after a poor night's sleep; if during day may be more Liver, other Heat signs. Tongue diagnosis: red w/yellow coat, red points on tip. Pulse diagnosis: full, rapid, overflowing (esp. in Heart position).

Kidney: Kidney pertains to water element; in relation to Heart, Kidney Yin/essence it provides the anchoring, cooling and calming force in the Heart-Shen-mind. With disharmony/imbalance between the Heart and Kidney, the Heart can be overheated by either excessive Fire in the Heart or a lack of cooling/anchoring from Kidney Yin-deficient Heat; the Heart-Shen-mind is therefore disturbed, unsettled or in severe cases depleted. The most common pattern of Kidney pathology is: Kidney Yin deficiency (leading to Heart-Shen-mind being unanchored).

Kidney Yin deficiency (Water-Fire disharmony): anxiety with dizziness, tinnitus, vertigo, sore back, constipation, may also have empty heat signs, malar flush, night sweats, five-palm heat, insomnia, a dry throat. Tongue diagnosis: red with or without coat, may have horizontal cracks, red tip empty Fire. Pulse diagnosis: floating, empty, rapid.

Liver: Liver pertains to wood element and is the mother element to Heart Fire. The Liver is in charge of emotional expressions—the emotions associated with the Liver are anger, frustration and stress, which can all affect the Heart-Shen-mind. The most common patterns of Liver pathology are: Liver Qi stagnation, Liver Fire (due to stagnant heat), Liver Blood deficiency (usually with underlying Liver Qi stagnation), Liver Yin deficiency (usually along with Kidney Yin deficiency).

Liver Qi stagnation: anxiety with chest distension, hypochondriac pain and/or distension, sighing, nausea, vomiting, poor appetite, diarrhoea, depression, moodiness, plum pit Qi, PMS, breast tenderness, painful and/or irregular menstruation. Tongue diagnosis: normal or slightly purple on sides of tongue. Pulse diagnosis: wiry.

Liver Fire: anxiety with headaches, irritability, explosive anger, dizziness, tinnitus, bitter taste in the mouth, red face, red eyes, dream-disturbed sleep, constipation. Tongue diagnosis: red, dry white or yellow coat, possibly redder around the Liver and gall bladder area. Pulse diagnosis: wiry, full, rapid.

Liver Blood deficiency: anxiety with numbness in the extremities, tics, tremors, dizziness, blurred vision, floaters, insomnia, dry skin/hair, scanty or lack of menstruation. Tongue diagnosis: pale, thin, dry. Pulse diagnosis: thin, choppy.

Liver Yin deficiency: anxiety and restlessness, cramps, with irritability, dizziness, dry eyes, blurred vision and floaters in eyes, scanty period or amenorrhoea, withered and brittle nails, dry hair and skin. Tongue diagnosis: slim tongue, red with little coating or rootless coating. Pulse diagnosis: thin/thready pulse, weak under moderate pressure.

Spleen: Spleen pertains to the Earth element. The Spleen is in charge of transformation and transportation of food and fluid in the body and is the key organ of Qi, Blood and body Jin Ye (liquid/fluid). Without a good support of Blood produce, the Heart and Liver will suffer. Therefore, anxiety could be a secondary consequence of Spleen deficiency. The most common patterns related to the Spleen are: dual Heart and Spleen deficiency, Spleen deficiency with Liver stagnation.

Dual deficiency of Heart and Spleen (Blood): anxiety or depression, with palpitations, dizziness, insomnia, poor memory, propensity to be startled, dull/pale complexion, pale lips, tiredness, weak muscles, loose stools with poor appetite, scanty periods. Tongue diagnosis: thin and pale tongue. Pulse diagnosis: thin or choppy pulse, weak under pressure, esp. on left cun and right guan.

Spleen deficiency with Liver stagnation: anxiety or depression with irritability, abdominal distension and pain, alternating diarrhoea and constipation, tiredness, stools sometimes dry and bitty (small pieces), sometimes loose, flatulence. Tongue diagnosis: light red or pale puffy tongue with white coating, dark or purple side with tooth marks. Pulse diagnosis: wiry on left guan, wiry thin but weak on right guan under pressure.

Gall bladder: Gall bladder is in charge of decision-making. A weak gall bladder makes people become timid and fragile; they frighten easily and are therefore restless and anxious. In addition, Shaoyang syndrome with gall bladder meridian disturbance presents restlessness and anxiety. The most common patterns related to the gall bladder are: dual deficiency of the gall bladder and Heart, and Shaoyang syndrome.

Dual deficiency of gall bladder and Heart: anxiety and restlessness or depression, feeling timid and fearful, inferiority complex and despair, with palpitations and becoming fatigued easily, difficulty with making decisions, insomnia and dream-disturbed sleep. Tongue diagnosis: light red tongue, with thin and white coating. Pulse diagnosis: deep, thin and weak, esp. on left cun and guan.

Shaoyang syndrome: anxiety or restlessness, with alternation of shivers (or cold feeling) and fever (or a feeling of heat), bitter taste in the mouth, a dry or tickly throat, blurred vision, hypochondrial fullness and distension, a lack of desire to eat or drink (loss of appetite), irritability, nausea, vomiting. Tongue diagnosis: unilateral thin white coating. Pulse diagnosis: thin/thready-wiry pulse.

Sanjiao/pericardium: Sanjiao suffering is a part of Shaoyang syndrome, the pericardium is the protector of the emperor Heart. Therefore, the treatment of the two is a supplementary method alongside the other organs, esp. the Heart.

16.3   General Acupuncture Treatment

Here we look at the most common complex patterns in clinic:

16.3.1 Liver Blood/Yin Deficiency with Liver Qi Stagnation

Signs and symptoms: patterns of Liver Blood/Yin deficiency + Liver Qi stagnation, sometimes with Liver heat/Fire (please refer to the above individual patterns for relevant signs and symptoms).

Treatment principle: Tonify Liver Blood/Yin, soothe the Liver Qi and reduce Fire/heat.

Points selection: LV-8 Ququan, SP-6 Sanyinjiao, LV-3 Taichong, LI-4 Hegu, LV-13 Qimen, GB-34 Yanglingquan, SJ-6 Zigou, DU-20 Baihui.

16.3.2 Shaoyang Syndrome with Chronic Spleen Qi Deficiency

Signs and symptoms: Shaoyang syndrome + Spleen Qi deficiency (please refer to the above individual patterns for relevant signs and symptoms).

Treatment principle: nourish Spleen Qi and soothe Shaoyang.

Points selection: SJ-5 Waiguan, GB-41 Zulinqi, SP-3 Taibai, REN-12 Zhongwan, REN-10 Xiawan, REN-6 Qihai, SP-15 Daheng, SP-9 Yinlingquan, SP-6 Sanyinjiao, BL-20 Pishu.

16.3.3 Heart and Gall Bladder Qi Deficiency

Signs and symptoms: pattern of dual deficiency of Heart and gall bladder Qi (please refer to the above individual patterns for relevant signs and symptoms).

Treatment principle: nourish Heart and gall bladder Qi, soothe and calm the mind.

Points selection: HT-7 Shenmen, REN-6 Qihai, GB-34 Yanglingqun, GB-40 Qiuxu, BL-15 Xinshu, BL-19 Danshu.

16.3.4 Dual Spleen and Heart Deficiency

Signs and symptoms: patterns of Spleen Qi deficiency + Heart Blood deficiency (please refer to the above individual patterns for relevant signs and symptoms).

Treatment principle: tonify Spleen Qi and enrich Heart Blood.

Points selection: DU-20 Bahui, HT-7 Shenmen, HT-3 Shaohai, SP-9 Yinlingquan, REN-6 Qihai, REN-12 Zhongwan, BL-15 Xinshu, BL-20 Pishu.

16.3.5 Dual Kidney and Liver Deficiency

Signs and symptoms: pattern of Liver and Kidney Yin deficiency (please refer to the above individual patterns for relevant signs and symptoms).

Treatment principle: tonify Liver and Kidney Yin.

Points selection: KI-10 Yingu, KI-3 Taixi, SP-6 Sanyinjiao, LV-3 Taichong, REN-4 Guanyuan, BL-15 Xinshu, BL-18 Ganshu, Ex-Sishencong (EX-HN1).

16.3.6   Dual Heart and Kidney Yin Deficiency

Signs and symptoms: pattern of Heart and Kidney Yin deficiency (please refer to the above individual patterns for relevant signs and symptoms).

Treatment principle: tonify Heart and Kidney Yin.

Points selection: KI-10 Yingu, KI-3 Taixi, SP-6 Sanyinjiao, HT-3 Shaohai, HT-7 Shenmen, BL-15 Xinshu, BL-23 Shenshu, Ex-Sishencong (EX-HN1).

Alongside the traditional organ-oriented differentiation principle for acupoint selection, the most recent recognized treatment protocols in modern China require more points on the head and face to be used as the leading points in the acupuncture treatment for anxiety. Among them, Yintang (EX-HN3), Sishenchong (EX-HN1), Shenting (DU-24) and Baihui (DU-20), are the most chosen in practice [12]. These points are believed to be the local points to the head and Brain, and the nervous system, and are more powerful in mental and neurological conditions.

16.4   Unique Brain Acupuncture Techniques

As we can see, the traditional acupuncture treatment for anxiety was mostly focused on the internal organs of the Liver, Heart, Spleen and Kidney, among others. The relevant treatments are called the "Zangfu differential treatment". Recently, thanks to the innovative development of TCM Brain theory, scalp or Brain-oriented treatment has started to attract more attention from practitioners of acupuncture. Acupoints located on the scalp or head, or specific zones/lines in modernized scalp acupuncture theory, are introduced more in the relevant treatments. Modern techniques, including electronic acupuncture and ear acupuncture, are becoming popular, and some pioneering methods, such as medicated oxygen therapy, are also being trialled.

16.4.1   Conventional Acupoints with Dao-qi Technique

DU-20 Baihui, DU-24 Shenting, Ex-Sishenchong, Ex-Yintang, all suitable for Dao-qi technique. Detail of Dao-qi technique on Du Mai and Ren Mai, points location and needling, please see Chap. 6.

16.4.2   Scalp Acupuncture Areas/Zones

As a new extension of modern acupuncture development, scalp acupuncture has a stronger effect on the Brain and the nervous system. Therefore, it is a good method to apply to go along with the traditional Chinese meridian system. The most commonly used points (zones) are: Foot-Motor Sensory Area, Spirit-Emotion Area and Mania Control Area. Detail of scalp acupuncture, location and needling, please see Chap. 5.

16.4.3   Other Techniques

Electronic acupuncture: low density/frequency electronic stimulation (1–50 Hz) is recommended in the treatment of anxiety, however there are no adequate researches on which exact frequency is the most effective in the treatment of anxiety. The figures vary across researches, as well as between different people.

Auricular acupuncture: Karst et al. [13] suggested that auricular points used effectively for anxiety treatment are relaxation, tranquillizer and master cerebral points. Other researchers also found that relaxation points along with Shenmen, or other points, namely lung, Shenmen, Kidney, subcortex and adrenal gland points, can be effective too [14].

Acupuncture with medicated oxygen therapy: this is still a new experimental method of treatment that has emerged in recent years in China. Application of this therapy involves medicated oxygen inhalation, either by nasal-feed pure oxygen gas or within a hyperbaric oxygen chamber during acupuncture treatment. It is believed to help increase the effect of acupuncture in influencing cerebral function.

16.5   Research

The interest of researchers in the treatment of anxiety disorders using acupuncture has become a worldwide trend. This trend is supported by several factors, such as growing knowledge about the anatomophysiologic mechanism of the action of acupuncture, empirical validation of acupuncture's benefits and results, and the growing interest of the general public in this therapy as a safe alternative, with fewer side effects than conventional pharmaceutical treatments, which present limited efficacy, toxicity, drug interactions and the risk of drug addiction.

Many researches have shown that acupuncture on its own, or integrated with Western treatment, has a better effect on anxiety, and presents fewer or no side effects.

In Sweden, Arvidsdotter and colleagues [15] conducted a randomized controlled clinical trial with 120 anxiety patients from primary care services, and found that integrative treatments and acupuncture therapies resulted in a statistically and clinically significant reduction of anxiety in patients. In four weeks, the differences between the groups were significant on IT-CT (integrated group, p = 0.005) and AT-CT (acupuncture group, p = 0.006). Similarly, both the AT and the IT improved significantly more than the CT (conventional group, both p < 0.001) in the eight-week baseline.

In their research, Wang and Kain [16] assess the effectiveness of acupuncture in reducing anxiety in volunteer adults before surgery, by randomizing them into three treatment groups: (a) Shenmen group—bilateral auricular acupuncture at the "Shenmen" point; (b) Relaxation group—bilateral auricular acupuncture at a "relaxation" point; and (c) Sham group—bilateral auricular acupuncture at a "sham" point. Press acupuncture needles were inserted in the respective auricular areas for 48 h. State anxiety, Blood pressure, Heart rate and electrodermal activity were assessed at 30 min, 24 h and 48 h after insertion. Analysing anxiety levels using repeated-measures analysis of variance has demonstrated a significant difference between the three treatment groups. *Post hoc* analysis demonstrated that patients in the relaxation group were significantly less anxious at 30 min and 24 h than patients in both the Shenmen group and the sham group, and less anxious at 48 h than patients in the Shenmen group. Repeated-measures analysis of variance performed for electrodermal activity, Blood pressure and Heart rate demonstrated no group differences. The authors conclude that auricular acupuncture at the "relaxation" point can decrease the anxiety level in a population of healthy volunteers.

The research of Wu and Liu [17] shows that both the EA group and the control/pharmacotherapy (Alprazolam) group presented a high success rate (> 80%) in the ability to decrease anxiety. However, only the control group presented several side effects, in contrast to EA, from which none was reported.

Zeng and colleagues [18] found that electro-acupuncture (EA) helps improve psychiatric symptoms induced by medicine (Methamphetamine MA) among addicts too. EA was able to effectively improve the symptoms of psychosis, anxiety and depression during abstinence in patients with MA addiction. In terms of PANSS (Positive and Negative Syndrome Scale) score, the scores for positive symptoms and general psycho-pathological symptoms in patients after receiving one to four weeks of treatment were significantly decreased compared with the control group, while the score for negative symptoms was significantly decreased after receiving two and four weeks of treatment. For the HAM-A (Hamilton Anxiety Scale) score, the psychotic anxiety scores in patients receiving one to four weeks of treatment were significantly lower than in the control group. In terms of HAM-D (Hamilton Depression Scale) score, there was a significant reduction in anxiety/somatization and sleep disturbance scores after the four weeks of EA treatment.

The biological mechanism and effect of acupuncture on anxiety in the Western context is the key bridge between the Chinese and Western world. We are inspired by what acupuncture can do to the body undergoing various types of anxious conditions measured with and explained by the Western context.

Arranz and co-workers [19] reported that their study found that chemotaxis, phagocytosis, lymphoproliferation and NK activity were significantly improved by acupuncture. Patients with abnormally high levels of superoxide anion and lympho-proliferation found that these parameters were greatly diminished after treatment. Overall, acupuncture brought the immune parameters closer to the control levels of healthy untreated women. More importantly, besides the proven stimulatory effect of acupuncture, it was also verified that it had a modulatory effect on the immune system-augmenting or reducing the levels of the immune parameters as needed to achieve healthy parameters.

The biochemical mechanism for anxiety is believed to be related to a neurotransmitter (5- hydroxytryptamine (5-HT) hyperfunction) and neuroendocrine function disorder (excessive excretion of adrenocorticotropic hormone (ACTH), corticosteroid (CS) and prolactin) [20, 21]. In the research of Yuan and co-workers [21], plasma CS and ACTH and platelet 5-HT levels were measured in patients to compare the efficacy of acupuncture to a control group administered with common pharmacological treatment and further compared to a group receiving combined therapy (acupuncture + pharmacology). They found out that, with all groups achieving effective results for anxiety in terms of the parameters, acupuncture not only had fewer side effects, but also helped prevent the side effects of the drugs in the combined therapy group.

Karst et al. [13] using heart rate and oxygen saturation measurements, observed a decreased Heart rate, but not oxygen saturation rate, for all treatment groups compared to the control group. Acar et al. [22] using a bispectral index electrode to measure cortical electrical activity, found that BIS values decrease significantly in relation to the sham acupuncture group and in comparison to baseline levels.

Shayestehfar et al. [14] observed heart rate and skin conductance following acupuncture treatment on anxiety patients. They describe a decreased rate of Heartbeat for the body acupuncture group relative to the sham acupuncture one. Furthermore, this study also measures skin conductivity and correlates skin sweat to the somatic manifestation of anxiety. They found a significant decrease in anxiety compared to both sham and control groups.

16.6 Conclusion

Anxiety is on the rise in the modern lifestyle throughout all cultures and countries. Western medicine's treatment for anxiety includes drugs and psychological therapies, with treatments either having a high risk of drug addiction, resistance and side effects or not being reliable in terms of recurrence and higher maintenance costs. The conventional TCM understanding of anxiety is based on the imbalance of internal organs, with the Heart, Liver, Kidney, Spleen and Gall bladder/Shaoyang being the leading pathological factors. The most common patterns of anxiety are related to: Heart and Kidney Yin deficiency, Heart and Liver Qi stagnation with Fire, Liver and Kidney Yin deficiency, Heart and Spleen Blood deficiency, and Heart and gall bladder deficiency. Persisting with the organ-focused differentiation as the core of TCM treatment, the modern TCM acupuncture practice has also now made progress by conducting a deeper investigation of the function and role of the Brain and therefore applying more thorough treatment involving the Brain, the nervous system or the scalp. Acupuncture integrated with modern methods like electric stimulation, ear reflexology and medicated oxygen is also presenting more potential nowadays. Researches on acupuncture treatment for anxiety indicate that acupuncture is promising to achieve a better effect in terms of controlling anxiety symptoms, and reducing or preventing the side effects of Western medication. And it has also been proven that acupuncture not only brings positive changes to indicators of physical body functions in patients but also presents solid evidence of biochemical improvements in patients suffering from anxiety. We are delighted to see that acupuncture as a strong alternative to the conventional treatment for anxiety is receiving more and more attention and enjoying more success in practice.

References

1. WHO ICD-11 for mortality and morbidity statistics, Version: 04 /2019. https://icd.who.int/browse11/l-m/en#/http://id.who.int/icd/entity/1336943699. Accessed 20 May 2020.
2. Borwin B, Sophie M. Epidemiology of anxiety disorders in the 21st century. Dialogues Clin Neurosci. 2015;17(3):327–35.
3. Martin-Merino E, Ruigomez A, Wallander MA, et al. Prevalence, incidence, morbidity and treatment patterns in a cohort of patients diagnosed with anxiety in UK primary care. Fam Pract. 2009;27(1):9–16.
4. Halliwell ED. In the face of fear. London: Mental Health Foundation; 2009. p. 5. https://www.mentalhealth.org.uk/publications/face-fear. Accessed 28 Apr 2020.
5. Fineberg NA, Haddad PM, Carpenter L, et al. The size, burden and cost of disorders of the brain in the UK. J Psychopharmacol. 2013;27(9):761–70.
6. McManus S, Bebbington P, Jenkins R, et al., editors. Mental health and wellbeing in England: adult psychiatric morbidity survey. Leeds: NHS Digital; 2014.
7. White A. A cumulative review of the range and incidence of significant adverse events associated with acupuncture. Acupunct Med. 2004;22(3):122–33.
8. Witt CM, Pach D, Brinkhaus BK, et al. Safety of acupuncture: results of a prospective observational study with 229,230 patients and introduction of a medical information and consent form. Forsch Komplementmed. 2009;16:91–7.
9. Samuels N, Gropp C, Singer SR, et al. Acupuncture for psychiatric illness: a literature review. Behav Med. 2008;34(2):55–64.
10. Unschuld PU, Tessenow H, Zheng JS. Huang Di Nei Jing Su Wen: an annotated translation of Huang Di's Inner classic–basic questions, vol. Vol. II. Berkeley, CA: University of California Press; 2011.
11. Maciocia G. The foundations of Chinese medicine. 2nd ed. Edinburgh: Elsevier; 2005.
12. Lu XY, Sun B, Wen Q. The exploration on point selection rules for acupuncture treatment of anxiety (article in Chinese only). Shanghai J Acu-Mox. 2018;37(4):474–9.

13. Karst M, Winterhalter M, Münte S, et al. Auricular acupuncture effectively reduces state anxiety before dental treatment: a randomised controlled trial. Clin Oral Investig. 2012;16:1517–22.
14. Shayestehfar M, Seif-Barghi T, Zarei S, et al. Acupuncture anxiolytic effects on physiological and psychological assessments for a clinical trial. Scientifica. 2016. 6 pages; https://doi.org/10.1155/2016/4016952.
15. Arvidsdotter T, Marklund B, Taft C. Effects of an integrative treatment, therapeutic acupuncture and conventional treatment in alleviating psychological distress in primary care patients: a pragmatic randomized controlled trial. BMC Complement Altern Med. 2013;13:308. 9 pages. https://doi.org/10.1186/1472-6882-13-308.
16. Wang S, Kain ZN. Auricular acupuncture: a potential treatment for anxiety. Anesth Analg. 2001;9(2):548–53.
17. Wu P, Liu S. Clinical observation on post-stroke anxiety neurosis treated by acupuncture. J Tradit Chin Med. 2008;28(3):186–8.
18. Zeng L, Tao Y, Hou WG, et al. Electro-acupuncture improves psychiatric symptoms, anxiety and depression in methamphetamine addicts during abstinence. a randomized controlled trial. Medicine. 2018;97:34. 7 pages, e11905. https://doi.org/10.1097/MD.0000000000011905.
19. Arranz L, Guayerbas N, Siboni L, et al. Effect of acupuncture treatment on the immune function impairment found in anxious women. Am J Chin Med. 2007;35(1):35–51.
20. Gerra G, Zaimovic A, Zambelli U, et al. Neuroendrocrine responses to psychological stress in adolescents with anxiety disorder. Neuropsychobiology. 2000;42:82–5.
21. Yuan Q, Li JN, Liu B, et al. Effect of jin-3-needling therapy on plasma corticosteroid, adrenocorticotrophic hormone and platelet 5-HT levels in patients with generalized anxiety disorder. Chin J Integr Med. 2007;13(4):264–8.
22. Acar H, Cuvas O, Ceyhan A, et al. Acupuncture on Yintang point decreases preoperative anxiety. J Alternative Compl Med. 2013;19(5):420–4.

Chapter 17
Bipolar Disorder

17.1 General Information on Bipolar Disorder

17.1.1 Basic Background

Bipolar disorder (BD) is a debilitating mental disease with alternating high and lower energy. Bipolar "highs" are characterized by periods of increased energy, minimal sleep and euphoric or delusional moods, which alternate with "lows" that can be depressive, sometimes leading to suicidal ideation [1]. BD is often undiagnosed and undertreated. Alcohol is a frequent choice for self-medicating patients, and, typically, manic depressive patients take some time and persuasion before they agree to treatment and compliance with treatment protocols [2]. It is estimated that BD afflicts between 1% and 3% of the world's population, and is disproportionately more common among those surveyed in Western populations, of higher socio-economic class, and among single and divorced individuals [3].

When milder subclinical presentations are included, the prevalence rate increases to approximately 4%. First-degree relatives of bipolar individuals are significantly more likely to develop the disorder than the population at large, and twins have a 70% risk of sharing the disorder [4].

This psychopathology represents a major psychiatric disorder that can have a significant negative effect on an individual who suffers from it and his or her social environment [5, 6].

BD has been associated with substantial disability in older adults. Remission of BD patients has been associated with significant but incomplete improvement in functioning, whereas psychotic and depressive symptoms and cognitive impairment seem to contribute to lower health-related quality of life and functioning (HRQoLF) [6].

BD is associated with higher rates of suicide than any other psychiatric disorder. Risk factors for suicide include a predominantly depressed presentation, substance and alcohol abuse or dependence disorders, being young and male, recent illness

© Springer Nature Switzerland AG 2021
T. Wang, *Acupuncture for Brain*, https://doi.org/10.1007/978-3-030-54666-3_17

onset, significant anxiety, impulsiveness, family history of suicidality, and social isolation. Recent life event stress also appears to be common before suicide [7].

Interestingly, BD is believed to be associated with elevated creativity and productivity: many famous artists, musicians, writers and politicians appear to have had the disorder [8].

17.1.2 The Aetiology and Pathogenesis

Although not yet fully elucidated, BD symptoms are probably caused by dysregulation of serotonergic and dopaminergic pathways, and diminished activity in the hippocampus and prefrontal cortex [7, 9]. It has been suggested that abnormal activity in hypothalamic circuits involved in maintaining normal circadian rhythms is manifested as affective and behavioural symptoms of BD [7]. Recurrences of mania or depression are a result of the mutually influential interactions between genes, neural pathways and socio-environmental influences. Special emphasis should be placed on new findings regarding the prognostic effects of psychosocial variables [7].

BD is among the most heritable of disorders. The concordance rates for identical twins average 57%, compared with 14% for fraternal twins [10]. The common susceptibility genes may predispose individuals to dopamine dysregulation and eventual psychosis. However, there are genes whose expression may affect neurodevelopment, illness-specific neurological changes and environmental factors. These factors distinguish the onset and course of BD from the onset and course of schizophrenia [11].

Researchers now focus on the functioning of neurotransmitter systems, such as increased sensitivity of the postsynaptic receptors in pharmacological challenges, neuroimaging or genetic studies. It is now widely believed that dysregulation in dopamine and serotonin systems interacts with deficits in other neurotransmitter systems, such as GABA and Substance P, to produce symptoms of mood disorders. Neuroimaging studies indicate that mood disorders are generally associated with decreased sensitivity of the serotonin receptors [12].

Three neurotransmitters have received the most attention in studies of mood disorders: norepinephrine, dopamine and serotonin. The original neurotransmitter models suggested that depression was tied to low levels of norepinephrine and dopamine, whereas mania was tied to high levels of norepinephrine and dopamine. Mania and depression were both posited to be tied to low levels of serotonin, which helps regulate norepinephrine and dopamine. Researchers initially believed that mood disorders would be explained by absolute levels of neurotransmitters in the synaptic cleft that were either too high or too low [7].

Many of the Brain regions involved when healthy people experience strong emotions have been implicated in the pathology of BD [13]. In functional studies, BD I disorder is associated with elevated activity in the amygdala, a key Brain structure involved in identifying the significance of emotionally relevant stimuli of both

negative and positive valences [14]. PET studies and functional MRI studies of
activity during cognitive or emotional tasks have both shown a pattern of amygdala
hyperactivity among people with BD I disorder [15, 16]. People with BD also demonstrate diminished activity of the hippocampus and prefrontal cortex [14].

Hence, one theory is that BD is related to dysregulation in Brain regions relevant
to emotion, including the amygdala, basal ganglia and dorsal anterior cingulate.
Hyperactivity in the basal ganglia may contribute to increased reward motiva-
tion [17].

17.1.3   Typical Clinical Symptoms

Below are the typical symptoms of the two main types of BD, and there are quite a
few similarities among them.

17.1.3.1   Depressive Episode

In bipolar I disorder (BD 1), a major depressive episode (one or more) usually
occurs, but not always. Bipolar II disorder (BD 2 involves one or more major depressive episodes. Common symptoms that occur in a major depressive episode include:
insomnia or hypersomnia, unexplained or uncontrollable crying, severe fatigue, loss
of interest in things the patient enjoys during normal times, and recurring thoughts
of death or suicide. Both disorders may include periods of euthymia—symptom-
free or "normal" states.

17.1.3.2   Mania Episode

Manic episode last at least seven days. An individual experiencing a manic episode
may experience: feelings of euphoria, less need for sleep, increased sexual desire,
hallucinations or delusions, a marked increase in energy. During a manic episode,
individuals may engage in risky or reckless behaviour. For example, someone may
indulge in risky sexual behaviour, spend excessive amounts of money or make
impulsive decisions.

It's important to note that experiencing mania does not automatically mean a
person will become violent or dangerous.

A meta-data analysis of qualitative studies that explored the experience of symptoms and the diagnosis of bipolar disorder noted "loss of control", "disruption,
uncertainty and instability", "negative impact of symptoms across life and the experience of loss", "negative view of self", "struggling with the meaning of diagnosis",
"stigma" and "acceptance and hope" as some of the themes that arose within the
lifelong process of living with bipolar disorder [18].

BD patients experience depressive symptoms three times more often than mania, and five times more often than rapid cycling or mixed episodes [19]. A diagnosis of BD is one of the highest risk factors for suicide [20]. BD usually presents in a rhythmic manner, oscillating between episodes of mania and depression, with several risk factors and triggers contributing to the rate of relapse and failed response to treatment [6]. That causes unusual shifts in mood, energy and activity levels, and an inability to carry out day-to-day tasks.

A substantial proportion of BD patients experience unfavourable functioning, other than mental disorders, suggesting that there is a significant degree of morbidity and dysfunction associated with BD, even during remission periods. Previous mixed episodes, current subclinical depressive symptoms, previous hospitalizations and older age were identified as significant potential clinical predictors of functional impairment [21].

17.1.4 Examination and Diagnosis

Bipolar disorder (BD) cannot be diagnosed like other illnesses where a blood test, X-ray or physical examination can provide a definitive diagnosis. The diagnosis is based on a set of criteria that a person must meet in order to be considered to have BD.

According to the *Diagnostic and Statistical Manual of Mental Disorders* by the American Psychiatric Association (DSM 5) [22], BD diagnosis is divided into two major types, bipolar disorder type I (BD 1) and bipolar disorder type II (BD 2), and three other types of BP, namely cyclothymic disorder, substance-induced bipolar disorder, BD 1 associated with another medical condition and bipolar disorder not elsewhere classified. BD 1 involves episodes of severe mania and often depression. BD 2 involves a less severe form of mania called "hypomania".

It can be differentiated from unipolar depression (major depressive disorder) by the presence of manic or hypomanic (lesser) episodes. A manic episode is a complex symptom pattern that may encompass disparate affective, behavioural and cognitive symptoms, including pressured speech, racing thoughts, euphoric or irritable mood, agitation, inflated self-esteem, distractibility, excessive or inappropriate involvement in pleasurable activities, increased goal-directed activity, diminished need for sleep and, in severe cases, psychosis. In both disorders, moderate or severe depressive episodes typically alternate with manic symptoms; however, in "mixed mania", symptoms of mania and depressed mood overlap. Another variant, called "rapid cycling", is diagnosed when at least four complete cycles of depressed mood and mania occur during any 12-month period.

A mild variant of BD, cyclothymic disorder, is diagnosed when several hypomanic and depressive episodes take place over a two-year period in the absence of severe manic, mixed or depressive episodes [22].

17.1.5   The Treatment of BD with Modern Medicine

The primary goal of treating BD is to bring a patient with mania or depression to symptomatic recovery and a stable mood. Once the patient's mood stabilizes, the goal will be moving to reducing subthreshold symptoms and preventing relapse into full-blown episodes of mania and depression [23].

The main treatments of BD with conventional medicine are pharmacotherapy and psychotherapy. Different drugs may have several purposes. The aim of some drugs is to reduce symptoms associated with acute manic or mixed mania/depression episodes, while for others it is to reduce acute depression symptoms, and for others it is to reduce acute symptoms, maintain relatively symptom-free periods and prevent relapsing into acute episodes. The commonly used non-drug therapeutic treatments range from psychoeducational, cognitive behavioural and family-focused therapies to interpersonal social rhythm therapy, and are provided both in individual and group therapy modalities. Acupuncture is listed as one of the non-drug treatment forms, which range widely from electroconvulsive therapy to treatments for circadian rhythms (such as light boxes), and repetitive transcranial magnetic stimulation by the systematic review prepared for the Agency for Healthcare Research and Quality USA 2018 [23].

Conventional pharmacotherapies are an important and often necessary treatment of both the depressive and manic phases of BD. First-line treatments of BD include mood stabilizers (e.g. lithium carbonate, carbamazepine and valproate), antidepressants, antipsychotics and sedative-hypnotics. On the hopeful side, uncontrolled studies find that lithium reduces long-term suicide risk, as does treatment with neuroleptics and antidepressants [2, 7].

A study observed that most of the effective pharmacological treatments for BD affect levels of dopamine and serotonin [24]. Current research on the action mechanisms of mood stabilizers centres upon signal transduction pathways responsible for communicating chemical signals from the postsynaptic receptors to the cell nucleus and nearby cells. Lithium and valproate both inhibit protein kinase C [25].

Side effects often occur with these medications, which have a mixed record of success due to their limited efficacy and high rates of treatment discontinuation. Partly due to the side effects, such as weight gain, fatigue and cognitive dysfunction, about 60% of BD patients stop their medications against medical advice. Non-adherence is a serious problem for all long-lasting medical conditions with intermittent symptoms [2, 26].

A recent review summarized that there was no strong evidence for any intervention to effectively treat any phase of any type of BD versus placebo or an active comparator. Lithium improved acute mania in the short term and resulted in a longer time to relapse in the long term versus placebo in adults with BD 1. Aside from low-strength evidence showing CBT and systematic/collaborative care having no benefit for a few outcomes, evidence was insufficient for non-drug interventions [23].

Current evidence supports the integrative treatment of BD using combinations of mood stabilizers and selected nutrients [2]. Complementary and alternative medicine, such as acupuncture, for the treatment of BD is needed.

17.2 TCM Understanding of Bipolar Disorder

The TCM foundation theory believes it is extremely important to maintain the relative dynamic balance between Yin and Yang. As described in "Huangdi Neijing Suwen Chapter 3-Shengqi tongtian luan (Discourse on how the Generative Qi Communicates with Heaven)", 'the [flow of] yin qi is interrupted. When the yin and yang are balanced and sealed, then essence and spirit are in order' [27, p. VI 78].

BP-related emotional disorder is equivalent to the "Dian-Kuang (madness-depression)" of Chinese medicine. The manic episode is equivalent to the "madness" of Chinese medicine, and the depressive episode is equivalent to the "depression". They were previously discussed in Huangdi Neijing, which was published 2000 years ago.

"Neijing-Lingshu Chapter 22-Dian Kuang (Mania-depression Syndrome described the aetiologies, symptoms and some acupuncture treatments of Mania-depression" [28, p. 614–617] "Neijing Suwen Chapter 74-Zhizhenyao Dalunpian (The Various Changes in the Dominations of the Six Energies and their Relations with Diseases)" states 'All the syndromes of irritability, uneasiness, mania and acting rashly are pertaining to the fire' [28, p. 458]. And "Neijing Suwen Chapter 49-Maijie (on Channel)" says 'The condition of mania is: The Yang energy is staying above exclusively, unable to combine the Yin energy below, the Yin energy asthenia below and the Yang energy asthenia above will cause mania' [28, p. 231]. Then same in the text "Suwen Chapter 30-Yangming Maijie (The Explanation on the Yangming Channel)" described the typical symptoms 'Some patients with the serious disease of Yangming take off their clothes and run about here and there, singing loudly as in a high place; sometimes they eat nothing for several days, jump up on the walls and roofs. They could not do such things usually, but they are able to do them when they are ill.' [28, p. 157].

There are no more deserving patients than those suffering from BP, whose energy swings from Yang to Yin, or from manic highs to depressive lows [1]. The key to successful treatment using Chinese medicine is accurate diagnosis of the pattern identifications of the patient in both the high and low parts of the cycle and the choice of acupuncture points, Chinese herbal medicines, etc. within contrast to Western medicine, Chinese medicine doctors treat all aspects of the BP patient rather than just one [2].

In addition, since it is difficult for a patient with BP to establish lifestyle regularity, practitioners treating these patients must take an active part in patient management, not just prescribing and treating. Co-morbidities are common and must be taken into account when prescribing and treating.

17.3   General Acupuncture Treatment for Bipolar Disorder

Acupuncture has been used for millennia in China and then some other Eastern countries for treating a range of illnesses, including various kinds of mental disorder. According to the TCM theory about BD classifications, the principle of general acupuncture treatment would follow the pattern identification as well. The patterns, symptoms and signs, and the points selection, are just sample suggestions. Practice in clinic should follow the real individual patient.

17.3.1   Manic Episode

17.3.1.1   Liver Depression with Phlegm Fire

Signs and Symptoms (SS): Emotional tension and agitation, excitement, impetuous behaviour, bitter taste, raving, bilateral rib side distension and pain, insomnia, profuse dreams, dizziness, headache, spitting yellow phlegm, red tongue, slimy yellow coat, wiry, slippery, rapid pulse.

Points selection: LV-2 Xingjian, LV-14 Qimen, ST-40 Fenglong, REN-12 Zhongwan, REN-17 Danzhong, HT-7 Shenmen, PC-8 Laogong, GB-20 Fengchi, DU-20 Baihui.

17.3.1.2   Qi Stagnation and Blood Stasis

SS: Emotional lability, changes in disease nature, sometimes agitated and impulsive, manic speech, predilection to unstable anger, constant crying, laughing, singing and swearing no matter who is present, dream-like confusion, aggression such as throwing of objects, chest region fullness and oppression, piercing lancinating headache, red bloodshot eyes, purplish tongue, possible static macules or engorged sublingual veins, wiry, choppy, possibly deep pulse.

Points selection: LV-3 Taichong, LI-4 Hegu, SP-10 Xuehai, BL-15 Xinshu, BL-17 Geshu, BL-18 Ganshu, GB-20 Fengchi, DU-20 Baihui.

17.3.1.3   Phlegm Fire Disturbing the Heart

SS: Acute onset with symptoms of manic and aggressive/destructive behaviour, red eyes and face, insomnia, complete loss of appetite. Agitated, irritable, distending headache prior to episode, increased thirst with preference for cold drinks, a dry mouth and throat, constipation, red tongue, yellow greasy coating, rapid, wiry, slippery pulse.

Points selection: DU-24 Shenting, DU-14 Dazhui, DU-16 Fengfu, DU-26 Renzhong, PC-6 Neiguan, PC-8 Laogong, PC-4 Ximen, ST-40 Fenglong, LV-3 Taichong, HT-7 Shenmen, GB-13 Benshen.

17.3.2   Depression Episode

17.3.2.1   Liver Qi Depression and Binding

SS: Low spirits, many worries, susceptibility to anxiety, sorrow, hopelessness, decreased movement, slowed reactions, rib-side distension and pain, abdominal distension, scanty eating, loose stools that are not crisp, pale tongue, wiry pulse.

Points selection: DU-24 Baihui, GB-13 Benshen, PC-4 Ximen, LV-3 Taichong, LI-4 Hegu, ST-36 Zusanli, REN-12 Zhongwan, LV-14 Qimen.

17.3.2.2   Heart-Spleen Deficiency

SS: Chronic depression, trance-like mental state, lack of interest, lack of contact with reality, self-blame, self-reproach, decreased activity, excessive thinking/worry, timidity and fearfulness, incoherent speech, insomnia, impaired memory, fatigue, exhaustion, pale white or sallow yellow complexion, scanty eating, palpitations, loose stools, pale enlarged tongue, tooth marks, white coat with thin and weak pulse.

Points selection: DU-24 Shenting, GB-13 Benshen, PC-4 Ximen, HT-7 Shenmen, SP-3 Taibai, SP-6 Sanyinjiao, ST-36 Zusanli, BL-15 Xinshu, BL-17 Geshu, BL-20 Pishu, REN-6 Qihai.

17.3.2.3   Spleen-Kidney Yang Deficiency

SS: Essence spirit listlessness, low spirits, desire to stay lying down, scanty movement, diminished willpower, sorrow, ennui, decreased sexual desire, impotence, seminal emission, clear/watery vaginal discharge and/or early menstruation, sombre white complexion, cold limbs, pale puffy tongue, white coat, teeth marks with deep and thin pulse.

Points selection: ST-36 Zusanli, SP-9 Yinlingquan, REN-4 Guanyuan, REN-6 Qihai, BL-23 Shenshu, BL-20 Pishu, DU-20 Baihui, DU-4 Mingmen. Moxa may apply.

The above pattern identifications may be used separately with general needling, or combined with the unique Brain acupuncture techniques outlined below. Some of the above patterns and points are referenced from Wingate [29, p. 554–561].

17.4   Unique Acupuncture Techniques for BD Disease

The above traditionally general acupuncture treatments, patterns and points, similarly to BD, have been practised for thousands of years and are still commonly practiced in many acupuncture clinics. In the last few decades, with the development of TCM Brain theory, it is believed that Brain has had a unique effect on BD, its ethology, pathology and treatment strategy. It is believed that internal and external pathological factors cause Brain Shen disorder, Brain channel stagnation, and Brain Yin and Yang imbalance, and may lead to damage of Brain marrow and result in BD. The main organ location of BD is no doubt in the Brain, and involves other Zangfu organs such as the Liver, Spleen and Kidney, among others.

In terms of the unique Brain acupuncture treatment, as the Brain is the main location of disease, the treatment principle will be more focused on rebalancing the Brain and regulating Du Mai (Governor vessel). Thus, scalp acupuncture and Du Mai Dao-qi technique are mostly used in acupuncture practice for BD.

17.4.1   Scalp Acupuncture for Treating BD (for Detail of Scalp Acupuncture, Location and Needling Please See Chap. 5)

- Commonly used scalp areas for BD are: Spirit-Emotion Area, Mania Control Area, Foot-Motor Sensory Area, and Central Area.

17.4.2   Du Mai Dao-qi Techniques (Detail of Dao-qi Technique on Du Mai, Points Location and Needling, Please See Chap. 6)

- DU-26 Renzhong, DU-24 Shenting, DU-20 Baihui, DU-16 Fengfu, DU-14 Dazhui, DU-11 Shendao, DU-10 Lingtai, DU-9 Zhiyang, DU-4 Mingmen, DU-3 Yaoyangguan

17.4.3   Ren Mai Dao-qi Technique (Detail of Dao-qi Technique on Ren Mai, Points Location and Needling, Please See Chap. 6)

- REN-12 Zhongwan plus two to four needles around it with 0.5–1 cm distance, REN-10 Xiawan, REN-6 Qihai, REN-4 Guanyuan, REN-17 Danzhong (Shanzhong).

The above unique Brain acupuncture techniques can be combined with syndrome differentiation treatment.

17.4.4 Brain Pattern Differentiation

The common clinical Brain patterns of BD and its possible symptoms are summarized below and are currently being developed and not perfect at the moment.

17.4.4.1 Deficiency of Brain Marrow

SS: Low spirits, many worries, susceptibility to anxiety, sorrow, hopelessness, decreased movement, slowed reactions, amnesia and dull facial expression, light-colored or light red tongue, thin and deep pulse.

Scalp acupuncture: Spirit-Emotion Area and Foot-Motor Sensory Area.

Points selection: DU-20 Baihui, DU-14 Dazhui, Ex-Bailaoxue, DU-4 Mingmen, KI-3 Taixi, GB-39 Xuanzhong and local area points. Techniques to be chosen include electric acupuncture, Dao-qi technique, etc.

17.4.4.2 Deficiency of Brain Yang Qi

SS: Essence spirit listlessness, low spirits, desire to stay lying down, scanty movement, diminished willpower, sorrow, decreased sexual desire, impotence, seminal emission, white complexion, shortness of breath and fatigue, sweating, palpitation, loose stool, swollen hand and feet, generally cold, light-colour tongue with white coat and teeth marks on sides, deep and thin pulse.

Scalp acupuncture: Spirit-Emotion Area, Central Area and Foot-Motor Sensory Area.

Points selection: DU-20 Baihui, DU-16 Fengfu, DU-14 Dazhui, DU-9 Zhiyang, DU-4 Mingmen, DU-3 Yaoyangguan, REN-12 Zhongwan, REN-10 Xiawan, REN-6 Qihai, REN-4 Guanyuan, Moxa could be applied, with Dao-qi technique on one or two key points.

17.4.4.3 Stagnation of Brain Collaterals

SS: Emotional lability, changes in disease nature, sometimes agitated and impulsive, manic speech, predilection to unstable anger, constant crying, laughing, singing and swearing no matter who is present, dreamlike confusion, aggression such as throwing of objects, chest region fullness and oppression, piercing lancinating headache, red bloodshot eyes, purplish tongue, possible static macules or engorged sublingual veins, wiry, choppy, possibly deep pulse.

Scalp acupuncture: Vasomotor Area, Spirit-Emotion Area and Mania Control Area.

Brain acupuncture points selection: DU-26 Renzhong, DU-20 Baihui, DU-16 Fengfu, DU-15 Yamen, DU-14 Dazhui, DU-9 Zhiyang, DU-3 Yaoyangguan, REN-12 Zhongwan, REN-10 Xiawan, REN-6 Qihai. Moxa could be applied, with Dao-qi technique, or electro-acupuncture.

17.4.4.4 Disorder of Brain Shen

Acute onset with symptoms of manic and aggressive/destructive behaviour, poor memory, lack of concentration, red eyes and face, insomnia, complete loss of appetite, agitated, irritable, distending headache prior to episode, light tongue, thin coating, wiry or slow pulse.

Scalp acupuncture: Spirit-Emotion Area and Mania Control Area.

Brain acupuncture points selection: DU-26 Renzhong, DU-24 Shenting, DU-20 Baihui, DU-16 Fengfu, DU-14 Dazhui, DU-11 Shendao, DU-10 Lingtai, Ex-Yintang, HT-7 Shenmen. Techniques to be selected include electric acupuncture, Dao-qi technique, etc.

Notes

- Bipolar disorder (BD), particularly when it is in the manic stage, can be quite severe. Sufficient knowledge and skill on both western medicine and Chinese medicine are essential.
- For treatment of BD, the earlier the involvement, the better the results.
- Treatment frequency: in the early stage, the more often the better. In Western countries, twice a week is suggested, then with time, slowing down to once a week followed by once every two to four weeks for maintenance. If possible, it may start with every day.
- Acupuncture can be combined with routine medications and other psychology therapy such as CBT, etc.
- The above Brain-related patterns and points for BD can be identified separately for severe BD, and combined with classic TCM pattern identifications.

17.5 Research

As a non-conventional therapy, acupuncture may have a potentially significant role in improving quality of life, reducing medication side effects, improving treatment adherence and reducing the severity of bipolar disorder (BD) symptoms [1]. Acupuncture is recommended as one of the Stage 6 options for treatment of BD in the TIMA BD Physician's Manual of Texas Implementation of Medication Algorithms [30, p. 14].

A clinical trial was conducted to examine the safety, effectiveness and acceptability of adjunctive acupuncture in the treatment of hypomania and depression associated with BD [31]. In the study, 20 patients experiencing symptoms of mood elevation were given targeted acupuncture (points specific to symptoms) versus "sham" acupuncture (non-acupoint needling) over 12 weeks, while for 26 patients experiencing symptoms of depression, targeted acupuncture was compared to (off the meridian) acupuncture for non-psychiatric health concerns over eight weeks. All patients experienced improvement over the course of their participation in the study. There was evidence that acupuncture treatment did target the symptom dimension of interest (mood elevation in Study I, depression in Study II). There were few negative side effects and no attrition directly associated with adjunctive acupuncture.

Acupuncture treatment stimulates the central nervous system, releasing endorphins that BD patients may not produce in high enough quantities normally. This process helps bipolar and depressed patients to enjoy a significant reduction in their symptoms of mania while following a regular course of acupuncture. Studies on acupuncture for depression have shown a reduction in symptoms, and there is increasing evidence that acupuncture may relieve symptoms of mania too.

Patients who received acupuncture with points specific to depression were able to lower their bipolar disorder medication doses when compared to patients who received a generalized acupuncture treatment. Recovering bipolar patients may not regain complete control of their lives immediately and may need a series of treatments in order to attain long-term benefits.

17.6 Conclusion

Bipolar disorder (BD) is a highly recurrent, debilitating mental illness. The main treatments for BD with conventional medicine are pharmacotherapy and psychotherapy. Due to weaker evidence of effectiveness and lots of side effects of the medication, there is a need to integrate non-drug therapy. Based on its long history, widespread practice and some clinical studies, acupuncture may play an important role in the treatment of BD. Brain acupuncture, including scalp acupuncture and Dao-qi needling technique, could work more directly on the Brain and thus benefit BD patients.

References

1. Post N. Challenging case in clinical practice; treatment of mood disorders in Chinese medicine: balancing high and low. Altern Complement Ther. 2017;23(2):49–50.
2. Sarris J, Lake J, Hoenders R. Bipolar disorder and complementary medicine: current evidence, safety issues, and clinical considerations. J Altern Complement Med. 2011;11(10):881–90.

3. Flaws B, Lake J. Chinese medical psychiatry. Boulder, CO: Blue Poppy Press; 2001.
4. Gurling H, Smyth C, Kalsi G, et al. Linkage findings in bipolar disorder. Nat Genet. 1995;10:8–9.
5. Merikangas KR, Jin R, He JP, et al. Prevalence and correlates of bipolar spectrum disorders in the world mental health urvey initiative. Arch Gen Psychiatry. 2011;68:241–51.
6. Depp CA, Davis CE, Mittal D, et al. Health-related quality of life and functioning of middle-aged and elderly adults with bipolar disorder. J Clin Psychiatry. 2006;67:215–21.
7. Miklowitz DJ, Johnson SL. The psychopathology and treatment of bipolar disorder. Annu Rev Clin Psychol. 2006;2:199–235.
8. Jamison KR. Touched with fire: manic-depressive illness and the artistic temperament. New York: Macmillan; 1993.
9. Konradi C, Eaton M, MacDonald ML, et al. Molecular evidence for mitochondrial dysfunction in bipolar disorder. Arch Gen Psychiatry. 2004;61:300–8.
10. Alda M. Bipolar disorder: from families to genes. Can J Psychiatr. 1997;42:378–87.
11. Murray RM, Sham P, Van Os J, et al. A developmental model for similarities and dissimilarities between schizophrenia and bipolar disorder. Schizophr Res. 2004;71:405–16.
12. Stockmeier CA. Involvement of serotonin in depression: evidence from postmortem and imaging studies of serotonin receptors and the serotonin transporter. J Psychiatr Res. 2003;37:357–73.
13. Phillips ML, Drevets WC, Rauch SL, et al. Neurobiology of emotion perception II: implications for major psychiatric disorders. Biol Psychiatry. 2003;54:515–28.
14. Kruger S, Seminowicz S, Goldapple K, et al. State and trait influences on mood regulation in bipolar disorder: blood flow differences with an acute mood challenge. Biol Psychiatry. 2003;54:1274–83.
15. Lawrence NS, Williams AM, Surguladze S, et al. Subcortical and ventral prefrontal responses to facial expressions distinguish patients with BPD and major depression. Biol Psychiatry. 2004;55:578–87.
16. Chang K, Adleman NE, Dienes K, et al. Anomalous prefrontal-subcortical activation in familial pediatric bipolar disorder: a functional magnetic resonance imaging investigation. Arch Gen Psychiatry. 2004;61:781–92.
17. Knutson B, Adams CM, Fong GW, Hommer D. Anticipation of increasing monetary reward selectively recruits nucleus accumbens. J Neurosci. 2001;21:RC159. [PubMed: 11459880]
18. Russell L, Moss D. A meta-study of qualitative research into the experience of 'symptoms' and 'having a diagnosis' for people who have been given a diagnosis of bipolar disorder. Eur J Psychol. 2013;9:643–63.
19. Judd LL, Akiskal HS, Schettler PJ, et al. The long-term natural history of the weekly symptomatic status of bipolar I disorder. Arch Gen Psychiatry. 2002;59:530–7.
20. Pompili M, Serafini G, Del Casale A, et al. Improving adherence in mood disorders: the struggle against relapse, recurrence and suicide risk. Expert Rev Neurother. 2009;9:985–1004.
21. Rosaa AR, Reinaresc M, Francoa C, et al. Clinical predictors of functional outcome of bipolar patients in remission. Bipolar Disord. 2009;11:401–9.
22. American Psychiatric Association. Diagnostic and statistical manual of mental disorders. 5th ed. Arlington, VA: American Psychiatric Publishing; 2013.
23. Butler M, Urosevic S, Desai P, et al. Treatment for bipolar disorder in adults: a systematic review. comparative effectiveness review No. 208. (Prepared by the Minnesota Evidence-based Practice Center under Contract No. 290–2012-00016-I.) AHRQ Publication No. 18-EHC012-EF. Rockville, MD: Agency for Healthcare Research and Quality; August 2018.
24. Goodwin FK, Jamison KR. Manic-depressive illness. New York: Oxford University Press; 1990.
25. Manji HK. The neurobiology of bipolar disorder. Econ Neurosci. 2001;3:37–44.
26. Vargas-Huicochea I, Huicochea L, Berlanga C, et al. Taking or not taking medications: psychiatric treatment perceptions in patients diagnosed with bipolar disorder. J Clin Pharm Ther. 2014;39:673–9.

27. Unschuld PU, Tessenow H, Zheng JS. Huang Di Nei Jing Su Wen: an annotated translation of Huang Di's inner classic–basic questions. Berkeley, CA: University of California Press; 2011.
28. Wang B, Wu LS, Wu Q. Yellow emperors cannon of internal medicine. Beijing: China Science & Technology Press; 1997.
29. Wingate DS. Healing brain injury with Chinese medical approaches: integrative approaches for practitioners. London: Singing Dragon; 2018. eBook
30. Suppes T, Dennehy E-B. Bipolar disorder algorithms manual. TIMA procedural manual. TIMA BD Physician's manual. 2002. eBook.
31. Dennehy EB, Schnyer R, Bernstein IH, et al. The safety, acceptability, and effectiveness of acupuncture as an adjunctive treatment for acute symptoms in bipolar disorder. J Clin Psychiatry. 2009;70(6):897–905.

Chapter 18
Post-traumatic Stress Disorder, Insomnia and Substance Abuse

Unlike the previous chapters on the most commonly seen psychotic disorders, i.e. depression, anxiety and bipolar, which explain the basic background, the aetiology and pathogenesis, typical clinical symptoms, examination and diagnosis, treatment with modern medicine, TCM understanding of the disease, general acupuncture treatment, unique acupuncture treatment and relevant research, among other things, this chapter will only focus on general information and unique acupuncture treatment for some sample psychological disorders.

These commonly seen psychological disorders are: post-traumatic stress disorder (PTSD), insomnia and substance abuse. In order to simplify the treatment principle and make it easy to follow for clinical practice, the Brain acupuncture treatment section of this chapter will start with general basic treatment and go on to look at several additional treatments.

18.1 Post-traumatic Stress Disorder

18.1.1 General Background of PTSD

Post-traumatic stress disorder (PTSD) is characterized by an exaggerated response to contextual memory and impaired fear extinction, with or without mild cognitive impairment, learning deficits and nightmares, which reduce the quality of life. PTSD is often induced by distressing traumatic events, especially life-threatening events such as war, terrorist attacks, natural calamities, etc. [1]. During a lifetime, a majority of the population, 60.7% of men and 51.2% of women, may be exposed to traumatic events that have the potential to trigger the development of PTSD [2].

© Springer Nature Switzerland AG 2021   249
T. Wang, *Acupuncture for Brain*, https://doi.org/10.1007/978-3-030-54666-3_18

If a person meets all of the following criteria—has experienced a potentially traumatic event at least a month ago; has at least one recurring symptom and one avoidance symptom and one hyper-arousal symptom; has difficulties in day-to-day functioning—then the person is likely to have PTSD [3, p. 16]. The after-effects of a stressful situation can cause a chronic complex of emotional and physical symptoms in which one re-experiences an overwhelming traumatic event. This causes intense fear, helplessness, horror and avoidance of stimuli associated with the trauma [4].

The current PTSD definition from the Diagnostic and Statistical Manual of Mental Disorders (DSM-V) includes four categories of symptoms: (1) intrusive symptoms, (2) physiological overstimulation, (3) avoidance and emotional dissociation, and (4) mood swings that appear after exposure to a trauma, including continued and excessive emotional distress, shame, guilt and anger related to the traumatic event and its outcomes [5].

It has been proposed that PTSD is characterized by an exaggerated amygdaloid response coupled with impairments in regulation of the medial prefrontal cortex, which fails to inhibit the heightened fear reactions of the amygdala. It has been further hypothesized that impairment of executive function due to injury of the frontal lobe increases the perseverance of the re-experiencing effect. Hippocampal atrophy has also been correlated to PTSD, as demonstrated by volumetric studies and magnetic resonance spectroscopy [4].

Neurochemical changes associated with PTSD involve many neurotransmitter pathways. There is a significant body of evidence indicating the role of serotonergic pathways in this process. The region's most sensitive to serotonin include the limbic system and frontal–subcortical circuits. SSRIs have often been used for PTSD symptoms, as benefits have been demonstrated. Endocrine changes associated with PTSD show that individuals tend to have low cortisol levels with high levels of corticotropin-releasing factor (CRF) [4, p. 593–608].

Animal studies suggest that the crucial Brain regions associated with PTSD symptoms are the prefrontal cortex (PFC), anterior cingulated cortex (ACC), amygdala and hippocampus, which are involved in the formation and retrieval of emotional and fear memory [1]. Moreover, both pharmacological and psychological therapies have been reported to increase the volumes of the hippocampus and/or ACC, in association with the improvement of PTSD symptoms. Due to its complexity, in order for treatment to be effective, the treatment approach should be individualized, integrated and multidisciplinary [6].

The two main types of traditional treatment of PTSD are pharmacological therapy and/or psychotherapy. Two commonly used medications for treating PTSD are Paroxetine (Paxil) and Sertraline (Zoloft). Both medications are SSRIs (selective serotonin reuptake inhibitors), a type of antidepressant medicine. The medications are used to help control PTSD symptoms such as sadness, worry and anger. However, more effective therapeutics are required for improving the quality of life in PTSD patients [1]. It is likely to take several weeks of treatment before a person feels any reduction in their PTSD symptoms [3].

However, mechanisms underlying increased susceptibility to impaired fear memory consolidation and extinction are not clear, and therefore there are limited effective therapeutics [1].

18.1.2 General Acupuncture for PTSD

Although classic TCM text does not mention the term "post-traumatic stress disorder" or PTSD, acupuncture is widely used in the treatment of mental disorders, such as stress, depression, anxiety, eating disorders, schizophrenia and sleep disorders, among others.

There are some clinical studies that have investigated acupuncture for PTSD as well as several systematic reviews [7, 8].

A randomized effectiveness trial of a brief course of acupuncture for PTSD compared acupuncture plus usual care with usual care alone. The results indicated that mean improvement in PTSD severity was significantly greater among those receiving acupuncture than in those receiving usual care only. Acupuncture was also associated with significantly greater improvements in depression, pain, and physical and mental health functioning. Pre-post effect sizes for these outcomes were large and robust [9].

A very recent clinical trial studied adult patients with psychological symptoms and musculoskeletal pain. Treatments were performed by experienced medical acupuncturists. A verbal/numerical scale was developed to quantify the effect of intervention. A Wilcoxon rank–sum test was used for comparing the scores before and after the acupuncture treatment. After three treatments performed in daily sessions, 54.05% and 60.6% of patients reported marked improvements in psychological and pain symptoms, respectively. No serious adverse events were reported. These results suggest that acupuncture could be a useful tool for reducing pain and psychological symptoms related to earthquakes [10].

An early randomized controlled pilot trial evaluated the potential efficacy and acceptability of acupuncture for PTSD. People diagnosed with PTSD were randomized into either an empirically developed acupuncture treatment (ACU) group, a group cognitive behavioral therapy (CBT) group or a wait list control (WLC) group. Compared with the WLC condition, acupuncture provided large treatment effects for PTSD, similar in magnitude to group CBT. Symptom reductions at the end of the treatment were maintained at three-month follow-up for both interventions. It was concluded that acupuncture may be an efficacious and acceptable non-exposure treatment option for PTSD [11].

The possible mechanisms of acupuncture in PTSD include: redirecting blood flow from the limbic system to the prefrontal cortex; balancing the sympathetic and parasympathetic responses; inhibiting the amygdala from alleviating hypervigilance; reducing epinephrine production to downregulate the sympathetic response and initiating endorphin secretion to reduce pain, etc. [4].

18.1.3   Brain Acupuncture for PTSD

Classic TCM and acupuncture treatment for mental disorders such as stress and depression, among others, was most focused on the internal organs of the Liver, Heart, Spleen, Kidney, etc. With the development of TCM Brain theory, it is believed that TCM Brain has played a unique role in mental occurrence, developments and recovery. The treatment principle will be more focused on regulating Du Mai and rebalancing the Brain. Thus the Du Mai Dao-qi technique and scalp acupuncture are mostly used in the practice of acupuncture.

18.1.3.1   Basic Treatment

Scalp acupuncture (SA) Spirit -Emotion Area, Foot-Motor Sensory Area, Manic Control Area, Central Area, plus DU-20 Baihui, DU-24 Shenting, DU-16 Fengfu (Dao-qi), REN-12 Zhongwan (Dao-qi or plus two to four needles), electric acupuncture may add on DU-24, DU-20 and DU-16. Auricular acupuncture point Shenmen may be added for some cases.

18.1.3.2   Additional Treatment

Deficiency of Brain Marrow

Signs and symptoms (SS): susceptibility to anxiety, stress, low spirits, many worries, sorrow, hopelessness, decreased movement, slowed reactions, dizziness and vertigo, poor memory and concentration, irritability, weak body or limbs, tinnitus, amnesia and dull facial expression, light-colored or light red tongue, thin and deep pulse.

Basic treatments as above plus below additional points/Areas:

SA Reproduction Area, Ex-Bailaoxue, DU-4 Mingmen (Dao-qi), REN-4 Guanyuan, KI-3 Taixi, LV-3 Taichong, GB-39 Xuanzhong, BL-23 Shenshu, etc.

Deficiency of Brain Yang Qi

SS: Hypervigilance, depression, insomnia, emotional disturbance, mental fatigue, low spirits, desire to stay lying down, palpitations, timidity, poor memory, poor appetite, sweating, loose stools, pale lips/complexion, dizziness, generally cold, light-coloured tongue with white coat and teeth marks on sides, deep and thin pulse.

Basic treatments plus below additional points/Areas:

SA Stomach Area, DU-14 Dazhui, DU-9 Zhiyang, DU-3 Yaoyangguan, REN-10 Xiawan, REN-6 Qihai, REN-4 Guanyuan, ST-36 Zusanli, SP-9 Yinlingquan, etc.

Moxa could be applied, with Dao-qi technique on one or two key Du Mai or Ren Mai points such as DU-16, DU-14, REN-12 and REN-6.

Stagnation of Brain Collaterals

SS: Hyper-arousal aggravated by suppressed emotions (anxiety, overthinking, anger, sorrow), depression, irritability, labile mood, distending pain in chest/hypochondria, insomnia, globus hystericus, possible abdominal masses, may be combined with limb paralysis, purple tongue with light or greasy coat, wiry or slippery pulse.

Basic treatments plus below additional Area/points:

SA Vasomotor Area, Head Area, DU-26 Renzhong, DU-15 Yamen, DU-14 Dazhui, REN-10 Xiawan, REN-6 Qihai, ST-36 Zusanli, SP-10 Xuehai, LV-3 Taichong, LI-4 Hegu, GB-20 Fengchi, etc. Moxa could be applied, maybe with Dao-qi technique on one or two key points, such as DU-16 and REN-12.

Disorder of Brain Shen

SS: Acute onset with symptoms of stress, manic and aggressive/destructive behaviour, poor memory, lack of concentration, insomnia, complete loss of appetite. Agitated, irritable, light tongue, thin coating, wiry or slow pulse.

Basic treatments plus additional points/Areas:

SA Head Area, DU-26 Renzhong, Ex-Yintang, DU-14 Dazhui, HT-7 Shenmen, PC-6 Neiguan, PC-7 Daling, BL-15 Xinshu, etc. Electric acupuncture may be added, along with Dao-qi technique on one or two key points, such as DU-16, DU-14 and REN-12.

18.2 Insomnia

18.2.1 General Background of Insomnia

Insomnia is the most prevalent sleep disorder, and is characterized by difficulty in initiating or sustaining sleep [12]. Insomnia is one of the most common diseases in modern society, with a prevalence of between 15% to 30% of adults and 10% to 23% of young people worldwide having different degrees of insomnia. It can lead to early awakening, short sleep, sleeplessness, dreaming, and poor sleep quality which causes a series of negative emotions, such as fatigue, inefficiency, cognitive decline, social interaction, tension and anxiety, which affect social harmony and stability. So insomnia has been attracting increasing attention [13].

Currently, because insomnia is a subjective complaint, we have not yet reached a consensus on its causes, so it is difficult to define and diagnose. Insomnia could be defined by its symptoms in terms of complaints of sleep disturbance, such as difficulty in falling asleep or disturbance of sleep maintenance, and/or early awakening. Patients with insomnia may feel tired, tense and/or lazy, or have delayed reactions, be easily distracted or suffer from headaches. The most serious consequence of insomnia may be mental illness, such as depression, anxiety, fatigue, retardation, memory loss and a general discomfort affecting many aspects of daytime activity, and the worst mental illness is schizophrenia [13, 14].

It is also a risk factor for arterial hypertension, myocardial infarction and chronic heart failure. It brings great psychological and economic burden [13]. Chronic insomnia (with symptoms for at least three nights a week for at least one month) presents a substantially increased risk factor for other psychiatric disorders as well as cardiovascular morbidity and mortality [15].

Evidence of hyper-arousal in insomniacs includes an elevated whole-body metabolic rate during sleep and wakefulness, elevated cortisol and adrenocorticotropic hormone during the early sleep period, reduced parasympathetic tone in heart rate variability and increased high-frequency electroencephalographic activity during non-rapid eye movement sleep. It has been proposed that genetic, environmental, behavioural and physiological factors contribute to the aetiology and pathophysiology of hyper-arousal-induced insomnia [15].

At present, there are three international diagnostic criteria for insomnia: The Diagnostic and Statistical Manual of Mental Disorders (DSM), the International Classification of Sleep Disorders and the ICD-10 Classification of Mental and Behavioural Disorders. The European Sleep Research Society has put forward three diagnostic criteria for insomnia [13].

The menopausal transition is often accompanied by insomnia, with about half of all menopausal and post-menopausal period women being estimated to be affected [12, 16]. Insomnia may occur in 60%–80% of patients with depression; it is one of the most frequent residual symptoms of depression, and may persist even after depressive mood symptoms have been relieved [17].

Currently, the first-line drugs available for clinical treatment of insomnia include benzodiazepines (BZs) and benzodiazepine receptor agonists (BZRAs), antidepressants, antipsychotics, antihistamines, phytotherapeutic substances and melatonin [13]. However, there is very limited evidence of their long-term treatment efficacy [15], and long-term use of these drugs will bring some side effects to patients, such as headaches, dizziness, a dry mouth and abnormal taste [15]. Cognitive-behavioural therapy (CBT) has been another first-line treatment. Although clinically effective, it is not widely used due to the intense labour and lack of trained therapists.

18.2.2   General Acupuncture for Insomnia

Acupuncture has been used to treat insomnia and some mental disorders since antiquity in China. It is still one of the commonly used non-drug therapies for patients with insomnia. According to the theory of traditional Chinese medicine, acupuncture provides balance to the body by stimulating specific acupoints, helping the body to achieve a state of relative equilibrium (the harmony of "Yin and Yang"), thereby restoring the normal sleep–wake cycle [15–17]. In modern medicine, acupuncture can increase the content of γ-amino butyric acid, and thus enhance sleep quality [18].

At present, there are many reports that acupuncture has a significant effect on insomnia [13]. Many studies have confirmed the efficacy of acupuncture for primary insomnia and related depressive disorders. An RCT study [14] investigated the six-week influence of acupuncture on sleep quality and daytime functioning in primary insomnia and found that verum acupuncture appeared to be more effective for increasing sleep quality and daytime functioning than sham acupuncture and Estazolam, a commonly used sleeping medication.

Based on the results of meta-analyses, the majority showed that compared with no treatment, sham acupuncture or medications, acupuncture was significantly better for improving parameters in terms of sleep quality and duration, and the combination of acupuncture and other interventions appears more effective than those interventions alone, though it was possible that the beneficial effect from acupuncture is overvalued because of the small sample size, the flawed methodology of the included trials and the short follow-up duration [18]. Another recent systematic review indicated that acupuncture could be effective against insomnia [15].

18.2.3   Unique Brain Acupuncture for Insomnia

18.2.3.1   Basic Treatment

Scalp acupuncture (SA) Spirit-Emotion Area, Foot-Motor Sensory Area, Central Area, plus DU-20 Baihui, DU-24 Shenting, REN-12 Zhongwan (Dao-qi or plus two to four needles), electric acupuncture may add on DU-24, DU-20 and DU-16. Auricular acupuncture point Shenmen may be added in some cases. For severe cases, DU-16 Fengfu with Dao-qi technique could be applied.

18.2.3.2   Additional Treatment

Deficiency of Brain Marrow

Signs and symptoms (SS): insomnia, difficulty falling asleep, irritability, restlessness, dizziness or dream-disturbed sleep, excess dreams, low energy, lower back ache, sore legs and feet, emaciation, poor memory and concentration, light-colored or light red tongue, thin and deep pulse.

Basic treatments as above, plus additional points/Areas:

DU-4 Mingmen (Dao-qi), REN-4 Guanyuan, KI-3 Taixi, LV-3 Taichong, GB-39 Xuanzhong, BL-23 Shenshu, Ex-Anmian, Ex-Yintang, etc.

Deficiency of Brain Yang Qi

SS: difficulty falling asleep, light sleep, frequent and vivid dreams, palpitations, forgetfulness, difficulty concentrating, dizziness, fatigue, pale complexion, lassitude of spirit, shortness of breath, disinclination to talk, nervous and moody, sleepy in the daytime, prefers to lie down, poor appetite, weight loss, reduced food intake, loose stools, generally cold, light-coloured tongue with white coat and teeth marks on sides, deep and thin pulse.

Basic treatments as above, plus additional points/Areas:

SA Stomach Area, DU-14 Dazhui, DU-9 Zhiyang, DU-3 Yaoyangguan, REN-10 Xiawan, REN-6 Qihai, REN-4 Guanyuan, ST-36 Zusanli, SP-9 Yinlingquan, etc. Moxa could be applied, with Dao-qi technique on one or two key Du Mai or Ren Mai points, such as DU-16, DU-14, REN-12 and REN-6.

Stagnation of Brain Collaterals

SS: insomnia, irritability, may be recurrent with palpitations, unpleasant dreams or nightmares, headaches, may have chest tightness, heaviness, or painful sensations, easily startled, wakes up at night, worse at night, may be exacerbated by emotional changes, long-term history of stress or emotional problems, purplish complexion, especially lips, purple tongue with light or greasy coat, wiry or slippery pulse.

Basic treatments as above, plus additional Areas/points:

SA Vasomotor Area, Head Area, DU-26 Renzhong, DU-15 Yamen, DU-14 Dazhui, REN-10 Xiawan, REN-6 Qihai, ST-36 Zusanli, SP-10 Xuehai, LV-3 Taichong, LI-4 Hegu, GB-20 Fengchi, etc. Moxa could be applied, maybe with Dao-qi technique on one or two key points, such as DU-16 and REN-12.

Disorder of Brain Shen

SS: insomnia, irritability, maybe stress or anxiety, dizziness, unpleasant dreams or nightmares, poor memory, lack of concentration, agitated, light tongue, thin coating, wiry or slow pulse.

Basic treatments plus additional points/Areas:

SA Head Area, DU-26 Renzhong, Ex-Yintang, DU-14 Dazhui, HT-7 Shenmen, PC-6 Neiguan, PC-7 Daling, BL-15 Xinshu, Ex-Yintang, Ex-Anmian, etc. Electric acupuncture may be added, Dao-qi technique on one or two key points such as DU-16, DU-14 and REN-12.

18.3   Substance Abuse

18.3.1   General Background of Substance Abuse

Substance abuse and substance use disorders (SUDs) have become a significant public health problem worldwide. At least 150 million people have used an illicit drug such as cannabis, opioids or cocaine, while individuals aged 15 or older drink

6.2 litres of pure alcohol on average per year. Substance abuse remains one of the most serious threats to our public health. Addiction can be defined as the loss of control over drug use, or the compulsive seeking and taking of a drug regardless of the consequences [19].

SUDs are associated with various physical health problems, such as infectious diseases, cardiovascular disease, Liver and pancreatic disease, neurologic impairment, diabetes, cancer and physical injury. People with SUDs also often have co-morbid psychiatric disorders, such as major depressive disorder, bipolar disorder and borderline personality disorder. In addition to health problems, SUDs are associated with significant social and economic consequences, such as interpersonal and relationship issues, lost productivity, homelessness, poverty, violent and property crime, and incarceration [20, p. 4–13] [21, p. 1–7].

One example is alcohol abuse, which leads to health and social problems [22]. Excessive alcohol consumption is an important risk factor for various medical diseases, such as cancers and cardiovascular disease, and can cause alcohol-related Liver disease and nutritional deficiencies. Moreover, some evidence suggests that sustained alcohol abuse may result in neural abnormalities and Brain damage. Individuals suffering from alcoholism can experience impaired neurocognitive functioning, including difficulties with executive functions and working memory, and dysfunction in several Brain regions, including the white matter, cerebellum, frontal cortex, hypothalamus and hippocampus. The harmful consequences associated with alcohol abuse and the high prevalence of alcohol use disorder require an effective intervention in a health-care setting.

Epidemiological data indicate that treating substance use disorders is known to be difficult [23]. Patients with alcohol use disorder are largely untreated despite the efficacy of treatment, which may reflect a need for treatment alternatives [22]. SUDs are mainly a policy problem due to their prevalence and societal impacts [19]. Available treatments for addiction remain inadequately effective for most individuals.

18.3.2 General Acupuncture for Substance Abuse

It has been recognized that acupuncture can play an important role in dealing with the opioid epidemic. The effects of acupuncture on opiate addiction have been investigated in many clinical trials [24].

In 1996, the World Health Organization (WHO) listed 64 medical problems that were considered suitable for acupuncture treatment, including the treatment of drug abuse [25]. There are three major advantages with using acupuncture to treat drug addiction. First, acupuncture therapy for opiate addiction is inexpensive, simple and has no side effects. Second, acupuncture can be used for preventing opiate relapse. Third, acupuncture therapy is safe for pregnant and parturient women.

The first recorded application of acupuncture in opiate addiction was from 1972 after serendipitous observation and was reported by a neurosurgeon in Hong Kong,

Dr. Wen, in 1975 [26]. Then, in 1977 and 1979, Wen followed up this unexpected finding and conducted a series of studies examining the effect of acupuncture on heroin addiction, and concluded that acupuncture relieved heroin withdrawal syndrome [27, 28]. The studies reported that acupuncture combined with electrical stimulation on four body acupoints and two ear acupoints greatly relieved the symptoms of opioid withdrawal in patients with opiate addiction and indicated that it was a relatively safe complementary and alternative medical approach. These protocols were developed in many Western counties, with the most widely practised being the National Acupuncture Detoxification Association (NADA) protocol, which only uses auricular acupuncture with five ear acupoints for addiction treatments [29, 30].

A development in this field came from Dr. Han of Peking University, China in 1990. The protocol in 2005 describes the placement of self-sticking electrodes to the skin over the acupoint followed by electrical stimulation to improve opiate withdrawal signs and prevent relapse into heroin use. The device used for this purpose was later named "Han's acupoint nerve stimulator" (HANS) [31].

Neurochemical and behavioural evidence have shown that acupuncture helps reduce the effects of positive and negative reinforcement involved in opiate addiction by modulating mesolimbic dopamine neurons. Moreover, several Brain neurotransmitter systems involving opioids and GABA have been implicated in the modulation of dopamine release by acupuncture. However, many unanswered questions remain regarding the basic mechanisms of action of acupuncture. Future research could better determine the influence of acupuncture therapy on the regulation of dopamine and other neurotransmitters [25].

A recent RCT demonstrated that acupuncture decreased the amount of morphine used by addicts in treatment and simultaneously improved sleep for patients. In addition, acupuncture addiction protocols can address acute and prolonged withdrawal symptoms, stress and anxiety related to drug withdrawal, and help prevent relapse [32].

Most studies from China used body acupuncture to treat opiate addiction whereas studies from other countries used auricular acupuncture for this purpose. The most frequently used points or sites for the treatment of opiate addiction by acupuncturists are grouped below based on their locations: Zusanli (ST-36), Sanyinjiao (SP-6), Hegu (LI-4), Neiguan (PC-6); Ex-Jiaji, Shenshu (BL-23), Ex-Sishencong, Baihui (DU-20), Dazhui (DU-14); and ear points: sympathetic, Shenmen, Kidney and lung.

A meta-analysis in 2017 demonstrated that an acupuncture intervention had a stronger effect on reducing alcohol-related symptoms and behaviours than did the control intervention [22].

A white paper published in 2017 concluded that acupuncture has emerged as a powerful, evidence-based, safe, cost-effective and available treatment modality suitable for meeting the need to decrease the public's opioid dependence with non-pharmacologic strategies [33].

18.3.3 Unique Brain Acupuncture for Substance Abuse

18.3.3.1 Basic Treatment

Scalp acupuncture (SA) Spirit-Emotion Area, Foot-Motor Sensory Area, Central Area, plus DU-20 Baihui, DU-24 Shenting, DU-16 Fengfu (Dao-qi), REN-12 Zhongwan (Dao-qi or plus two to four needles), electric acupuncture may add on DU-24, DU-20 and DU-16. Auricular acupuncture point Shenmen may be added in some cases.

18.3.3.2 Additional Treatment

Deficiency of Brain Marrow

SS: yellowish or pale face, dizziness, palpitations, insomnia, dreaminess, forgetfulness, a dry throat and dry mouth, a dry cough and less phlegm, susceptibility to anxiety, stress, low spirits, irritability, weak body or limbs, tinnitus and amnesia, light-colored or light red tongue, thin and deep pulse.

Basic treatments plus additional points/Areas:

SA Reproduction Area, Ex-Bailaoxue, DU-4 Mingmen (Dao-qi), REN-4 Guanyuan, KI-3 Taixi, LV-3 Taichong, GB-39 Xuanzhong, BL-23 Shenshu, etc.

Deficiency of Brain Yang Qi

SS: easily tired, lack of energy or laziness, low voice, fatigue and spontaneous sweating, coughing, wheezing, weight loss, body or local chills, cold limbs, pale face, trembling, frequently nocturnal, loose stools, spermatorrhea, impotence, irregular menstruation, insomnia, low spirit, desire to stay lying down, palpitations, timidity, poor memory, poor appetite, light-coloured tongue with white coat and teeth marks on sides, deep and thin pulse.

Basic treatments plus additional points/Areas:

SA Stomach Area, Reproduction Area, DU-14 Dazhui, DU-9 Zhiyang, DU-3 Yaoyangguan, REN-10 Xiawan, REN-6 Qihai, REN-4 Guanyuan, ST-36 Zusanli, SP-9 Yinlingquan, etc. Moxa could be applied, with Dao-qi technique on one or two key Du Mai or Ren Mai points, such as DU-16, DU-14, REN-12 and REN-6.

Stagnation of Brain Collaterals

SS: whole body pain (tingling, long-term pain, night pain, soreness, worm-like sensation, refusal to press), purple black on face, lips, gums and around eyes, wrong skin, numbness of limbs, mental mania, irritability, insomnia, bluish or dark tongue with purple petechiae, tortuous sublingual veins, astringent or nodal pulse.

Basic treatments plus additional Areas/points:

SA Vasomotor Area, Head Area, DU-26 Renzhong, DU-14 Dazhui, REN-10 Xiawan, REN-6 Qihai, ST-36 Zusanli, SP-10 Xuehai, LV-3 Taichong, LI-4 Hegu, GB-20 Fengchi, PC-6 Neiguan, etc. Moxa could be applied, maybe with Dao-qi technique on one or two key points, such as DU-16 and REN-12.

Disorder of Brain Shen

SS: mental depression, up and down, painful expression, negative thinking, easily upset, sighing, poor appetite, poor memory, lack of concentration, insomnia, full chest and rib region, low sexual desire, irregular menstruation, even amenorrhea, light red tongue, thin coating, wiry or slow pulse.

Basic treatments plus additional points/Areas:

SA Head Area, DU-26 Renzhong, Ex-Yintang, DU-14 Dazhui, HT-7 Shenmen, PC-6 Neiguan, BL-15 Xinshu, etc. Electric acupuncture may be added, Dao-qi technique on one or two key points such as DU-16, DU-14 and REN-12.

Brain Yang Hyperactivity

SS: mental mania, anxiety, irritability, fever, distending headache, hallucinations or delusions, marked increase in energy, instability, restlessness, restless sleep, blurred vision, dream-disturbed sleep, flushed face, red eyes, chatter, bitter taste in the mouth, thirst, a dry throat, constipation, red tongue, yellow and scanty coat, fast and wiry pulse.

Basic treatments plus additional points/Areas:

SA Mania Control Area, DU-26 Renzhong, DU-24 Shenting, DU-20 Baihui, DU-14 Dazhui, Ex-Yintang, REN-6 Qihai, REN-4 Guanyuan, Ex-Shixuan. One or two key points maybe with Dao-qi technique. Bleeding needling may apply for DU-14, Ex-Shixuan, etc.

Notes

Acupuncture may offer some advantages over existing pharmacological interventions for substance abuse: it is safer, has fewer side effects and is cheaper. Acupuncture may help in treating various conditions related to drug addiction, such as withdrawal symptoms, drug craving, anxiety and depression.

References

1. Yabuki Y, Fukunaga K. Clinical therapeutic strategy and neuronal mechanism underlying post-traumatic stress disorder (PTSD). Int J Mol Sci. 2019;20:3614. 20 pages. https://doi.org/10.3390/ijms20153614.
2. Foa EB, Gillihan SJ, Bryant RA. Challenges and successes in dissemination of evidence-based treatments for posttraumatic stress: lessons learned from prolonged exposure therapy for PTSD. Psychol Sci Public Interest. 2013;14:65–111.

3. WHO. World Health Organization and United Nations high commissioner for refugees. assessment and management of conditions specifically related to stress: mhGAP Intervention Guide Module (version 1.0). Geneva: WHO; 2013.
4. Wingate DS. Healing brain injury with Chinese medical approaches: integrative approaches for practitioners. London: Singing Dragon; 2018. eBook
5. American Psychiatric Association, editor. Diagnostic and statistical manual of mental disorders. 5th ed. Washington, DC: American Psychiatric Association Publishing; 2013.
6. Ravid S, Shorer S, Reshef A, et al. Treatment of post-traumatic stress disorder using integrative medicine: case history. J Chin Med. 2019;119:5–12.
7. Grant S, Colaiaco B, Motala A, et al. Needle acupuncture for posttraumatic stress disorder (PTSD): a systematic review. Santa Monica, CA: RAND Corporation; 2017.
8. Kim YD, Heo I, Shin BC, et al. Acupuncture for posttraumatic stress disorder: a systematic review of randomized controlled trials and prospective clinical trials. Evid Based Complement Alternat Med. 2013. Article ID 615857:12 pages. https://doi.org/10.1155/2013/615857.
9. Engel CC, Cordova EH, Benedek DM, et al. Randomized effectiveness trial of a brief course of acupuncture for posttraumatic stress disorder. Med Care. 2014;52(12 Suppl 5):S57–64.
10. Moiraghi C, Poli P, Piscitelli A. An observational study on acupuncture for earthquake-related post-traumatic stress disorder: the experience of the Lombard association of medical acupuncturists/acupuncture in the world, in Amatrice, central Italy. Med Acupunct. 2019;31(2):116–22.
11. Hollifield M, Sinclair-Lian N, Warner T, et al. Acupuncture for posttraumatic stress disorder: a randomized controlled pilot trial. J Nerv Ment Dis. 2007;195(6):504–13.
12. Bezerra AG, Pires GN, Andersen ML, et al. Acupuncture to treat sleep disorders in postmenopausal women: a systematic review. Evid Based Complement Alternat Med. 2015. Article ID 563236, 16 pages; https://doi.org/10.1155/2015/563236.
13. Zhang MM, Zhao JW, Li X, et al. Effectiveness and safety of acupuncture for insomnia. Medicine. 2019;98:45.e17842. 5 pages. https://doi.org/10.1097/MD.0000000000017842.
14. Guo J, Wang LP, Liu CZ, et al. Efficacy of acupuncture for primary insomnia: a randomized controlled clinical trial. Evid Based Complement Alternat Med. 2013. Article ID 163850:10 pages. https://doi.org/10.1155/2013/163850.
15. Guo J, Huang W, Tang CY, et al. Effect of acupuncture on sleep quality and hyperarousal state in patients with primary insomnia: study protocol for a randomised controlled trial. BMJ Open. 2016;6:e009594. 7 pages. https://doi.org/10.1136/bmjopen-2015-009594.
16. Li SS, Yin P, Yin X, et al. Effect of Acupuncture on insomnia in menopausal women: a study protocol for a randomized controlled trial. Trials. 2019;20:308. 8 pages. https://doi.org/10.1186/s13063-019-3374-8.
17. Yin X, Dong B, Liang TT, et al. Efficacy and safety of electroacupuncture on treating depression-related insomnia: a study protocol for a multicentre randomised controlled trial. BMJ Open. 2019;9:e021484, 9 pages. https://doi.org/10.1136/bmjopen-2018-021484.
18. Cao HJ, Pan XF, Li H, et al. Acupuncture for treatment of insomnia: a systematic review of randomized controlled trials. J Altern Complement Med. 2009;15(11):1171–86.
19. Grant S, Kendrick R, Motala A, et al. Acupuncture for substance use disorders: a systematic review and meta-analysis. Drug Alcohol Depend. 2016;163:1–15.
20. WHO. Global status report on alcohol and health. Geneva: World Health Organization; 2018.
21. National Drug Intelligence Centre. The economic impact of illicit drug use on American Society. Washington, DC: US Department of Justice; 2011.
22. Shin NY, Lim YJ, Yang CH, et al. Acupuncture for alcohol use disorder: a meta-analysis. Evid Based Complement Alternat Med. 2017., Article ID 7823278, 6 pages; https://doi.org/10.1155/2017/7823278.
23. Stuyt EB. Ear acupuncture for co-occurring substance abuse and borderline personality disorder: an aid to encourage treatment retention and tobacco cessation. Acupunct Med. 2014;32(4):318–24.
24. Gong C, Liu W. Acupuncture and the opioid epidemic in America. Chin J Integr Med. 2018;24:323–7.
25. Lin JG, Chan YY, Chen YH. Acupuncture for the treatment of opiate addiction. Evid Based Complement Alternat Med. 2012;2012:739045. 10 pages. https://doi.org/10.1155/2012/739045.

26. Wen HL. Role of acupuncture in narcotic withdrawal. Med Pr. 1975;2:15–6.
27. Wen HL. Fast detoxification of drug abuse by acupuncture and electrical stimulation (AES) in combination with naloxone. Mod Med Asia. 1977;13:13–7.
28. Wen HL. Acupuncture and electrical stimulation (AES) outpatient detoxification. Mod Med Asia. 1979;15:39–43.
29. Serafini K, Bryant K, Ikomi J, et al. Training psychiatry addiction fellows in acupuncture. Acad Psychiatry. 2016;40:503–6.
30. Motlagh FE, Ibrahim F, Rashid RA, et al. Acupuncture therapy for drug addiction. Chin Med. 2016;11:16. 20 pages. https://doi.org/10.1186/s13020-016-0088-7.
31. Cui CL, Wu L, Luo F. Acupuncture for the treatment of drug addiction. Neurochem Res. 2008;33:2013–22.
32. Chan YY, Lo WY, Li TC, et al. Clinical efficacy of acupuncture as an adjunct to methadone treatment services for heroin addicts: a randomized controlled trial. Am J Chin Med. 2014;42(3):569–86.
33. Fan AY, Miller DW, Bolash B, et al. Acupuncture's role in solving the opioid epidemic: evidence, cost-effectiveness, and care availability for acupuncture as a primary, non-pharmacologic method for pain relief and management—White Paper 2017. J Integr Med. 2017;15(6):411–25.

Index

Name of Channel and Point

The book "A Manual of Acupuncture" by Deadman et al (Deadman P, Al-Khafaji M, and Baker K. A Manual of Acupuncture. Second edition. East Sussex: JCM publications. 2003.) has been widely used as the key text of acupuncture education in western countries. This book "Acupuncture for the Brain" will mostly follow its principles of the name of acupuncture channel and acupoints, with some exemptions.

LU: The Lung channel of hand Taiyin, sample point: LU-1 Zhongfu
LI: The Large Intestine channel of hand Yangming, sample point: LI-2 Erjian
ST: The Stomach channel of foot Yangming, sample point: ST-3 Juliao
SP: The Spleen channel of foot Taiyin, sample point: SP-4 Gongsun
HT: The Heart channel of hand Shaoyin, sample point: HT-5 Tongli
SI: The Small Intestine channel of hand Taiyang, sample point: SI-6 Yanglao
BL: The Bladder channel of foot Taiyang, sample point: BL-7 Tongtian
KI: The Kidney channel of foot Shaoyin, sample point: KI-8 Jiaoxin
PC: The Pericardium channel of hand Jueyin, such as PC-9 Zhongchong
SJ: The Sanjiao channel of hand Shaoyang, sample point: SJ-10 Tianjing
GB: The Gall Bladder channel of foot Shaoyang, sample point: GB-11Touqiaoyin
LV: The Liver channel of foot Jueyin, sample point: LV-12 Jimai
REN: The Ren Mai, or the Conception Vessel (CV), sample point: REN-13 (CV-13) Shangwan
DU: The Du Mai, or the Governing Vessel (GV), sample point: DU-14 (GV-14) Dazhui
Ex: Extraordinary channel, such as Ex-Shixuan

Easy Confused Acupoints, or with Other Pinyin Names

CV = REN, Conception Vessel, Ren Mai, Ren meridian,

© Springer Nature Switzerland AG 2021
T. Wang, *Acupuncture for Brain*, https://doi.org/10.1007/978-3-030-54666-3

GV = DU, Governor Vessel: Du Mai, Du Meridian or supervisor vessel, Governor
   Meridian
LIV = LV, or LR
SJ = TB (Triple Burner channel) or TH (Triple Heater channel)
GB-39 Juegu, another Pinyin name Xuanzhong
REN-17 Danzhong, other pinyin names Shanzhong, or Tanzhong
DU-26 Renzhong, another Pinyin name Shuigou

The Translations of the Name of Huangdi Neijing (黄帝内经)

- Huangdi Neijing
- The Yellow Emperor's Internal Classic
- Yellow Emperor's Classic of Internal Medicine
- Yellow Emperors Cannon of Internal Medicine
- Inner Classic of the Yellow Emperor
- Neijing
- Inner Classic

Suwen (素问): Part One of Huangdi Neijing, or NJSW

- Plain questions
- Simple questions
- Essential questions

Lingshu (灵枢): Part Two of Huangdi Neijing, or NJLS

- Spiritual Pivot
- Spiritual Axis

T. Wang, *Acupuncture for Brain*, https://doi.org/10.1007/978-3-030-54666-3

Index

Printed in the United States
by Baker & Taylor Publisher Services